T0367365

PRAISE *FOR THE HIDDEN PSYCHOLOGY OF PAIN*

The Hidden Psychology of Pain is a fresh and welcome look at the problem of chronic pain. In this well researched book, Dr. James Alexander offers his readers a new paradigm backed up by relevant information, results of recent research, case studies from his own professional experience, and also a handbook of self-help suggestions readily accessible to those living with chronic pain. He offers readers hope through new knowledge, better understanding, and the opportunity to see themselves as whole beings rather than as a collection of symptoms.

As a Physiotherapist, I found that the treatments I had to offer for chronic pain would sometimes only give short-term symptomatic relief, falling short of the true needs of the person. This timely book tells us that a more holistic approach is not only possible, but is already proven to have helped many people.

CHRISTABEL STREHIE – PHYSIOTHERAPIST.

Most of us know someone whose life is limited by chronic pain. *The Hidden Psychology of Pain* clearly describes why we have this form of pain, and how we can free ourselves of it. This book provides an evidence-based argument from pain research into why the techniques described can work so effectively. The scope of the book is not limited to physical pain, but it also provides useful information and instruction about the psychological pain of Post-Traumatic Stress Disorder and chronic depression. The book is easy to read and would be of benefit to professionals as well as to their clients and patients. I have personally tried the techniques to manage arthritic back pain and have found that they work.

ROWENA HARDING-SMITH

MA, M ED, BA (PSYCH), DIRECTOR OF THE WORKING MEMORY
INSTITUTE.
AUTHOR OF *PROCRASTINATE NOW!*, AND
TEACHING CREATIVE WRITING TO RELUCTANT WRITERS.

I believe that the information in *The Hidden Psychology of Pain* is vital to unlocking the mystery of chronic illness and the pain-body, as well as helping us evolve emotionally as a culture. Healing = Hearing.

DR JACQUELINE BOUSTANY –
GENERAL PRACTITIONER. MBBS, DIP. PEADS. MPH.

In *The Hidden Psychology of Pain*, Dr James Alexander guides us through the labyrinth of previously-hidden information with clarity, expertise and profound knowledge on the subject of chronic pain. The subject is so relevant to current issues, as we move from a place of 'educated guess work' to an actual understanding of the true origins of chronic pain. Dr Alexander has produced a book of crucial information for all health professionals. As I read each chapter, I was nodding my head in agreement. I have been working with chronic pain and trauma for many years, and I know the premise of *The Hidden Psychology of Pain* to be absolutely true. I thoroughly enjoyed reading this book.

DEIRDRE MIDDLEHURST. CLINICAL PSYCHOLOGIST

This is a very good book. I wish it had been one of the text books when I trained to be a physiotherapist in the 1980's. It should be a required text for present students studying to be doctors or allied health workers. I feel that the true nature of what is going on for the majority of chronic pain sufferers is not being understood by most doctors and allied health workers. This failure of understanding results in ongoing frustration for the sufferers and the earnest people trying to assist them. I feel that my 25 year career as a physiotherapist, with a special interest in back and neck problems, would have been much more rewarding if those chronic pain patients were directed towards the knowledge available in *The Hidden Psychology of Pain*. This could have prevented some of them being labelled malingers, becoming depressed, or continuing with manual treatment and/or medication, sometimes for many, many years without resolution of their chronic pain. This book finally helps me to understand some of the inconsistencies, and affirms my belief that the majority of these people were neither malingering or crazy.

TERRY PAGE. BACHELOR OF APPLIED SCIENCE (PHYSIOTHERAPY).

As Dr James Alexander stresses throughout his book, *The Hidden Psychology of Pain,* providing solid information is what the pain sufferer needs first. He has succeeded at this goal brilliantly. By first introducing the Hidden Psychology of Pain as having purpose, he normalizes what all humans do: having pain distracts us from unconscious emotional dilemmas. He then offers many approaches that can help people work toward eradicating chronic pain and dealing with emotional issues that if suppressed, maintain the pain. There are many self help techniques, as well as solid information about psychotherapy, often needed to deal with serious, underlying trauma. This book is a comprehensive guide to the understanding of the central role of emotion in the development and maintenance of pain.

CAROL FORGASH, LCSW, BCD. PAST PRESIDENT: EMDR HAP BOARD
OF DIRECTORS; EMDR INSTITUTE CONSULTANT & FACILITATOR
SMITHTOWN, NY. CO-AUTHOR: *HEALING THE HEART OF TRAUMA AND
DISSOCIATION WITH EMDR AND EGO STATE THERAPY.*

A "Doctor" is a teacher. Dr James Alexander is a gifted, erudite healer who straddles several disciplines to explain why the medical model, a bio-chemical-mechanical model, does not elucidate chronic pain. Nor do anatomy, pathology or radiology explain its origins or mechanisms. *The Hidden Psychology of Pain* provides take home messages, insights and gems. It also has essential insights for psychologists, pain therapists, and those who want to heal and be healed. It is not just a self-help book. It is an education. Understanding one's pain can make a difference.

DR YOLANDE LUCIRE. PHD MBBS DPM FRANZCP.
FORENSIC PSYCHIATRIST.
AUTHOR OF *CONSTRUCTING RSI: BELIEF AND DESIRE.*

The Hidden Psychology of Pain is a comprehensive psychological textbook which heralds a new paradigm shift in the way we can look at chronic pain. This book challenges the readers to change their beliefs and understanding about chronic pain as we explore the psychological basis of pain. The author presents a theory that chronic pain is psychologically based in the unconscious mind. Fortunately readers are also given the psychologically based solutions to eliminate chronic pain, or radically reduce it. This book is hugely relevant today in a world where we find many suffers with chronic pain, depression, poor sleep, anxiety and stress related disorders that are not being adequately treated by current therapeutic practices. *The Hidden Psychology of Pain* gives psychologists, medical practitioners and the suffering patients a new pathway to treat chronic pain.

DR KAREL HROMEK, PRESIDENT OF ACNEM
—AUSTRALASIAN COLLEGE OF
NUTRITIONAL AND ENVIRONMENTAL MEDICINE.

The Hidden Psychology of Pain is an engaging and information-rich exposition on how to heal chronic pain. Dr James Alexander skilfully weaves together his own healing journey from chronic pain, and the history of Western philosophy and medicine. He shows how the latter relate to cultural assumptions about pain, and explores the meaning and unconscious purpose of pain, that, as sufferers know, often exists independent of a defined physical cause. Dr James examines chronic pain myths and various healing modalities, some of which may be new to readers. As an ex-sufferer of decades-long chronic pain, I highly recommend this book to any who wish to take responsibility for their own health. I know from personal experience that the information presented provides an invaluable opportunity for healing and wholeness.

CATHERINE—FORMER SUFFERER OF CHRONIC PAIN

I honestly don't know how to thank you enough for putting me on to these ideas. After seven months of pain, and two months of disability, in only four weeks, I am back to normal. I'm riding my bike again, studying full time at uni, essentially doing everything I used to do, and also more. As terrible as the pain was, getting over it psychologically has also given me the opportunity to address a number of other areas in my life which I was neglecting. Through the EMDR therapy, I have been able to look at a number of childhood events which I hadn't properly dealt with, and essentially reprogram my brain into adult mode. All of this has given me a dizzying sense of control over my own life which I now realize I had been lacking. So, thank you, thank you, thank you. All of this has really given me a new start at my life.

'REBECCA'—FORMER SUFFERER OF CHRONIC PAIN

The
HIDDEN
PSYCHOLOGY
of PAIN

THE USE OF UNDERSTANDING TO HEAL CHRONIC PAIN

2ND EDITION

DR. JAMES ALEXANDER
www.drjamesalexander-psychologist.com

BALBOA.
PRESS
A DIVISION OF HAY HOUSE

Balboa Press books may be ordered through booksellers or by contacting:

Balboa Press
A Division of Hay House
1663 Liberty Drive
Bloomington, IN 47403
www.balboapress.com.au
1-(877) 407-4847

ISBN: 978-1-4525-0680-7 (sc)
ISBN: 978-1-4525-0681-4 (e)

Because of the dynamic nature of the Internet, any web addresses or links contained in this book may have changed since publication and may no longer be valid. The views expressed in this work are solely those of the author and do not necessarily reflect the views of the publisher, and the publisher hereby disclaims any responsibility for them.

The author of this book does not dispense medical advice or prescribe the use of any technique as a form of treatment for physical, emotional, or medical problems without the advice of a physician, either directly or indirectly. The intent of the author is only to offer information of a general nature to help you in your quest for emotional and spiritual well-being. In the event you use any of the information in this book for yourself, which is your constitutional right, the author and the publisher assume no responsibility for your actions.

Any people depicted in stock imagery provided by Thinkstock are models, and such images are being used for illustrative purposes only.
Certain stock imagery © Thinkstock.

Printed in the United States of America

Balboa Press rev. date: 09/19/2014

To my parents, Lindsay and Noel Alexander. They are the inspirational examples who taught me the virtue of giving back to the world according to one's means and abilities.

CONTENTS

ACKNOWLEDGMENTS xiii
INTRODUCTION xv
Epidemic of chronic pain. xviii
Pain Questionnaires xxiv

Chapter 1: PSYCHOLOGY & PAIN 1
Opening to the unconscious. 6
The Mind/Body Syndrome 15

Chapter 2: PHYSICAL PERSPECTIVES ON PAIN. 20
Western philosophy & medicine. 20
The split between psychology and medicine 23
Medical explanations of chronic pain. 26

Chapter 3: BIO-PSYCHO-SOCIAL MEDICINE 34
A role for psychology 36
"Holism" and health care. 40
Psychological studies of chronic pain. 41

Chapter 4: CHRONIC PAIN MISUNDERSTOOD. 47
Chronic pain does not equate with damage 47
Pointing the bone in a scientific culture. 53
RSI as a case example 55
The transition from acute to chronic pain 58
Pain following an injury 60
Chronic pain sufferers with no structural pathology 61
When no pain results from injury 62
Multiple factors 67

The physicality of pain 71
Chronic pain myths. 73

Chapter 5:   THE PHYSIOLOGY OF CHRONIC PAIN 76
The role of oxygen and ischemia 76
The pain pattern & psychological overlay. 81
Additional muscle problems. 83
Nerve pain 87
Tendon/ligament pain. 93

Chapter 6:   CONSCIOUS & UNCONSCIOUS FACTORS. 96
Conscious stressors. 96
The unconscious purpose of chronic pain 98
Unacceptable feelings. 104

Chapter 7:   THE DEPTHS OF THE UNCONSCIOUS 113
Childhood attachment patterns. 113
Thoughts, feelings & the body. 118
The hidden side of success 121
Classical conditioning. 123
The "why there?" of pain 128
Cultural influences. 134

Chapter 8:   GETTING BETTER 140
Thinking psychologically. 144
Exceptions as clues 154
Information as the best treatment. 157
Getting active again. 166
Readiness for pain relief. 171

Chapter 9:   SELF-HELP STRATEGIES. 174
Self-analysis questions 174

Chapter 10: PSYCHOLOGICAL TRAUMA & DEPRESSION 195
The medical notion of depression. 195
The study of trauma 199

Chapter 11: THE HEALING POWER OF DREAMS...............208
    Healing emotions with dream awareness 221
    Dream-seeding...224
    Dream rescripting 225
    Cognitive Control Training 228

Chapter 12: THE PROMISE OF ENERGY PSYCHOLOGY.........236
    Acupuncture & acupressure 237
    Emotional Freedom Techniques (EFT) 240
    EFT & pain 248
    Plasma Ball model 251

Chapter 13: IMPROVING YOUR SLEEP 262
    EFT for sleep...270
    Circadian problems....................................275
    Sleeping tablets......................................278

Chapter 14: EFT, ANXIETY & STRESS....................283
    Fight/Flight/Freeze response 283
    EFT as exposure therapy...............................290
    Calming the amygdala with EFT........................291

Chapter 15: PSYCHOTHERAPY FOR PAIN...................299
    Psychologists...306
    Psychiatrists, psychotherapy & drugs..................308
    Pharmacogenetics 311
    Social workers and counselors 316

Chapter 16: EYE MOVEMENT DESENSITIZATION
    & REPROCESSING 318
    A chance observation 319
    Comparison with antidepressants & CBT 321
    Bilateral stimulation 324
    Possible therapeutic mechanism.......................328

Chapter 17: MINDFUL AWARENESS
OF THE PRESENT MOMENT 334
Acceptance of what is 336
The right understanding 341
The Power of Now 342
Psychological & clock-time..........................356
Icon of suffering 359
Acceptance & Commitment Therapy 364

APPENDICES 367

Appendix 1:   Pain Questionnaires (I) 367
Appendix 2:   A neurological understanding........................370
Appendix 3:   Anatomy of the spine 384
Appendix 4:   Standard medical treatments for chronic back pain 386
Appendix 5:   The value of physical therapies?......................389
Appendix 6:   The evolution of psychology.........................397
Appendix 7:   Sample of research demonstrating structural
              pathology in pain-free populations 405
Appendix 8:   EFT on a Page..409
Appendix 9:   Process for staying in the present moment 411
Appendix 10: Testimonials from the Hidden Psychology
              of Pain clients 412
Appendix 11: Pain Questionnaire (II) 418
Appendix 12: Placebo treatment? 421

BIBLIOGPRAPHY...................................425
INDEX 435

ACKNOWLEDGMENTS

THIS BOOK WAS INSPIRED BY the confusing problem of chronic pain which is prevalent in our culture. I suffered a form of it for eighteen years. Over the years, I have worked with countless numbers of people who also suffer chronic pain. Perhaps due to the valiant attempts to train psychologists in a scientific approach to our subject matter, over all these years, I have looked for and retained scientific information which I thought was relevant to this widespread problem. The conclusions that I came upon seemed to require justification, especially in relation to the standard ways of making sense of chronic pain which our culture offers. Consequently, when my son and his friend (who were both studying exercise physiology at university) made enquiries about my "odd" views on chronic pain, I decided that I would like to be able to furnish them with a collection of the information which I had been collecting over many years. I could have just suggested that they just read the ground-breaking books by Professor John Sarno. However, while incorporating many of Sarno's views, I found that I had added to these with many years of searching out other sources of information which complemented his basic propositions. I also found that several of the approaches I had been using in my psychology work with distressed and traumatised people were entirely relevant to working with chronic pain. If I was to present all the information which I thought was relevant to successfully making sense of and treating chronic pain, I would have to write my own book. As such, I thank my son and his friend for their enquiring young minds that "pushed" me into this venture.

I would also like to thank a range of other people who, without their efforts and support, this book would not have been possible. Firstly, my wife, Karen. She has given me the space, time and understanding required to approach this project as a second job. My children Will, Emily and Taylor have also had to make allowances over the last few years. Rowena Harding-Smith provided me with invaluable structural editing advice, turning what was a modest family sedan into the Porsche you now hold. Susan Gumley created the illustrations which grace these pages, from very inadequate rough ideas that I presented her with. Ollie Dean and Luke Caddaye offered valuable feedback from reading various manuscripts of this book. And finally, the many clients who I have worked with over the years have each taught me valuable lessons in life, slowly adding to the accumulation of knowledge and experience which one would hope to find in a mid-career psychologist. As such, this book is essentially a team effort, with all of the above adding their necessary elements over a long period of time. Ultimately, it is an expression of our culture, and my own peculiar place in it as a psychologist (not forgetting the well-built twenty-something year olds who, in enjoying smashing into an old bloke on the football field for seven seasons, taught me not only that that my body was actually quite resilient, but that great psychological aliveness is to be gained by using our bodies vigorously). Thank you to all involved.

INTRODUCTION

THIS BOOK IS ABOUT THE experience of chronic pain, and more importantly, about the proposition that you can do something to either eliminate or radically reduce it. You will be presented with a theory of chronic pain which, although novel in the current era, actually has a long history. With the sophistication of modern biological science, we are now at a point in time where it is possible to verify much of this theory with current research based evidence. Everything in this book is supported by scientific evidence. No doubt, despite the various forms of evidence presented, there will still be detractors—people who cannot or will not be open to what the evidence is suggesting. However, for those sufferers who are open to these possibilities, the potential for healing arises.

Research has made it clear that how we make sense of any particular health condition actually has a large role in determining our level of disability from it, the degree of pain we experience, and the ultimate outcome.[1] While this finding is true for a broad range of health conditions, it is perhaps no more true than it is for chronic pain. Further, research demonstrates that how you view your condition is actually *more* important in determining the outcome than is the actual severity of the condition. The sense that we make of chronic pain, our beliefs about its causes, and our expectations of its course can be modified through straightforward psycho-educational processes, such as this book. Evidence confirms that information alone can have a positive impact on, and lead to improvements with many health conditions. Chronic pain is a particularly good example of this.

---

[1] Petrie & Weinman (2012). "Patients' Perceptions of Their Illness: The Dynamo of Volition in Health Care." *Current Directions in Psychological Science.*

What is presented in this book is the notion that psychological factors, of which we are often unaware, can have a large role to play in causing chronic pain. The Hidden Psychology of Pain refers to these unconscious psychological factors.

Just how out of step with cutting edge medical thinking is the suggestion that psychology could have a large role to play in the causation of chronic pain? Professor of Psychological Medicine at the University of Oxford, Michael Sharpe, advocates that psychological factors must be taken into account when approaching the broad range of medically unexplained symptoms. He suggests that medical researchers, and health care funding bodies such as governments, are now recognising the need to go beyond the traditional separation of psychological and physical issues. This dichotomy has simply failed up to one quarter of all people seeking medical treatment who do not to get better with psychology being left out of the treatment approach.[2]

In discussing the role of psychological factors, former convener of the Australian Pain Society and Professor of Medicine David Cherry, recently acknowledged that the psychological factors which are relevant to chronic pain are often operating at an *unconscious* level.[3]

Even authors of popular books on the neurophysiology of pain recognize that both physical *and* emotional trauma can make the mind/brain more vigilant towards potential threat. For example, Butler & Moseley state that recurrent or multiple traumatic events give the mind/brain more reason to protect the body, and pain is a method of doing this.[4] Psychological and social factors are estimated to explain around 70% of the differences between an injury that eventually result in chronic pain, and one that the person recovers from.[5]

Although regarded as a 'new' proposition within medicine, this is actually a *rediscovery* of accepted wisdom from past eras. Hopefully, such recognition of unconscious psychological factors can again enter the therapeutic enterprise—this book is a step in that direction.

---

[2] Sharpe (2012) *Unexplained Medical Symptoms*. ABC Radio National The Health Report, 28th August.

[3] Cherry (2009). "Managing Chronic Non-malignant Pain." *Medicine Today*.

[4] Butler & Moseley (2003) *Explain Pain*.

[5] Burton et al (1995) "Psychosocial predictors of outcome in acute and subchronic low back trouble". *Spine*. 20 (6).

I will run the risk of alienating some readers at the very start of this book by suggesting that although your pain is unwanted, it actually presents you with the possibility of emotional healing. Despite chronic pain posing a crisis in many people's lives, seen for what it really is, it actually creates an opportunity for healing of the whole person. This is not to glorify pain and suffering—my intention is to help you overcome it. But in so doing, an opportunity for the healing of deep wounds is presented. As a result, I am usually excited by the possibilities when I meet a new client who is suffering from chronic pain. They are often on the verge of some important self-discoveries, and the recovery process presents an opportunity to heal both physical and psychological hurts.

In discussing pain, we must firstly distinguish between acute pain and chronic pain (or persistent pain as it is often called). Acute pain usually results from traumatic injury. Body tissue, hard or soft, has been damaged, and pain is the typical response when the injury is substantial enough. We don't like acute pain, but if we didn't feel it, we would probably not survive beyond infancy. Acute pain has both great evolutionary value for our species, and greatly adaptive value for individuals. We tend to not repeat actions which result in such pain. This is positive, as such actions are likely to be dangerous for us, and we have a greater chance of surviving by not repeating incredibly dangerous behaviours. Most soft tissue injuries tend to repair in a few weeks, depending on the ability to rest the injury. Hard tissue injuries can take up to three months to repair, give or take some time due to other factors such as age, and general state of health.

A diagnosis of chronic pain should not be made until at least *three months* after an injury, when most forms of physical damage have actually been long healed. Regardless of the type of tissue you have damaged, the physical healing process is usually the same. The damaged tissue becomes inflamed, which bring the body's immune and rebuilding cells into the afflicted area. An "inflammatory soup" is released into the damaged area which contains potassium, bradykinins, histamine, calcitonin, substance P, prostaglandins, as well as other products of arachidonic acid metabolism.[6] Scar tissue forms on the damaged area, with the tissue being remodeled so as to make it a close match to the original tissue. The same process is utilized whether your body

---

[6] Siddall, P. & Cousins, M. (1997) "Spinal Pain Mechanisms". *Spine.* 22(1)

is healing your liver or gut, or joints and muscles.[7] Due to having a poorer blood supply, tissues such as vertebral discs and ligaments take longer to heal than do other soft tissues abundant in blood, such as the skin and muscles. Pain generally diminishes once the healing is complete.

Like many other people, I have fractured several bones and can testify to the healing capacities of the physical body. When I fractured three vertebrae in my neck a few years ago, the treating specialist said it would take around three months for the bones to heal and return to a full range of movement without pain. The first couple of weeks were very painful, and I was capable of little neck rotation. But sure enough, around the three month mark, my neck was back to a near full range of movement with no pain. X-rays showed the bones had healed. The internal inflammation, lack of rotation and the experience of acute pain kept me relatively still in the early weeks, and I only gradually increased my activity level as the weeks marched on towards the three month mark. These unpleasant symptoms gave my bones time to heal, allowing them to knit back together by keeping me somewhat inactive.

During this acute phase of recovery, pain is rarely considered a medical mystery. It is obviously related to an injury, and serves some kind of useful function in terms of slowing us down so that healing can occur.

Chronic pain is a different story—it lasts for much longer than the healing process requires. This book is about chronic pain, which is still often viewed as something of a medical mystery.

Epidemic of chronic pain

My country, Australia, is fairly typical for industrialized Western countries in regards to chronic pain statistics. One in five people here suffer from chronic pain. It afflicts people from all walks of life and employment groups. For the people who suffer the most, with each day taken off work due to chronic pain, many more days suffering with the pain at work will have to be endured. The total cost to the Australian economy from lost workdays, as well as health care costs, is nearly 4% of the GDP.[8] While ongoing pain

---

[7] Butler & Moseley (2003) *Explain Pain*.
[8] The Kolling Institute of Medical Research.

is experienced by a sizable minority, up to 70% of people report significant episodes of back pain during their lives.[9]

These figures reflect the same trends for most Western societies. Statistics from Europe show that one in every six Europeans suffer from chronic pain[10], and the US Institute of Medicine of the National Academies reports that 116 million Americans are afflicted by this condition—this equates with around one in every three people.[11]

It is apparent that chronic pain is a *large scale* human problem, and there are no signs of it abating yet. Curiously, chronic pain has not reached the same epidemic proportions in non-Western and non-industrialised countries, where plenty of heavy lifting still happens.

John Sarno, recently retired Professor of Rehabilitation Medicine at New York University Medical Centre, states that chronic pain is amongst the most painful conditions that physicians can be confronted with over their medical careers.

Like most people in our society, I have experienced occasional bouts of extreme lower-back pain, in addition to other forms of chronic pain. As such, I am fully aware of how excruciating and disabling this condition can be. At times, the pain has been so extreme that, had I not known better, I could have sworn that my back was literally '*broken*'. As is the case for most people experiencing this kind of pain, nothing could have been further from the truth, despite how it feels.

But why yet another book about chronic pain? While no one professional seems to have all the answers, each is adding more pieces to the overall jigsaw puzzle of chronic pain. For all health professionals, any experience of life in general, and treatment of chronic pain in particular, is necessarily limited. When considering some of the experts in this field, this statement may seem odd. John Sarno, a pain-physician whose experience this book will be drawing on, worked in rehabilitation and pain medicine from 1965 until 2012. During that time, he worked with many thousands of people in chronic pain.

---

9 Barnsley (2010). "The Significance of Chronic Back Pain." *Medicine Today*.

10 Luo et al (2012). "Presynaptically Localized Cyclic GMP-Dependent Protein Kinase 1 Is a Key Determinant of Spinal Synaptic Potentiation and Pain Hypersensitivity." *PLoS Biology*.

11 American Academy of Pain Management. http://www.aapainmanage.org/

My experience, while not quite as extensive as his, is also thorough. I am well into my third decade of practising psychology, including much work in chronic pain rehabilitation, and have many clients with wide variations of this disabling condition. In addition, having been a suffering of chronic pain myself, I am able to bring a firsthand knowledge of the experience to my work.

Even so, both Sarno and myself only know what we know by virtue of our experiences, and no practitioner's experience is all encompassing. Neither of us have seen *all* people in pain, and individual differences can be significant. Moreover, as a psychologist, I am familiar with some treatment approaches that will differ from his general approach as a physician.

Other psychologists working with chronic pain clients would also be able to add to my list of useful interventions. As such, I do not suggest the contents of this book are the only approach that will work with chronic pain. Rather, this book contains interventions which I have seen work well in my clinical practice—many of my clients have become better as a result. By 'becoming better' I mean they experience a reduction in pain, usually sufficient to allow the client to come off all pain medications; and many are able to return to pre-pain vocational and recreational activities. As such, I am confident in recommending these ideas and approaches to assist you with reducing or overcoming your chronic pain.

There are some other excellent books on the market already about chronic pain, and I have personally seen many people resolve their pain simply by using some of these resources as well. My favourites are books written by John Sarno (*Healing Back Pain* and *The MindBody Prescription*), as well as *When the Body Says No* by Dr. Gabor Maté, and I commend these to you. Research continues to demonstrate that for highly motivated people with less intensive cases of distress, self-help books are often as effective as professionally guided treatment.[12]

The more good information you have about the causes of much of the chronic pain which is currently afflicting our society, the greater your chances of recovery. In fact, our beliefs about the causes of chronic pain are perhaps the main factor which can either intensify the pain until it becomes

---

[12] Scogin (2003). "The Status of Self-Help Administered Treatments." *Journal of Clinical Psychology.*

chronic, or alleviate it. This book will challenge many of your beliefs about chronic pain. The experience of many of my clients is that this informational process is a key to recovery.

I did not invent the ideas presented in this book, and try to give due acknowledgement to others who have discussed these notions and approaches before me. Most importantly, however, you should be aware these ideas really emerged from within our culture over the last 300 years at least, and perhaps even longer. All researchers, practitioners and thinkers stand on the shoulders of their predecessors, with knowledge accumulating over decades, and even centuries. The history of medical literature is dotted with ideas similar to those presented in this book.[13] Approaches similar to these were probably part of our culture and healing practices long before medicine emerged as the social phenomenon it is today. The difference today is that state of the art science can inform and support the propositions of this approach.

Psychology, as a discipline, is a relatively new enterprise. But humans have been 'doing' psychology ever since we learned to talk and think. Sympathetic priests in ancient Greece would comfort wounded warriors as they returned from battles with harrowing accounts.[14] Formal psychology emerged from a combination of philosophy, scientific research and clinical medicine. Two hundred years ago, before such a discipline was named, what we may now call psychological therapy was being 'done' by philosophers, physicians, and the clergy. Academic psychology began in the late 19th century laboratories of Wilhelm Wundt in Germany, and William James in America. This new discipline immediately entered the long cultural conversation about human experience, including issues such as health, illness and chronic pain.

Each psychologist will interpret and blend various approaches in a unique manner, and will be in a different position to see possible areas of confluence amongst different approaches where the additive effect can increase success rates. As such, my particular way of going about this will be different to that of other psychologists. We are all part of this ongoing

---

[13] For example, Cullen (1710-1790) suggested a role for emotions in some chronic pain conditions (in Lucire 2003 *Constructing RSI*).

[14] Forgash & Copeley (2008). *Healing the Heart of Trauma and Dissociation with EMDR and Ego State Therapy.*

long-term process of better understanding and treatment, and we each stand in different places within this evolutionary endeavour.

Around 300 conditions come under the term 'chronic pain'. While I won't focus exclusively on back pain, it is the prime example of chronic pain at the end of the 20th century and the beginning of this one. After respiratory infections, back pain is the most common reason for people seeking help from GPs. Next to headaches and colds, it is also the most common reason for taking time off work. Back pain is the most prevalent cause of work related disability in people under forty five, and in regards to workers compensation and medical expenses, it is the most costly cause of work related disability.

While around 90% of us will recover from back pain within four weeks or so, around 30% of people with back pain will experience a recurrence at some time in the future. A smaller group experience the pain as ongoing, becoming chronic. These people can be so adversely affected that they often become extremely disabled by the pain, and their entire life changes as a result.

The second and third groups, sufferers of reoccurring and/or chronic pain, are the focus of this book. However, anyone who experiences back, neck or shoulder pain at all needs to be equipped with accurate information concerning its causes, otherwise they may also progress on to repeated bouts of pain, which can then become chronic.

Other forms of chronic pain and health conditions have also become commonplace, including musculoskeletal complaints, Repetitive Strain Injury (RSI); respiratory, dermatological, gastrointestinal problems; fibromyalgia and chronic fatigue syndrome. John Sarno suggests that all of these conditions (and many more) are related to the underlying psychological realities of every person's functioning.

Types of chronic pain or health conditions seem to come and go in an epidemic-like fashion. As long as we focus only on the specific symptoms of a new pain or health epidemic, we risk failing to understand the causes which underpin many if not all of them.

People rarely experience just one chronic pain or health problem in isolation from others. Such health problems tend to emerge in 'clusters'. People suffering from one will usually suffer from others as well. The Hidden Psychology of Pain is relevant for nearly all chronic pain problems across the board, with the exception of pain caused by cancer and spinal infections. At the very least, where there may be a range of contributing factors, psychology is relevant as one of these factors to many ongoing health problems.

No one can seriously doubt the role which biology plays in chronic pain, however the dominant view of pain has for decades neglected the role which psychology also plays in this debilitating condition. An important point of this book is that we are not simply biological beings, but are very much psychological and social beings as well.

The chronic pain and ill-health trends will continue to change over time with various epidemics, such as RSI, rising and falling in turn. We can only be equipped to deal with each of these if we look for the underlying cause beneath all of them. In this way, we can avoid having to reinvent the wheel each time a new pain or chronic ill-health epidemic emerges. This may prevent decades wasted on looking in all the wrong places for causes and exploring useless, expensive and potentially dangerous 'cures'.

Without an appreciation of the Hidden Psychology of Pain, the natural inclination is to view most chronic pain conditions as being unrelated, as different systems or areas of the anatomy may be involved. Although the prevalent tendency, it is a mistake to see different aspects of the human organism in isolation. When it comes to chronic pain, we need to look for the realities underlying all of them.

The widespread failure to treat chronic pain successfully is something of a medical and social failure. Emeritus Professor at the University of Virginia in the Departments of both Medicine and English, David B. Morris, states that chronic pain is the "invisible crisis at the center of contemporary life."[15] Our health professions seem to struggle to make a sense of what is going on. Two disciplines lead inquiry into the problem of chronic pain. Medicine (including physical sciences and health practices such as physiotherapy, chiropractic), and, from a different perspective, psychology.

"What has psychology to do with pain?" is a valid question to ask. The standard view is that psychology can contribute little to analysing causation or treatment of chronic pain. Usually, psychology is asked only to help sufferers merely *adjust* emotionally to the pain. This book will help you to understand the role which psychology plays in *causing* chronic pain.

---

[15] Cited in Lucire (2003). *Constructing RSI: Belief and Desire.*

The basic contention, that often hidden psychological factors and processes have the power to cause pain, will be explored in detail. A program to use this information will be presented to help you convert this information into healing. With this framework in mind, we can now explore the various aspects of this program.

Some of what is written in this book is purely informational, detailing relevant research and scientific findings. As a reader suffering from ongoing pain, you are probably more interested in just jumping straight to the chapters which discuss what to do about it. While entirely understandable, my suggestion is that you do process the factual information as much as possible, as this is actually part of your 'cure'.

We have been so inundated with phoney ideas relating to chronic pain that, essentially, we need a new education about it. The wrong ideas feed directly into the psychological issues which maintain the pain, and as such, need to be directly addressed and challenged with accurate information.

You may still want to jump straight to the chapters which discuss interventions, but I would urge you at the very least to return to the more informational chapters for clarification. Again, how we make sense of most health conditions, including chronic pain, has a direct impact on the severity of the condition, the level of disability, and its outcome. The beliefs about chronic pain, in which we have been instructed and conditioned, are a significant part of the problem. The flip side of the coin is that the different sense of chronic pain, which this book presents, is a significant part of the solution.

Pain Questionnaires

Two questionnaires have been demonstrated through research to be highly associated with levels of pain and disability, as well as psychological distress from chronic pain—the Pain Catastrophizing Scale[16], and the Pain Vigilance

---

[16] Sullivan, Bishop, & Pivak, J (1995). "The Pain Catastrophizing Scale represents a range of catastrophizing thoughts and feelings in response to the experience of pain . . . This scale has good construct and criterion validity, and has been associated with levels of disability in patients with soft tissue injuries, even when controlling for levels of depression and pain intensity."

and Awareness Questionnaire.[17] Taken together, these questionnaires are able to indicate whether your way of thinking about, and psychologically responding to the pain, is a significant contributing factor to the impact which the chronic pain is having on you. Professor of Psychology at Auckland University, Keith Petrie and his colleagues have demonstrated that how we respond to and make sense of health conditions can be as powerful in determining the outcomes (e.g whether the condition is short lived or becomes chronic) as is the seriousness of the condition itself.[18]

Take ten minutes now to complete these two questionnaires, which can be found in Appendix 1. Complete them again after couple of months of engaging with the ideas presented in this book. Appendix 11 has an additional copy of each questionnaire for completion at a later date.

The Pain Catastrophizing Scale assesses people's differing tendencies towards a highly emotional focus on the awfulness of pain. The overall score has been linked with levels of disability in people with soft tissue injuries.

The Pain Vigilance and Awareness Questionnaire assesses people's level of 'hypervigilance' in regards to the pain—how focused you are on every aspect and variation in it. High scores on this scale have been linked in research to pain intensity, psychological distress from the pain, as well as high levels of psycho-social disability from the pain.

High scores on these questionnaires would suggest a significant psychological contributor to chronic pain, and/or a risk of pain becoming even more entrenched. The Pain Catastrophizing Scale has a maximum possible score of 52. If your score is more than the mid-point of 26, then you are in the higher end of the dimension of catastrophizing about your pain. The Pain Vigilance and Awareness Questionnaire has a maximum possible score of 80, so if your score is above 40, then you are in the higher end of the dimension of hypervigilance to your pain.

---

[17] McCraken (1997). "The Pain Vigilance and Awareness Scale measures the extent to which people focus on or attend to that pain ... The total scale has good internal reliability and construct validity . . . High scores are associated with pain intensity, psychological distress, psychosocial disability, and physician visits."

[18] Moss-Morris et al (2007). "Patients' perceptions of their pain condition across a multidisciplinary Pain Management program: Do they change and does it matter?" *Clinical Journal of Pain*.

If you score high on these questionnaires, the ideas presented to you in this book will aid you in counteracting many of the psychological risk factors for chronic pain. If you score low on these questionnaires, reading this book and internalising its messages could protect you from a pain syndrome becoming entrenched and therefore chronic. Most forms of chronic pain firstly begin their lives as short-term acute pain. In a sense, the ideas presented here can 'inoculate' you against pain today evolving into long-term chronic pain tomorrow.

Chapter 1 provides an overview of the role which psychology can play in both the causation and the cure of chronic pain. The case examples presented throughout this book are all real people, with only their identifying information changed to protect their anonymity. Chapter 2 looks more closely at the medical treatment of chronic pain. Confusion between and amongst health professionals have added to the current epidemic of chronic pain. It is important to understand the guiding philosophy underlying the medical treatment of this condition, as gaining such an understanding is part of the treatment process—knowledge is power. Conventional medical treatments of chronic pain will also be discussed, as well as the new understanding of pain which is developing within medicine. Chapter 3 introduces a more expanded model of medicine, which incorporates both psychological and social, as well as physical factors. This bio-psycho-social approach to medicine is viewed as an important development, and is in essence entirely compatible with The Hidden Psychology of Pain. Chapter 4 discusses the range of misunderstandings which abound with chronic pain. These misunderstandings are not simply benign, but play an important role in creating and perpetuating the current epidemic. Chapter 5 introduces some of the biological pathways, triggered by psychological issues, which can result in chronic pain. Some basic physiology, in relation to parts of the anatomy which are vulnerable to chronic pain, is presented. Chapter 6 discusses the unconscious psychological factors which can trigger chronic pain in more detail. As you will read, by virtue of being unconscious, these are often not the most obvious ones. Chapter 7 presents more in-depth discussion of unconscious psychological factors, which range from childhood experiences to broad cultural issues. Chapter 8 discusses many of the strategies and changes in thought that are required to overcome chronic pain. You will be taught to 'tune into' what your experience is telling you as a tool to helping you in your recovery. Chapter 9 begins the presentation of self-help strategies. It will come as no surprise that these are psychological. Many of the helpful activities can be done by you at home with no professional help. Chapter 10 involves a discussion about depression, as this is a common experience for people in chronic pain. Again, how we make sense of this experience has a major role to play in regards to what we do about it, and the subsequent likelihood of recovery. Unfortunately, our culture provides as many blind-alleys with depression as it does with chronic pain, so being a well-informed consumer of health services is vital. Chapter 11 examines the healing potential which dreams hold. Learning how to harness their healing potential will take your further on the path of physical and emotional recovery. Chapter 12 presents an approach to 'energy psychology' (EFT) which I have seen work wonders for many sufferers. It can be thought of as 'psychological acupuncture', although a more neurological explanation aids in the understanding of how it achieves results. As it is a self-help strategy, you can begin using it on a range of issues as soon as possible. Chapter 13 addresses another common problem for people in chronic pain—the inability to sleep well. A range of strategies to improve sleep are presented, and you will be taught how to use EFT to assist in overcoming this problem. Chapter 14 discusses the application of EFT to stress and anxiety. Most people who suffer chronic pain feel stressed by the condition, and will often be highly anxious in regards to flare-ups, or actions associated with the pain. EFT is a very useful means of reigning in these anxieties. The value of psychotherapy in the treatment of chronic pain is discussed in chapter 15. Like any other health service, psychotherapy is a market place of ideas and differing approaches. Some types of psychotherapy are especially useful for treating chronic pain, while others can offer little. Chapter 16 presents a particular type of psychotherapy, EMDR, which is especially effective in dealing with both trauma and chronic pain. Chapter 17 discusses the importance of finding greater acceptance of chronic pain. This is deliberately left as the final chapter. The basic thesis of this book is that there is much you can do to radically decrease your experience of chronic pain. However, cultivating an attitude of acceptance towards all challenges allows you to minimise your stress response to the pain. You will learn that emotional pain, such as 'stress', is highly related to the experience of physical pain, so decreasing one is likely to have a flow-on effect to the other.

There are two streams of information running throughout this book. On the one hand are the case studies and information which are there to help you work out how to alleviate your pain. On the other hand are segments of information which present research-based information and other more academic points. Rather than write two books, one for sufferers and one for professionals, I have decided to incorporate both of these streams in the one book. Many sufferers are also interested in the some of the more academic information, and many health professionals also suffer from chronic pain. Much of the technical information can be found in the Appendices. Appendix 2 discusses some of the basics of the brain as well as the neurology of pain. It is essential that you read this Appendix early on, as the brain is repeatedly discussed throughout the book. While pain is clearly *not* all in your head, what happens in the head is just as central to the experience chronic pain as it is to the pain derived from stepping on a nail—in both cases, brain processes are fundamental. Appendix 3 presents the anatomy of the spine, while Appendix 4 details standard medical treatments for chronic back pain. Following on from this, Appendix 5 reveals what the evidence says about the value of physical therapies such as chiropractic and physiotherapy manipulation. As psychology is a disparate field of endeavor, Appendix 6 presents the evolution of psychology. With this, readers can appreciate some of the theoretical differences in approaches, and why not all approaches to psychology are the same when it comes to treating chronic pain. In support of some of the major contentions of this book, Appendix 7 reviews a sample of research relating to structural pathology in the spine, clearly demonstrating that spine pathology is not relevant to most cases of chronic pain. Appendix 8 presents the self-help EFT procedure, while Appendix 9 details a process for remaining in the present moment. You will be referred to these appendices where they become relevant throughout the book. Appendix 10 presents some testimonials from people who have benefited from this program. Appendix 11 gives you the opportunity to complete the Pain Questionnaires after undertaking this process. And finally, Appendix 12 addresses the question of whether *The Hidden Psychology of Pain* is merely a placebo treatment. My suggestion is that you read the book in the order it has been prepared and presented so that you are able to answer this question for yourself.

CHAPTER 1

Psychology & Pain

I WAS FIRST ALERTED TO THE true nature of chronic pain from the experience of a friend whom I had known since my early teenage years. As a young man, he had suffered for months from such intense back pain that a surgeon had advised him to undergo a fusion of what were believed to be the offending vertebrae. Nothing else had helped up to that point. Desperate for relief, he made arrangements for the surgery. I rang him a few days later to see how he was after the operation. He told me he ended up not having the procedure at all. On the day of the surgery, he simply woke up with no back pain, and had concluded that it was not necessary. He experienced a spontaneous remission, and has remained largely pain-free ever since. Many years later, now a middle-aged man, this friend regularly trains for and runs half-marathons.

What had happened here? Was he a malingerer who, having achieved the sympathy he figured he deserved, simply decided to drop the issue? This explanation simply did not hold with my knowledge of his character. Something else had happened to remove his pain, but at the time I had no idea that psychology could be part of the answer.

Years later, a similar thing happened with a different friend who complained of chronic rhinitis, asthma and food allergies. I saw her after she had just come back from a weekend of "spiritual development" at a quasi-religious workshop. Over the weekend, she had simply realized that she no longer "needed" to have these respiratory complaints or the associated food allergies. From then on, she was symptom-free. As with my other friend, I had no way of understanding this experience at the time, but nor could

1

I deny the reality of it. It was not until several years later that I was able to make any sense of these two puzzling reports.

Let's look now at another sufferer—this time, experiencing a chronic groin pain. At its worst, the pain in his left groin was excruciating, barely allowing him to walk normally. At other times, he was able to run and even play tennis, but the pain could return without any notice or warning. As an otherwise fit and healthy young man, being stuck with a limiting pain was inevitably depressing. Fortunately, his occupation did not require heavy lifting or vigorous movement, as that would have left him unemployable around 50% of the time. Regardless of its fluctuations, the pain was a constant in his life for eighteen years.

A physiotherapist tried manipulation and traction to treat him. She diagnosed that a lower back nerve was being pinched as a result of a car accident he'd had a few years earlier, producing a referred pain in his groin. She placed him in traction a couple of times a week, which according to the bio-mechanics, would stretch the offending vertebrae apart, allowing more room for the nerve and thereby reduce the pain.

The traction helped to alleviate the pain, but it usually returned immediately after the treatment—often, as soon as he got into his car in the physiotherapist's car park. Then he tried a highly regarded chiropractor who said the pain came from a twist in his hips, again sending a referred pain into his groin. Like the physiotherapist, the chiropractor viewed the physical trauma from the car accident as the likely cause of the problem.

In addition to vigorous manipulation, the chiropractor had him lay flat and placed blocks under one hip and the opposite buttock. As did the physiotherapist's traction, the blocks relieved the pain during the treatment, but it generally returned again soon afterwards. He became resigned to having this pain for the rest of his life, due to the impact of the car accident. All he could do was to attempt to manage the pain with using blocks he made for himself, and replicating the treatment each day at home. For years, he tried to come to grips with this pain being with him for life. In fact, he suspected it was likely to get worse with age as his body naturally deteriorated, and the best he could do was to accept the fact.

After eighteen years of pain, he came across the notion that psychological distress and traumatized emotions could play a role in the causation of chronic pain. In his case, accompanying the physical trauma from his car accident was a high level of emotional trauma. He had been hit in a head-on car accident, with the front of his van collapsing in on his legs. He was trapped in the car wreck for the next two and half hours, with broken bones protruding from his body, and bleeding profusely. For the most part, in the laudable medical attempts to heal his body, the distressed emotions were ignored by the treating health practitioners. He, in turn, suppressed and ignored the emotional trauma as well.

The Hidden Psychology of Pain details the role which suppressed psychological distress plays in the causation of chronic pain—usually, so suppressed that for all intents and purposes, it is hidden from the sufferer's awareness.

For this man with chronic groin pain, discovering these well-hidden emotions, and seeing the role which they played in his pain, resulted in the same type of symptoms elimination which the other two people detailed above experienced. This breakthrough gave him the physical freedom he believed would never again be possible, even allowing him to play amateur Australian Rules Football after a twenty-year absence.

How do I know about his experience? That sufferer of chronic pain was me. After struggling with it for nearly two decades, I have now been free of that pain for more than 15 years. What brought about this seemingly miraculous cure? Nothing other than the information you will find in this book.

It is possible to cure yourself of chronic pain; however, the ideas in this book are not "conventional." For the most part, the contemporary "pain industry"—the medical and associated professions, and even psychology—do not subscribe to these ideas. They are, however, ideas with a very long history and a very well-demonstrated track record. They have been on the edges of medicine and psychology for many decades, however, in previous eras they were regarded as conventional therapeutic wisdom. The time has come for these notions to again take center stage if we seriously want to relieve the chronic pain epidemic currently gripping our society.

Some readers of this book will respond with *"Of course!"*—you will find the approaches described as merely reinforcing views which you have long held, and always suspected were relevant to chronic pain. For many others, these ideas will be radical and challenging—so challenging for some people that they will dismiss the notions out of hand, despite the evidence presented. This is each person's prerogative. Perhaps such people may come back to these ideas at a later time in their lives.

For professionals reading this book, especially physicians and psychologists, my hope is that you are able to go beyond what have become standard concepts of chronic pain. This may also require that you go beyond the views with which your training equipped you. If you do so, many of your patients and clients will ultimately thank you for having the insight and the courage.

My early 1980s academic training in psychology treated "depth-psychology" and the highly related "Freudian psychology" more as an historical artifacts than viable approaches to the study of human psychology. Certainly, many of Freud's psychoanalytic notions can now be seen as reflecting 19th century European beliefs and thoughts, and as such, are now quite dated. However, one of the lasting contributions which Freud and his predecessors made is the notion that when it comes to human psychology, there is usually more going on than meets the eye. It is quite common for people to show a lack of awareness of psychological factors operating within them at a level below their conscious awareness.

Freud's approach—psychoanalysis—left psychology with an emphasis that we are aware of only a small portion of our psychological realities at any one time. Much of what is actually dictating our emotions, thoughts and behaviors are factors which are operating at an unconscious level. By definition, we are largely unaware of these.

Rather than learning from the depth-psychology tradition, contemporary psychology has overwhelmingly opted for the cognitive-behavioral model, which emphasizes the role of our conscious thoughts in producing our feelings and actions. For many people, such an approach may prove quite adequate, especially when they are suffering from problems other than chronic pain. This book will argue, however, that chronic pain often requires a different approach.

We like to think that our rational mind is in charge of the show; however, Freud suggested that this is merely a vain fantasy. As a European, he was profoundly affected by the mass-murder on his doorstep which was WWI. Industrial society was so convinced of its own rationality that it came as a bewildering shock to most people that racially and culturally similar people could slog it out for years on end, killing countless millions in the process, in order to temporarily gain small parcels of land. This did not strike Freud as an example of rationality dictating our actions, or as evidence that humans are an essentially logical and reasonable species. Rather, he suggested that our behavior is largely instinctively driven by factors outside of our conscious awareness, and our mind will go to almost any lengths to ensure that the real causes remain hidden from us.

However, to many contemporary psychologists, the importance of psychological factors operating at an unconscious level is seen as irrelevant at best, and as a ridiculous insult at worst. Originators of the currently very popular cognitive therapy, such as psychiatrist Aaron Beck and psychologist Albert Ellis, spent their careers arguing that a focus on what occurs in the conscious awareness is all one needs attend to in order to progress psychologically.

Ellis viewed suggestions of unconscious factors creating behavior and feelings as utterly incorrect. His goal was to have us fully utilize our capacity to think rationally by the very conscious endeavor of arguing sense to ourselves. Beck's goal is to teach us how to avoid typical thinking errors, and instead use scientific methods for arriving at rational conclusions through gathering evidence. As such, Beck and Ellis argue that our conscious thoughts are both the problem as well as the potential solution.

This is the mindset in which I was trained as a psychology student around thirty years ago. As such, I was scornful of the entire depth-psychology enterprise until, when in my early 30s, I attended a weeklong residential workshop in a therapy called "re-birthing." This was not an approach that I would ever have voluntarily chosen, however my wife had participated in the workshop a couple of months earlier and strongly urged me to do so as well. On the first night of the workshop I was brought face-to-face, against all of my expectations, with material that was clearly of an unconscious nature.

Many years earlier, I had been nearly killed in a head-on car accident as an eighteen-year-old whilst attempting to travel around Australia. My journey was brought to a sudden halt one night when the VW Kombi van I was driving was hit by a drunk driver. This experience, and the associated trauma, was so powerful that within a year it had led to my decision to become a psychologist, so that I could help other people who had been similarly damaged.

For around six months after the accident, I was clearly in a bad way psychologically. This lasted until I began to recover physically. Six months later, around the time I came off crutches, I discovered in my father's library his psychology books on meditation, self-hypnosis and other forms of personal development and self-help. This was the beginning of my recovery. A year and a half after my accident, I was studying psychology, and my indoctrination into the contemporary psychological worldview commenced.

By the time I had completed my post-graduate training and became a trainee psychologist, I was convinced that any form of depth-psychology was interesting as a theory, but essentially a load of bumpkin as far as its practical applications were concerned. Upon graduation, I proceeded to practice the cognitive-behavioral psychology that I had been trained in, and never gave another thought to notions of the unconscious, unless it was dismissive. Applying the rationality of Ellis, and Beck's CBT notions of thinking errors to myself, I proceeded to get on with life, and viewed my accident as something akin to a bad movie I had seen years earlier.

Opening to the unconscious

When, in my early 30s, my wife urged that I attend the week long re-birthing workshop, no approach could have sat worse with where I was as a psychologist (although as a husband, I had been married long enough to know that it was highly advisable I attend). More than feeling that it was a complete waste of time, I resented the money involved, as well as the "fruitcake" notions that I would have to endure over the week. I was wrong, however, and the whole experience opened my eyes to the reality of the unconscious mind.

The term "re-birthing" suggests that it involves re-experiencing one's birth. It may include this, but the process is more commonly used for working with any upsetting experience, especially traumatic ones.

On the first night, with little introduction to what was involved in the re-birthing process, we were paired up with other participants. In my pair, I was to be the "subject" first. I lay on the ground and began rapid, shallow breathing as instructed. The only thought repeatedly going through my mind was "*What an outrageous waste of time and money it's costing me to lie here and breathe!*"

Before too long, other participants in the workshop were "going off," with shouts, howls, and much screaming. "*Great*'," I thought, "*and it's costing me money to lie here and breathe, and listen to this!*"

A short time later, I became cold and started shivering. My thoughts quickly incorporated this complaint into the growing list. Then my body began gyrating, and I couldn't believe my stupidity, a cognitive-behavioral psychologist, getting caught up in this madness. Before I had time to complain internally any further, with a *whoosh*, I was transported into a virtual-reality scene of when the medical team were examining me in the emergency room after finally being freed from my car wreck. I was reliving the moment when I began to cry from the shock of what I had been through. As an eighteen-year-old, even in such a serious state, I noticed that many of the medical staff attending to me were attractive young nurses. On realizing this, I felt embarrassed and stifled my crying. People can die from shock from the type of injuries I had. Not giving in to my emotions may have been a survival instinct, or it may have just been the dumb shame of a teenage boy.

In the re-birthing session, without any programming or expectation—in fact, with only very negative expectations—I re-experienced the emergency room scene, and this time bellowed like a wounded bull. Part of me was listening to the noise that I was producing, and was shocked by the intensity of it, as well as the lack of control which "I" had over it.

"I," being my conscious mind, was clearly not choosing to do this. In fact, "I" did not even believe it was possible, as up until that moment I believed that the unconscious was an elaborate and outdated myth. But then where was this howling coming from, if not from my unconscious? While on a conscious level, I firmly believed that I had dealt with my trauma (reciting positive mantras, changing my thinking errors, learning to cope, etc.), there was something obviously a lot deeper within me that was howling. A part of my psyche was still carrying the trauma, and was now giving expression to it. All of this was happening without any conscious choice or control.

I howled like a broken record for perhaps twenty minutes, until the workshop leader came and talked me through the experience. I didn't stop being a cognitive-behavioral psychologist in that moment, but I certainly did become one who appreciated the reality of the unconscious mind, and the distress that could be deeply buried within. Despite my training, the reality of the unconscious had become suddenly and dramatically undeniable to me. With this experience, I became a cognitive-behavioral psychologist who is open to notions of depth-psychology.

The depth-psychology model recognizes that our present experience of life is often highly influenced by our experiences of the past. Early childhood experiences, both positive and negative, are stored away in our psyche and the ensuing psychological patterns can have massive ramifications for our current thoughts, feelings and behaviors as an adult. Cognitive-behavioral psychologists like Ellis and Beck are highly critical of this notion, preferring to believe our emotions and behaviors result purely from our thoughts about the current situations in which we find ourselves. They generally agree we have patterns of cognition learnt as children, but they give priority to current perceptions of events or situations. Beck and Ellis suggest that rational thinking can actually free people from the damaging effects of the past. If it were only that easy.

I now find it implausible that my behavior as a young adult in my 20s and 30s was not at least in part attributable to the trauma which I experienced as an eighteen-year-old. The re-birthing experience made me aware of a "reservoir" of distress within me, of which I previously had only the vaguest notion. But, despite my best cognitive-behavioral attempts to cope, my past could not be merely "disappeared" by the optimistic theorizing of contemporary psychology.

I wasn't inspired to become a re-birther as a result of my profound experiences (which kept happening over the course of the week-long workshop). It was still too far removed from all I had done and learned as a psychologist. The experience did, however, open me up both intellectually and emotionally to a range of other realities which I had dismissed many years earlier.

Years later, while working as a rehabilitation psychologist with people in chronic pain, a friend gave me a copy of *Spontaneous Healing,* by the "alternative" medical doctor, Andrew Weil. In this book, Weil refers to the astonishing claims of John Sarno, which had me following up with the latter's books. In addition, I also sought out the sources of Sarno's approach in the historical depth-psychology literature.

What I was read was a startling revelation to me. At this time, I was still plagued by the reoccurring pain in my left groin that had bothered me for the previous eighteen or so years. It felt like a permanently torn muscle that just refused to heal. A chiropractor I saw within a couple of months of the crash assessed that vertebrae were out of place as a result of the impact of my car accident. By suggesting this, he planted a seed which allowed me to explain my chronic pain in light of the physical trauma. Over the next few years, each of the treating professionals further nurtured this seed with their diagnoses.

The depth-psychology approach to chronic pain initially excited me because of the benefit it may have for my clients. My academic training, however, made me suspicious of introducing to suffering people an approach that I had only read about in books and articles.

Though Sarno's and Maté's case studies were very impressive, the skeptical part of me didn't actually know whether they were of *real* people, or just a clever marketing strategy. Over the next few months, I slowly opened to trying depth-psychology ideas with myself in regards to my groin pain. I read several relevant books, spoke to friends about what they were saying, and generally chewed over the possibilities. However, it was still difficult to be confident about the possibility that unconscious psychological issues could be producing my persistent groin pain.

Around this time, my wife and I took our kids on a family holiday to the area where my accident had happened when I was younger. I wanted to show them the place where I *hadn't* died. Although not consciously aware of it at the time, it happened to be around the anniversary of the accident. In the preceding week, the pain in my groin steadily grew to the most intense I had ever experienced. I was barely able to walk, and felt I was dragging my left leg behind me as I struggled just to move. As we came closer to both the anniversary of the accident, and visiting the accident site, the pain intensified to the worst level of disability I had ever experienced.

It was then that the penny finally dropped. I became aware of the coincidence of the dates and where I found myself. Now, the extreme pain seemed to be not so much a random fluke as an event with a psychological cause. It became obvious to me that the pain was related to emotional trauma from my accident, and not, as I had been led to believe, to the physical trauma. The pain persisted on the day we visited the crash scene, but over the next week, it gradually diminished to virtually nothing. Now, after more than fifteen years, the pain that bothered me for nearly twenty years has never returned as more than a very occasional, very slight reminder of what it once was. And this rare slight "tweak" of pain only ever occurs now at times of heightened emotional stress.

Needless to say, I was extremely impressed with this relief. I began to feel some credibility in introducing the "Hidden Psychology of Pain," as I came to call it, to clients suffering from chronic pain. Although I was a sample-size of only one, a single case experiment, it had worked for me, and the results were certainly impressive. But just because I had this positive response did not mean it would work for anyone else. However, I was willing to tentatively give people the information and allow them to decide for themselves. Over the past fifteen or so years, this approach has made an enormous difference to many of my clients who were suffering a far greater level of disability than I ever had.

The following is a genuine case study of man whom I will call Max. I saw him several years ago whilst working in the pain management unit of a hospital. Max was a forty-five-year-old father of two young children who had suffered extreme back pain for around five years. His job entailed heavy lifting, and having done this work for most of his adult life, it was logical to assume the demands of the job were causing the pain. As the pain got progressively worse, he had to leave the job and had not yet returned five years later, although his employer was keen to get him back if ever possible. Max's medical reports showed some minor degenerative changes in his spine, but according to the medical specialists, nothing that should produce the debilitating pain he was clearly experiencing.

On meeting him, I learned that he was also very depressed about being in constant pain for so many years. He was distressed by his "failings" as a husband, and believed himself to be an inadequate father who had little tolerance for, or joy in his children. At times, he was so depressed that he felt suicidal, and had been placed on antidepressant drugs. Fortunately, his wife was very supportive, despite his impatience and constant sour mood.

I introduced the Hidden Psychology of Pain to him during our second consultation, raising the idea that unconscious distressed emotion could play a role in his chronic pain. Like most clients, he listened politely and ended the session with few questions, and stated that he would think it all over. When I next saw him a week later he nervously ventured to me, "There are some things that happened to me as a kid which I have never told anyone about. It could have something to do with my pain." He then proceeded to tell me that his older brother had sexually abused him throughout most of his childhood. He had vaguely alluded to the abuse to his wife, although he had never disclosed the details. He had just mentioned to her that his brother should not be trusted with their children, as he wanted to protect them if he should ever die unexpectedly.

The brother lived with their mother, the father having died a few years earlier. On one occasion, when younger, Max confronted him when they were both drunk. The brother said nothing but hastily withdrew from Max while crying. It had never been discussed since. Max maintained relatively normal family relations with his brother, going to family dinners and, incredibly, to football matches together each weekend. But comments like, "I know what he did was wrong, but I can't bring myself to hate him," showed his internal distress and dilemma. Max described himself as having been a problem teenager and young adult, drinking to excess and misbehaving as a result of the emotional turmoil that he was in. He certainly suffered emotionally from what had been done to him, yet Max was unable to articulate this distress to anyone, or to resolve his upset feelings.

Suspecting that his back pain could indeed be related to his emotional pain, I asked Max what was happening in his life when the pain began. He told me about two significant events: "My first baby was born, and at around the same time, my brother got a job at the same place where I worked. Everyone, especially my mum, was so happy that my brother and I could work together. It cut me up inside, but I just kept on pretending that I was happy to be with my brother each day."

As a new parent, he found himself suddenly responsible for the safety of a vulnerable little human being, as he knew only too well how vulnerable little human beings could be. "I wasn't safe as a kid, so then I started to worry that I might not be able to protect my young son." His daily contact with the perpetrator of the sexual abuse inflicted on him throughout childhood reinforced his feelings of helplessness and responsibility.

As Max had maintained a positive relationship with his brother on the surface, he couldn't bring about a sudden change without offering an explanation. He believed that telling his mother would simply kill her. All this was complicated by his brother living with his elderly mother so as to look after her. Max was under intense pressure to enjoy his brother's company at work, but at a deeper level, it is conceivable that he wanted to kill him. The obvious psychological quandary, which had been present since his childhood, was made even more intense and inescapable. Unable to admit to himself his intense feelings of rage and hatred towards his brother, much less than to anyone else, Max developed the chronic back pain which forced him to leave work within just a few months of his brother starting there.

None of this was a conscious ploy, and Max had no awareness of it as a possible cause of his pain. Until I introduced Max to the Hidden Psychology of Pain, the connection had never previously occurred to him. Although he discussed the assault with me without any great detail, Max did talk about the effects it had had on his life.

Three weeks after our first session, Max told me that revealing the abuse had taken an enormous weight off his shoulders. "Just telling someone about it was a huge relief. I guess I blamed myself for so many years. What he did to me made me feel so guilty and dirty—I just always felt ashamed of myself." Over the week following his disclosure of the abuse to me, his pain began to diminish until it was not present at all. Five years of crippling pain virtually disappeared within just one week of revealing his trauma.

Max attributed the improvement to disclosing the abuse after years of having to repress the negative feelings. This remains one of the fastest improvements from a chronic pain condition I have ever seen. As his pain continued to diminish over the next few weeks, he became more tolerant with his family, was able to play with his children, and started to be the type of family man he had always wanted to be. Needless to say, his depression lifted as well, all without any attempt on my part to treat his emotional state.

Max remained pain-free for a six-week period. Then his favorite aunt died unexpectedly, and the back pain returned with ferocity. In addition to the grief at the loss of his aunt, he was also distressed by being in pain again. As before, I assumed the pain was happening for a reason, rather than just being a random occurrence. When I asked Max about the significance of his aunt's death, he revealed, "I used to stay with her every second weekend when I was a kid. I don't know why, but my brother never came and stayed there with me, so it was just me and her family. It was the only place I was safe from the abuse throughout my whole childhood, the only place I could relax and be off-guard."

A week later, after discussing the possible connection between his aunt's death and the re-emergence of his back pain, Max reported that the pain began to diminish again, back to the level where it ceased to be problematic. Again, this was a remarkable improvement.

The next challenge for Max, after around two months of being pain-free, was the prospect of returning to work. Max revealed, "My boss told me that if I ever got over the pain, my job would always be waiting for me, and the job is still there for me. Now my GP is saying that he can't keep signing me off as unfit for work because I've been telling him how much better I am. The problem is that my brother still works there, and I don't think I can put myself back in that situation again." The prospect filled him with so much anxiety that, at some level, he was reluctant to get too much better—in fact, his back pain had returned again.

Beginning to see a pattern emerging, we again discussed the possible connection between his distressed feelings and his experience of back pain. The relief of his back pain had actually created another dilemma for Max. If he refused to go back to the same job, when deemed fit for work by his GP, he would be ineligible for government financial assistance and his family would suffer. Yet, if he went back to the same job, he knew that he would suffer emotionally, and most likely physically again as well.

Max was now well aware of the relationship between emotional factors and the experience of his physical pain. He could not, realistically, put himself back in that situation again. We discussed informing his mother of the abuse, and demanding that his brother leave the workplace. Max decided against this course for a range of reasons. Primarily, he was worried about the effect it may have on his aged mother. Ultimately, he opted for facing the financial challenge and retraining for different work, and gratefully did this with his wife's support.

This case study shows the complexity of what chronic sufferers of pain can face. It was not a straightforward case of Max revealing the abuse, seeing the connection, and then getting better for all time. Although his physical improvement was dramatic, he obviously had further psychological work to do if he wanted to remain pain-free. This case is not a typical example (as most people don't get better so quickly), but is an example of *what is possible*. I have also successfully worked with many people who were not abused as children, but nevertheless wound up with chronic pain for other reasons. Abuse is not a necessary ingredient, although it is certainly overrepresented in the chronic pain population.

I have since had conversations with physiotherapists who said this dramatic improvement, and other ones just like it were simply *"not possible."*

Their response reminds me of reports of indigenous people simply failing to "see" the tall ships of Europeans for the first time. I was reporting events so far out of their frame of reference that they insisted it was not real. To these physiotherapists, either the client was lying, or I was lying. Let me assure you that my clients and I are telling the complete truth. The cases I present in this book are all entirely real, with only identifying information altered to protect their anonymity.

Chronic pain is very real physical pain which is generated by our own mind/brain in order to prevent us from having to confront and deal with psychological pain. This reality is "hidden" in that the pain is being generated within us in an unconscious manner, with no conscious choice, and usually very little awareness. The issues leading to such psychological pain are often known to us, in the form of traumatic memories of terrible or hurtful events which we have experienced. With Max, this was clearly the case: he knew that he had been sexually abused by his brother. However, the hidden element of this was how deeply disturbing the abuse was, and how much ill-feeling towards his brother he had to repress in order to maintain a civil relationship with him.

In other cases, the hidden element is an impossible dilemma, or an unsolvable problem, which our mind would prefer to keep from our conscious awareness. Sometimes it can even be hidden fears in relation to positive events in our lives. And it can also be self-doubts and insecurities which we would prefer not to be aware of, or aspects of our personalities of which we are ashamed. All of these examples share the common thread of being threatening to our conscious awareness, particularly to our sense of who we are. As such, our mind/brain will go to great lengths to prevent this unconscious material from erupting into our conscious awareness, fearing the consequences were it to emerge. An unconscious 'part' of us is able to create chronic pain in order to protect us from upsetting realities, be they internal or external realities. This unconscious emotional part is able to utilise biological pathways to result in physical pain as an attempted 'solution' to what it perceives to be an even greater problem than the pain. For example, according to a particular emotional position within Max, having his attention focused on being in chronic back pain was an attempted solution to awareness of the reservoir of rage which he felt towards his brother, a preferable option to becoming fully aware of this rage with potentially murderous consequences.

Chronic pain, generated by our own mind/brain, is an excellent way in which our conscious attention can be monopolized in order that we remain unaware of deep psychological distress. It's intention is usually protective, shielding our conscious awareness from deep emotional pain and dilemmas. That is its purpose, and the mind/brain can use a range of biological pathways in the body to generate very real physical pain. These pathways will be explored in a later chapter.

The Mind/Body Syndrome

John Sarno calls psychologically induced chronic pain the Tension Myositis Syndrome, or TMS for short. Here, "tension" refers to the role that emotional tension plays in causing pain—this refers to "both anxiety and to the state of defensive hyper-vigilance and guardedness in perception of danger."[1] "Myositis" refers to pain in the skeletal muscles due to changes in lactic acid metabolism and episodic muscle spasm. And "syndrome" refers to the cluster of symptoms that tend to go together. In more recent years, he has referred to TMS as "The Mind/Body Syndrome," in recognition that the syndrome can entail more than just muscular pain.[2]

The syndrome involves not just the initial emotional distress, which the pain is unconsciously designed to protect us from, but also the additional contributions of various elements of "psychological overlay." This includes all the fears and anxieties, the anger and despair and the grief associated with being in constant pain. Also, the range of debilitating thoughts, negative beliefs about oneself and the future, and the restricted social worlds which people find themselves in. In addition, certain bodily movements and postural preferences evolve over time, which become entrenched, and can create extra problems through the imbalances that are created.

---

[1] Sarno & Coen (1989, p.361). "Psychosomatic Avoidance of Conflict in Back Pain." *Journal of the American Academy of Psychoanalysis.*

[2] Sarno (1998) *The Mindbody Prescription.*

These additional elements of "overlay" also feedback into the syndrome, constantly adding to the emotional and physical distress. As such, the syndrome becomes like hardened cement, set in a solid pattern that traps the person in unchanging and painful emotional and physical constriction.

There are a wide range chronic pain and health conditions that fall under the term TMS, and they all share a common purpose- to protect the person from having a conscious awareness of deep emotional hurts and dilemmas. Sarno observes that the skin, the gastrointestinal system, the genitourinary system, the circulatory system, the immune system, and the cardiac system can all be affected by TMS.

The following is a comprehensive list of such conditions that he includes under TMS, many of them using different physiological pathways to produce different symptoms, but all for the same purpose of protecting us in some important way. This protection may be in the form of distracting our attention, so that we are shielded from awareness of painful emotional material, or it may be to prevent us from engaging in certain activities. While the distraction purpose gets considerable attention in this book, please note that this is just one potential 'solution' which chronic pain can offer—others may become more apparent to you in the self-help sections. Some of these conditions, especially ones that do not involve chronic pain, can have other medical causes, so a thorough medical examination is highly suggested before considering them as equivalents to TMS.

- Low back pain, diagnosed with one or more of the following: Sciatica, Osteoarthritis, Spinal stenosis, Herniated/bulging/ degenerated lumbar disc, Scoliosis, Spondylolysthesis, Piriformis syndrome, Weak/inflexible torso or hip muscles, Spina bifida occulta, Spondylolysis, Transitional vertebra.
- Neck/shoulder pain, diagnosed with one or more of the following: Osteoarthritis, Pinched nerve, Herniated/bulging/ degenerated cervical disc, Whiplash, Thoracic outlet syndrome, Weak/inflexible neck, shoulder girdle, or rotator cuff muscles, Rotator cuff tears, Bursitis, Tendonitis.
- Knee pain, diagnosed with one or more of the following: Tendonitis, Torn meniscus, Chondromalacia, Unstable patella, Muscular imbalances around the knee joint, Osteoarthritis

- Elbow pain, diagnosed with one or more of the following: Tennis elbow, Tendonitis, Muscular imbalances around the elbow joint, Osteoarthritis
- Foot/lower leg pain, diagnosed with one or more of the following: Tendonitis, Plantar fasciitis, Plantar metatarsalgia, Neuroma, Flat feet, Calcium deposit/heel spur, Shin splints, Muscular imbalances around the ankle or foot joints, Osteoarthritis
- Wrist/hand pain, diagnosed with one or more of the following: Carpal tunnel syndrome/repetitive stress injury, Tendonitis, Muscular imbalances around the wrist or hand joints, Osteoarthritis
- Nerve dysfunction, diagnosed with one or more of the following: Sciatica, Carpal tunnel syndrome/repetitive stress injury, Trigeminal neuralgia/tic douloureux, Bell's palsy
- Temporal mandibular joint syndrome (TMJ)
- Fibromyalgia
- Myofascial pain syndrome
- Tension myalgia
- Gastrointestinal disorders: Heartburn/acid reflux,
- Hiatus hernia, Gastritis, Ulcer, Nervous stomach, Spastic colon, Irritable bowel syndrome, Colitis
- Circulatory disorders: Tension headache, Migraine, Reynaud's phenomenon (excessively cold hands/feet)
- Genitourinary disorders: Frequent urination, Urinary tract infections, Prostatitis
- Cardiac disorders: Rapid pounding heartbeat (paroxysmal auricular tachycardia), Extra (ectopic) heartbeats
- Immune system disorders: Allergies, Asthma attacks, Frequent infections, Skin disorders, Epstein-Barr syndrome
- Miscellaneous disorders: Dizziness/vertigo, Tinnitus (ringing in the ears), Chronic fatigue syndrome, Laryngitis/spasmodic dysphonia

You will gather from the comprehensiveness of this list that such conditions are pervasive in our society—very few people will go through life without experiencing at least one of them. In fact, these conditions are so pervasive that they can rightly be said to simply reflect the human condition. The good news is that these conditions are all treatable with information and greater awareness as promoted in this book.

This list would not be surprising to most depth-psychology oriented psychologists or psychiatrists. In fact, some mind/body health practitioners would extend it even further to include extreme health conditions such as cancer and heart disease. At the start of the twenty-first century, there are also more physicians who would acknowledge the above list than in the previous few decades.[3]

Allan House, Professor of Liaison Psychiatry at the University of Leeds in the UK, reports to using ideas similar to the Hidden Psychology of Pain in assisting people suffering from "hysterical" paralysis.[4] When he began working as a young physician, he was referred to many people with medically unexplained symptoms such as those listed above. With psychiatry over the second half of the twentieth century having become largely drug-focused, there was no framework of understanding which his psychiatric or medical training had given him. Like myself and Sarno, House also had to revert back to depth-psychology in order to understand what was happening with these people.

Hysterical paralysis refers to a condition whereby sufferers are, for all intents and purposes, paralyzed; however, no physical pathology can be found that would explain the paralysis. House reports that several of the patients he treated were so adversely affected that they were confined to wheelchairs. However, extensive medical assessments concluded that the only physical problem they displayed was muscle wastage associated with not walking. Far from malingering, if these people were trapped in a house

---

[3] In a book edited by Sarno (*The Divided Mind*), and written for a professional audience, a range of medical specialists contribute chapters describing how they have used the mind/body notions described here to work successfully with their patients. These specialists include rheumatologists, heart specialists, orthopaedic surgeons, dermatologists, rehabilitation specialists as well as general practitioners. All agree that emotions play a key role in the chronic conditions which they treat.

[4] House, A (2005). *Blind through the Mind – Contemporary Cases of Hysteria*. ABC Radio National.

fire on their own with no assistance, they would not be able to get out of their wheelchairs and walk to safety in order to save their own lives. Their level of paralysis is so great that they would be more likely to die a horrible death engulfed in flames than be able to walk to safety. Clearly, the paralysis is not a result of a conscious choice they are making.

House has successfully treated such people, enabling them to walk again after as many as twenty years of paralysis, by psychologically treating them with notions akin to those in The Hidden Psychology of Pain. He assisted them to work out what may be the deeply hidden sources of distress in their unconscious minds, and over the course of the treatment, helped them to bring these to conscious awareness in a safe and supported therapeutic environment. As a result, and with the assistance of appropriate physical therapy to recondition their weakened muscles, his patients have learned to walk again. These sorts of stunning outcomes make overcoming chronic pain with psychological awareness sound like a less impossible endeavor.

The possibility of overcoming chronic pain with psychology will be explored in great detail in the following chapters. In order to understand this approach, to such an extent that it helps you overcome your chronic pain, you will need to learn about how medicine usually makes sense of chronic pain, and the limitations of this approach. Some basic information about spine anatomy and the neurology of pain will also be useful, and these will be presented in Appendices.

You will benefit from reading about the various forms of evidence which support the basic contention of this book. We have been so brainwashed by misinformation about chronic pain that only substantial amounts of evidence can hope to break through the prevailing myths. We will also need to explore depth-psychology further, as it plays a vital role in the resolution of chronic pain for many people.

The types of improvements as seen with Max are entirely possible for many people in chronic pain. I have seen many examples of them in my work, and there is every reason to expect that you can experience the same type of relief as well.

CHAPTER 2

Physical Perspectives on Pain

Western philosophy & medicine

In overcoming chronic pain, it is important to understand how it is that medicine and other physical approaches, such as chiropractic and physiotherapy, have arrived at the treatment approaches that they have. Rather than just being some form of "natural" explanation which reflects reality, the physical perspective of chronic pain has evolved from a certain historical and social context. It is important to understand this context so as to be able to effectively dispute the pain myths which are prevalent. It is also important to have a basic grasp of anatomy in order to be clearer about what does and does not cause chronic pain. Appendix 2 presents the neurological processes involved in the experience of pain, and Appendix 3 presents the anatomy of the spine.

One of the oldest references to ancient medical practices is from the four thousand year old Indian text, The Mahabharata, which states:

> "There are two classes of disease—bodily and mental. Each arises from the other. Neither is perceived to exist without the other. Mental disorders arise from physical causes, and likewise physical disorders arise from mental causes."[1]

---

[1] Cited in Eysenck (1991 p. 230). Two thousand years ago, Hippocrates was suggesting notions similar to the Indian sage quoted, and was thereby promoting

What is suggested in this quote is a philosophy of monism as opposed to dualism, or perhaps better stated as a "holistic model" of medicine. The West, however, also has a history of what may be referred to as holistic medicine. Even though it was centuries in developing, the separation of psychological factors from medical issues only gained dominance in the West over the last century. In the long history of Western medicine, ancient physicians such as Hippocrates and the Roman physician Galen both argued for a role of psychology in ill-health.[2] This appreciation of psychological factors in medicine was maintained well into the 18th and 19th centuries.[3] The traditional holistic view appears to have prevailed in Western medicine until the beginning of the 20th century. Sir William Osler, often referred to as the Father of British medicine, stated in 1906,

---

a non-dualistic model of illness. Specifically, Hippocrates suggested that the bodily fluids were causal in the aetiology of various mental disorders, and that personality factors, e.g. melancholia, were relevant in the aetiology of physical illnesses. In the second century AD, the Roman physician Galen, viewed as being the last of the "classical physicians," promoted the notion of personality as being a relevant factor for physical ailments, specifically, the formation of neoplasm.

[2] In a review of literature from 1701-1893, Eysenck (1985) states that there were 14 anecdotal studies cited in the medical literature which suggested a link between extreme emotional stress and/or loss and the development of cancers. For example, Gendron in 1701 was amongst others from the next two centuries who suggested that stress, leading to feelings of helplessness, hopelessness and depression was an important factor in the onset of cancer. Other observations suggested that temperaments that were of a more sensitive and easily frustrated nature were more susceptible, as were those who suppressed their emotions. Information from another quarter, the Pavlovian school of physiology, demonstrated early on that acute stress induced in dogs would create not only behavioral disturbances, but also chronic diseases. Petrova, a student of Pavlov, demonstrated that spontaneous tumors could be created in dogs undergoing such experimentally induced stress.

[3] The implications of the standard biomedical model are both physicalistic reductionist (i.e. reducing all phenomena down to its smallest physical components), as well as dualistic wherein the mind is viewed as being distinct from the body (Russell 1961). In terms of physicalism, the guiding assumption is that the language of chemistry and physics will ultimately explain all biological phenomena with "the philosophic view that complex phenomena are ultimately derived from a single primary principle"(Engel 1977 p.130).

"It is many times much more important to know what patient has
the disease than what kind of disease the patient has."[4]

It would seem, however, that this type of sentiment was shortly to be
eclipsed by the ascending biomedical model of medicine. Perhaps at the
time, Osler's comment was one of the last statements of a traditional wisdom
that had been developed through careful observation over the preceding
centuries. But, that wisdom had run its course, and was soon to be disparaged
as a quaint relic of the pre-scientific age.

In the history of Western culture, the separation of mind and body
(referred to as "dualism") can be seen as a general trend in philosophy from
the ancient Greeks to Christian philosophers. Following the Greek lead,
Christian theology later added to this division of mind and matter. Around
five centuries ago, the body was viewed by the Church as an imperfect
vehicle for the transmission of the soul from this to the next world. As such,
the Church approved the study and dissection of the human body, however
it did not approve of the study of the mind, as this was seen as the rightful
domain of religion. This trend culminated in the doctrine espoused by
French philosopher Rene Descartes, whereby the worlds of physical reality
and mental reality were presumed to be independent from each other.

As seen in the work of scientist Isaac Newton, the universe became
viewed as an elaborate machine, not unlike the highly complicated clocks
that were also being developed at the time. Before the rise of this view, the
universe (including the world, and all things in it) was viewed almost as a
living organism, imbibing an essential "life-force." As an expression of this
life-force, humans and our bodies were viewed as a manifestation of nature
and/or God.

Until the end of the 17th century, when science was beginning to emerge
as the new explanatory system, the world and all living things were viewed
from this organic perspective, i.e. as growing life-forms, rather than as
cleverly built machines. With the rise of a materialistic science, the human
organism also came to be viewed and treated as a machine, albeit a highly
complex one, but a machine nevertheless. This mechanistic view of the

---

[4] In Eysenck (1991). "Science, Racism, and Sexism." *Journal of Social, Political &
Economic Studies.*

human is alive and well today, as seen in this statement from a contemporary book on neuroscience: "We may accept rationally that we are machines, but we will continue to feel and act as though the essential part of us is free from mechanistic imperatives."[5]

When the mind/brain is today presented in a pictorial form, it is usually with nuts, bolts and cogwheels within the skull. However, it would be more accurate to symbolically present it as something like a tree, growing and alive, complete with a root system and branches with twigs growing above.

With mind-body dualism being the Church-approved doctrine, early medicine developed the mechanistic metaphor of the body, disease being the breakdown of the machine, and the physician's job being the repair of the machine. Over the centuries, the Western world has become perhaps the greatest example of a "mechanistic" culture, in which only physical realities are given the status of being "real." Within this view were the seeds of the crisis of modern medicine, evidence of which is the current chronic pain epidemic. This crisis is a logical conclusion to the definition of medical disorders as concerning only physical factors, with psychosocial issues being of no interest or consequence to a biomedical model of medicine.

The split between psychology and medicine

Isaac Newton and Rene Descartes were central figures in this transformation from an organic world view to a mechanistic one. Modern medicine is a product of this split between physical and non-physical matters, as the new life sciences became busy dissecting the world (and the human body), looking for its basic nuts and bolts—the physical building blocks.

Psychology is also a product of this split, and it has focused almost exclusively on the non-physical aspects of human functioning and experience, largely to the exclusion of many relevant physical factors. No doubt, many of the advances of modern medicine can be attributed to this focus on the human organism as an elaborate and complicated machine, so it certainly has not been a waste of time—many lives are routinely saved by medicine as a result of this approach. And psychology's almost exclusive focus on

---

[5]   Carter (2010). *Mapping the Mind.*

mental phenomena has also borne fruit, but these developments have come at a cost as well.

While early medicine and the physical sciences were developing in the universities of Europe and Britain, philosophy departments were grappling with non-physical subject matter. Towards the end of the 19th century, philosophy combined with the relatively new scientific experimental method in order to address compelling age-old questions, ultimately producing psychology as a new discipline.

Humans have always "practiced" psychology in the sense that the need to make sense of our experience is a defining characteristic of our species. However, the notion of *scientifically* observing human behavior and experience, utilizing concepts of objectivity and rationality, and performing controlled experiments to answer many questions about human experience was a new development, and occurred under the term psychology—the logic (science) of the psyche.

Within the dominant mechanistic mind-set of medicine, there is a tendency to dismiss anything to do with psychology, as psychological factors can't be 'seen', and usually cannot be measured with anything like the level of accuracy as can physical factors. A dismissal of psycho-social factors has come to characterize not only the health care system, but also our entire culture. The notion that non-physical factors may play a role in the human organism is sometimes seen as an affront to the commonly held mechanistic view of the universe. An appreciation of non-physical realities is often dismissed with the greatest of all modern slurs, that it reflects an unscientific superstition, or some other form of hocus-pocus.

In Western medicine, the mechanistic approach to human health is reflected in the purely biological medical model. Western medical theory understands the body in anatomical, physiological and biochemical terms.[6] The notion of "disease" is understood as untoward changes in body cells which are identified through their clinical manifestations. "Roughly agreed upon norms" are used as the criteria by which physiological, biochemical and radiological deviations may constitute evidence of illness.

Towards the end of the 19th century, Pasteur discovered the role of microbes as infectious agents, with the implication that diseases came to

---

[6]   Lucire (2003). *Constructing RSI: Belief and Desire.*

be viewed as specific entities, each with a specific germ cause. This was a watershed moment in the history of Western medicine, however it took some time for the full impact to be felt. As can be seen with the quote from Osler, many physicians still maintained a belief in the contributing role of emotions towards the development and course of illnesses until early in the 20th century, but this awareness began to diminish as time went on.

The stunning advances in medical technology and the successful treatment of many conditions suggest that the physicalist tendencies of the biomedical model have been worthwhile. Treatments of serious conditions that were only imagined a generation ago, such as heart transplants, are now possible thanks to a mechanistic medical science. However, these extraordinary breakthroughs have no parallels in the medical treatment of chronic pain. As neuropsychiatrist Stephen Porges (2011) states,

> Contemporary medicine, especially over the past century, has focused on mechanisms of disease. Medical advances have been largely technical. The natural mechanisms underlying health and healing remain remarkably poorly understood.[7]

Despite having reached epidemic proportions over the last few decades, there have been no serious advances in the physical treatment of chronic pain, or even in the medical understanding of it. From a medical perspective, chronic pain is still commonly viewed as a mystery, although a range of inadequate theories are regularly offered.

The biomedical model of medicine has become contemporary culture's popular "folk model" of medicine rather than a scientific model. It often operates as a cultural dogma wherein its limitations are rarely questioned. In contrast to science, dogmas require that non-supporting data are either excluded from the discussion, or are modified to fit the existing model. With the dominance of the physicalistic view within medicine over the last hundred years, those who subscribed to the views that included non-physical realities became ignored, discredited, and ultimately excluded.

---

[7] Porges (2011 p.295). *The Polyvagal Theory. Neurophysiological Foundations of Emotions, Attachment, Communication, Self-Regulation.*

Medical explanations of chronic pain

As an example of chronic pain, lower back pain, provides many clues as to the true nature of the problem afflicting our society, and will receive some special attention in this section. The following statement from the Australian Government National Occupational Health and Safety Commission presents a conventional understanding and explanation of back pain:

> Most people do not exercise on a daily basis and few of us relax when we are not on the move. Sometimes your work may require you to hold yourself in postures that make movement difficult and unnatural. This can lead to lower back pain. Any posture that compromises the natural curvature and muscular balance of the spine places strain and tension on the supporting muscles and ligaments, weakening them. Without proper support, the joints of the vertebrae are forced to carry weight they are not meant to carry. This leads to premature spinal degeneration and pain.[8]

Implied in this statement, which is accepted and promoted by most professionals working with those in chronic pain, are a range of erroneous and potentially harmful ideas which can actually promote the very condition they are trying to help to alleviate. The view that most cases of chronic back pain are due to unspecified mechanical dysfunction of the spine is the prevailing belief in medicine.

As a further example of the conventional wisdom regarding causes of back pain, the following quote is from an information sheet provided by The Australian Divisions of General Practice, intended to educate the public. In answering "What causes back pain?", discs are suggested to be the problem:

> The most common cause of back pain is a crack in one of these discs. A crack allows fluid from the middle of the disc to squeeze

---

[8] "Managing Back Pain" statement from the Australian Government National Occupational Health and Safety Commission (2005).

into the outer, pain sensitive part of the disc. This movement
of fluid results in muscle spasm in the large back muscles. This
spasm leads to pain and stiffness in your back.

In yet another variation of the conventional back-pain wisdom, the
ABC (Australian Broadcasting Commission) "Health Matters Back Pain
Fact File" suggests that the problem with our backs is that as a species we
came down from the trees sometime between one and two million years
ago.[9] The proposition is that the development of *Homo erectus,* moving on
two legs rather than four, came at a huge price. Standing erect meant that a
lot more weight was carried by the spine, hips, knees and ankles. (Perhaps
the advocates of this notion should spend a day on their all fours to discover
what *is* the natural position for humans?) The fact that four-legged animals
also suffer from spinal conditions should limit this theory. Enthusiasts for
such a view also have no explanation as to why the "design faults" in the
anatomy of *Homo erectus* should only have become apparent in the last few
decades, rather than being a constant feature over the last million or so years
of humans being bipedal.

A significant part of the problem of chronic pain is misinformation,
albeit well-intended. Just a little thought will reveal that humans have always
engaged in work which required the straining of bodies and the holding of
difficult positions. If these positions or movements were 'unnatural," then
we wouldn't be able to do them—it is unnatural for us to fly, so we don't. If
we can actually carry a weight, how can it be said that we are not "meant"
to carry it?

Even extremely fit people, such as professional athletes who are strong
and exercise on a daily basis, are prone to experiencing chronic back and
other pains. The body is designed for vigorous use, much of which over the
course of a lifetime will produce harmless degenerative changes in soft tissue
such as spinal discs. As you will read, this is actually normal and is found in
most people, even in those who do not experience pain.

In addition to structural pathologies of the spine, the "pain industry"
also attributes chronic pain to disease or incompetence of the muscles and
ligaments surrounding the spine, however there is scant evidence of this.

---

[9] Lavelle (2005). "Back Pain Fact File." *ABC Health Matters.*

Humans have always had a capacity to lift weights (in varying degrees), and in the past this fact has not produced epidemics of chronic pain such as we are currently witnessing. People in developing and agrarian societies still lift similar weights as did our grandparents, but chronic pain epidemics are not evident in those countries. Researchers have found that the prevalence of disc abnormalities differ little between people who have a sedentary or a heavy workload.[10] As such, it is not at all clear that chronic back pain is caused by heavy lifting. In addition to heavy lifting, other risk factors for back pain are said to be twisting, bodily vibration, obesity and poor conditioning. The problem is that back pain is common in people *not* exposed to these risk factors as well.[11]

Despite such conventional statements regarding physical causes of back pain, research clearly demonstrates that it is usually impossible to identify a specific physical cause for most back pain. Structural pathologies of the spine are so common amongst people without pain that their role in causing pain must be seriously questioned.[12] Although pain researchers state that "Perhaps 85 percent of patients with isolated low back pain *cannot* be given a precise anatomical diagnosis,"[13] this lack of knowledge does not seem to dent the confidence shown by some medical experts in suggesting a precise anatomical cause. It is apparent that results of scientific research do not greatly inform the conventional wisdom regarding chronic pain.

[10] Jensen et al (1994) found that the prevalence of disc abnormalities differed little with physical activity score in terms of sedentary or heavy workload.
[11] Deyo & Weinstein (2001). "Low Back Pain." *New England Journal of Medicine.*
[12] In Jensen et al's MRI study of 98 people with *no back pain*, the majority (64%) were found to have structural pathologies of their spines. The studies of many eminent researchers in this field suggest that the occurrence of structural pathology of the spine and back pain appears to be mostly coincidental (see Nachemson 1976; Magora & Schwartz 1980; Borenstein & colleagues 2001; Deyo 2002; Weisel & colleagues 1984 & 1990; Stadnick & colleagues 1998; Jensen & colleagues 1994; Bigos and colleagues 1991).
[13] Deyo & Weinstein (2001). "Low Back Pain." *New England Journal of Medicine.*

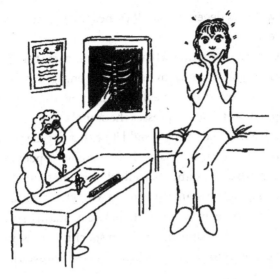

Despite the evidence, structural pathology of the spine is still routinely blamed for chronic back, neck and shoulder pain.

As can be seen, the variety of physical explanations offered to explain chronic pain usually involve notions of physical strain. One of the glaring problems with all of these explanations is that in the last couple of decades, most people in the developed world have stopped working physically for a living. We are exerting ourselves far *less* than ever before in human history, at a time when there are far *more* reports of chronic pain. The amount of laboring jobs that used to be prevalent in Western society has radically diminished as our work places have become increasingly automated. As such, the physical explanations of chronic back pain have also had to adapt to this changing reality.

Rather than emphasize how dangerous hard physical work is, spokespeople for the pain industry are now choosing to emphasize how dangerous it is to *not* do physical work. Our sedentary lifestyles, with long hours of sitting, are now blamed for the epidemic of chronic back pain. "Despite what you think, sitting is actually one of the hardest positions to maintain for a long time," according to the latest physical explanation. Generations of hard working laborers may be surprised to learn that *sitting* in front of a computer all day is now viewed as being "hard work" for the spine—in fact, amongst the hardest work. "It stresses the soft tissues and, done repeatedly, causes degeneration,"[14] comes the recent warning from a physiotherapy lecturer.

The problem with this notion is that exactly the same things were being said of hard physical work when many people were engaged in that. Although fewer people actually exert their bodies for a living now, the same explanation is still being applied—sitting compresses the spinal discs, as does the more active bending, twisting and lifting. Could it be that degeneration of spinal discs is basically normal, regardless of the type of work people engage in? Further, could it be that the spine typically degenerates with age, and that this natural process rarely has anything to do with chronic back pain?

The medical views seem to alternate between stating specific causes for chronic back pain, and admitting that no specific causes are known in most cases.[15] The most informed views in medicine, however, have come to

---

[14] "Increase in Back Pain is Hitting us Where It Hurts." Health and Beauty section of *The Northern Star*, Saturday, April 23 2010, p.53.

[15] In a *Medicine Today* article titled "The Significance of Chronic Back Pain," Barnsley (2010 p.18) confidently states that "Most cases of back pain are *due to unspecified mechanical dysfunction* and not to serious underlying medical disorders such as infection of malignancy"(italics added). This statement would not seem to accord with the current state of scientific research which clearly demonstrates that no precise anatomical diagnosis can be made in the vast majority of cases— how then can Barnsley (2010) possibly know that most cases are due to mechanical dysfunction? As an example of the medical opinion of chronic pain in general, he goes on to have a bet each way in the same paragraph, this time sticking more to what the science actually suggests. "It is usually *not possible* to determine the specific structure or pathology responsible for back pain in a given individual"(Barnsley 2010, p.18. italics added). Barnsley then cites American research in which around forty to forty five percent of a back-pain sample of people were found to have pain arising from either disc pathology or sacroiliac or zygapophyseal joints—this sounds pretty much like a presumption of specific mechanical dysfunction having been found. That is, the observed structural pathologies are assumed to be causing the pain. However, the remainder of the sample did not have an anatomical source of their pain identified. A purely physical medicine remains unable to explain these seemingly contradictory findings. As a result, sufferers are often treated as malingerers at worst and as medical mysteries at best. Barnsley's apparently contradictory comments above are really just an indicator of the confusion and ambivalence that contemporary medicine displays in regards to chronic

support the notion that back pain does not necessarily mean that anything has been, or is being damaged, or that the back is now weakened. When viewed as a purely physical condition, back pain will often seem to just come and go for no apparent reason, further adding to the sense of mystery. However, when a broader view is taken, as in *The Hidden Psychology of Pain*, the reasons usually become more apparent and often comprehensible for the first time. Being able to make accurate sense of what is going on is an essential element of the solution to chronic pain.

You will read in this book evidence which suggests that something other than the presumed physical explanations is going on to produce such widespread chronic pain in all its various forms. All of the above explanations are inadequate accounts of the causes of chronic pain, but they inform the conventional treatments used. Treating chronic back pain, when guided by inadequate explanations, tends to produce inadequate outcomes. What constitutes standard medical treatment for a condition like chronic back pain? The interested reader is referred to Appendix 4, where the conventional medical treatments for chronic back pain are reviewed and evaluated.

Despite the best intentions, medical interventions are clearly of limited use with chronic pain. Appendix 5 reviews the evidence relating to the equally poor efficacy of other physical therapies such as chiropractic and physiotherapy for chronic pain. This lack of treatment success is further compounded by a sense of hopelessness within the conventional approach, as seen in the following expert statement: "Unfortunately, chronic pain is much harder to cure because the injury is so severe or because the underlying condition is a degenerative one that can't be reversed."[16]

With statements like this, it is no wonder that most sufferers become quite helpless in response to treatment failures and unremitting pain. On hearing such views, it makes sense that the average sufferer will arrive at a state of hopelessness, as they will typically experience repeated treatment failures, *and* internalize the view that these failures are due to the inherently untreatable physical condition causing the pain.

---

pain—we are witnessing the transitional mid-way point between an old view and a more progressive one, as demonstrated by Cherry (2009) with the bio-psycho-social model.

[16] Lavelle (2005). "Back Pain Fact File." *ABC Health Matters.*

This hopelessness is taken to an extreme when a person in excruciating pain also works physically for a living, as a great deal of anxiety about their employment and financial situation can follow. This just worsens with each aborted attempt to push through the pain so as to earn an income. Unfortunately, such people are generally told that the pain results from their physical workload, and that if they want to avoid pain, they need to find different work—more easily said than done, especially for people with limited education or vocational training.

However, an important error is being made in the conventional treatment approach. Just because physical therapy fails to effectively treat chronic pain does not mean that it is essentially untreatable. It may just mean that physical therapists are treating the problem with the wrong approach, despite all the best intentions. Fortunately, other viable treatment options are available.

One of the few current medical acknowledgements of psychological factors having a role to play in chronic pain is in the concept of "somatization." Lucire states,

> Somatization theory looks at how symptoms are influenced and delineated by what a patient believes or fears is wrong. It explains how popular beliefs affect a body part that the patient believes to be diseased, whether it is or not. Somatization is a central phenomenon, mediated by the mind and those entities that impinge on the mind, ideas and beliefs, needs and desires. Pain is conceptualized as referred onto the affected part: general hypersensitivity follows and random clinical signs are to be found, most commonly those of disuse.[17]

Somatization is not a concept embraced and utilized by contemporary medicine, and is the only hint of psychosomatic medicine that remains today, even in psychiatry. However, it differs from The Hidden Psychology of Pain in that somatization theory assumes there to be no physical basis to chronic pain. You will learn that there is often an identifiable basis to the

---

[17] Lucire (2003 pg.153). *Constructing RSI: Belief and Desire.*

physical pain, but it is simply not what the majority of the pain industry would have us believe is responsible.

Clearly, a new model of medicine is required to adequately explain and treat contemporary problems like chronic pain. The next chapter will explore such a new approach.

CHAPTER 3

Bio-Psycho-Social Medicine

IN RECENT YEARS, MEDICAL SCIENCE has developed what is referred to as the bio-psycho-social model, taking into account psychological, social and physical factors. George Engel, Professor of Medicine at University of Rochester, was an early advocate for this development in which psychological and social factors are viewed as relevant for the causation of both positive health, as well as health problems. *The Hidden Psychology of Pain* is well supported by the development of the bio-psycho-social approach to medicine.

Within this "new" approach, such aspects of life as a person's beliefs and attitudes, their level of social support and degree of love experienced, as well as the environmental stressors to which they are exposed, are all viewed as important predictors of health and illness. As a perennial irony, the truth of "what is old is new again" can be seen in what is essentially a rediscovery of the importance of psychosocial factors. This view was held by many previous generations of physicians prior to the 20th century. Nevertheless, the bio-psycho-social model is credited with having advanced the management of many forms of chronic illness in the last 30 years.[1]

As its title suggests, the bio-psycho-social model attempts to integrate both psychosocial and biological models of ill-health in order to develop a comprehensive picture of human functioning. This has been a necessary adaptation in light of compelling research evidence which suggests a role for psychosocial aspects of functioning, and an "Information Age" which

---

[1] Cherry (2009). "Managing Chronic Non-Malignant Pain." *Medicine Today.*

has disseminated these findings to the general public. The Internet is being increasingly used by general medical patients as a rich source of information. As the public becomes more educated, the need to incorporate psychosocial factors into medical explanations and treatments of health problems becomes more compelling—patients are generally very aware of their own psychosocial realities, even if their health practitioners have not been.

The message of the bio-psycho-social approach to medicine is that no one system of thought is adequate to reflect the complexity of the human organism in the context of its physical, emotional, social, political and economic environment. No single model or approach on its own is capable of capturing the larger and interconnected realities of the human organism, as this reality, which operates as a whole, is simply beyond the theories and models used to represent it.

The standard biomedical model is based on a model of science derived from 17th century physics, whereas the "new" bio-psycho-social model is based on both a traditional wisdom as well as a more contemporary approach to science. Where technology based on a 17th century models of physics is useful in medicine, this approach is entirely relevant and valid. However, there are many health issues, such as chronic pain, where the relevance of such an approach becomes far less valid and a broader focus needs to be incorporated.

Medical students are now introduced to the bio-psycho-social model, and this must be considered a great advance in the approach to contemporary medicine. As such, there are certainly more physicians today that are practicing this broadened approach to health and well-being. As an example, a recent article in an educational publication for GPs, *Medicine Today* represents something of an advance in that it highlights the role which psychological factors play in the causation of chronic pain.[2] In fact, the article goes so far as to state that psychological treatments are the *most* appropriate option for pain disorders. This is a significant breakthrough in regards to the medical views of chronic pain that have been dominant for several decades.

Despite this important recognition of the role of psychology in regards to chronic pain, the question is how much bio-psycho-social medicine is

---

[2] Cherry (2009). "Managing Chronic Non-Malignant Pain." *Medicine Today.*

actually being practiced when it comes to dealing with real life clinical issues, or whether many physicians still fall back on the biomedical model? This is not intended as a criticism—it is very difficult for anyone to transcend the emphasis of their training and branch out into areas for which they have not been adequately equipped. Innovative physicians often face ridicule from both patients and colleagues, and sometimes exclusion from the medical fraternity if they swim too hard against the prevailing current.

When the bio-psycho-social approach becomes genuinely widespread and informs conventional day-to-day medical practice, it will lead to cultural change not only within the medical profession, but also in the public's expectations about medical services. In order for this approach to gain traction in the way that some medical educators desire, medicine will have to seriously consider views such as those expressed in this book, and incorporate them into their clinical practice. However, as a reflection of where contemporary medical practice still is, the notions provided here are often disparaged and ignored by those practitioners in the pain industry.

The issue of chronic pain is perhaps the subject in which this Western tendency to think mechanically becomes the most relevant—*"We are talking about* physical *pain, so why are you talking about psychology?"* Our culture's way of making sense of chronic pain is one of the contributing factors to this wide-spread problem, and may play a large role in your experience of chronic pain.

A role for psychology

More than 50% of patients seen in medical specialties such as cardiology, neurology, gynecology, gastroenterology, dentistry and rheumatology have symptoms for which there is no clear-cut physical explanation.[3] In addition to chronic pain, there is a long list of conditions which are referred to as "perplexing disorders with unexplained physical symptoms," including chronic fatigue syndrome, fibromyalgia, tinnitus, irritable bowel syndrome, pre-menstrual syndrome and atypical chest pain.[4] The U.K. Royal College

---

[3]   Royal College of Psychiatrists' 2001 Press Release.
[4]   Ibid.

of Psychiatrists suggests that psychological intervention for these conditions is the treatment of choice. Such conditions only remain incomprehensible and mysterious when the wrong explanatory system is used to make sense of them. What follows is that chronic pain is only resistant to treatment when the wrong treatments are being applied. My experience is that for many people chronic pain is highly treatable when the right approach is used. As will be explained throughout this book, much chronic pain can be explained in terms of psychological distress, unconscious dilemmas and tensions, and traumas. In addition to being explained by psychology, much chronic pain can be successfully treated with psychological information and approaches.

When I state that psychology has a role in healing chronic pain, there is no suggestion that your pain is imaginary or *"all* in your head." Please understand that there is no suggestion of malingering, whining or imagining of chronic pain. The brain needs to make sense of nerve messages, and can conclude from these messages that pain is the appropriate experience to have. This is as true for the pain associated with stepping on a nail as it is for chronic pain. As such, pain is a function of both the nerve sensations from the afflicted part of the body *and* the sense which the brain makes of these messages.

My years of experience in working with people in chronic pain has taught me that for most people, the pain is entirely real. Unfortunately, some people have had the harmful experience of being told by health care professionals that as no adequate physical explanation for the pain can be found, they must be making it up. This represents a very poor understanding of the psychology of chronic pain (in fact, a complete lack of understanding), and shows little compassion towards people's suffering. No one with a good understanding of the psychology of pain would make such a statement, unless they were confronted with a clear case of pain having a secondary gain, e.g. to increase an insurance pay-out. While this *can* happen, it is simply not the norm for most people in chronic pain. A full understanding of chronic pain, however also requires that we understand the sense which the brain makes of nerve messages. As you will read in this book, the brain can also generate very real physiological changes in body tissues which will be perceived as painful.

If you choose to see a psychologist at random, there is a better than average chance that you will not be exposed to the ideas in this book. For the last thirty or so years, my profession has been in awe of cognitive-behavioral therapy (CBT). My intention here is not to suggest that CBT has nothing useful to offer— like many approaches in psychology, it can be useful for certain people and certain situations. The problem in psychology as a profession is that it has developed an almost exclusive preference for CBT. This is often, or usually, at the expense of all other approaches, many of which are actually very relevant and helpful when it comes to chronic pain. Research shows very clearly that most higher level psychology degrees offered in clinical psychology are by and large training in CBT.[5] This trend is replicated in the most of the English-speaking world, such that applied psychology has been largely reduced to the almost exclusive practice of this approach only. (see Appendix 6 for a brief review of the history of psychology)

Cognitive-behavioral psychology takes the common sense notion that our thoughts affect our feelings, and extends this to *all aspects* of human experience. This philosophical contention was espoused by the Stoic philosophers, and also has parallels in philosophies from other parts of the world, such as Buddhism. There is no need to dispute the basic notion that our thoughts affect our feelings—our normal lived experience tells us that it has a ring of truth to it. But CBT takes this observation and turns it into the *only* useful observation of human functioning, reducing all human problems down to a problem with the messages we are telling ourselves, and the behaviors we engage in.

The CBT notion that thoughts cause feelings is an extreme oversimplification. Research suggests that the actual relationship between thoughts and feelings is highly complex and not uni-directional at all, i.e. feelings affect thoughts just as much as thoughts affect feelings. Just because an observation, such as the importance of thoughts, can be *relatively* true in some or many circumstances does not mean that it is *absolutely* true in all circumstances. And it certainly does not mean that this observation is the sum total of all useful observations relating to human emotions or experience.

If the only tool modern psychology has is CBT, it will treat everything that it comes across as though it is a problem in thinking style or thought

---

[5] Pachana, O'Donovan &Helmes (2006). "Australian Clinical Psychology Training Program Directors Survey." *Australian Psychologist.*

errors. As such, nearly all contemporary human psychological problems are now, for the main part, viewed as being amenable to CBT—square pegs are regularly being forced into round holes. However, this zealous picture of CBT as being superior to all other approaches in psychology, is simply not borne out by the research evidence.[6] I would like to open you up to other psychological possibilities, especially as they pertain to chronic pain. We live in a marketplace of ideas, and many of the ideas developed within psychology have tremendous potential to help people, even if they are not the current flavor of the month.

The psychological contribution to most pain management programs that operate within state funded health systems in the Western world is predominantly CBT. The focus of this psychology input is generally to help people accept the pain that they are in so as to minimize reactive anxiety and depression, and to assist in the increase of activity levels. The most recent development in cognitive-behavioral therapy for chronic pain management is Acceptance and Commitment Therapy, otherwise known as ACT.[7] No doubt, there are many benefits to this approach, but if there were no other option than "learn to live with it," then this approach to pain management would make more sense. However, when there are viable and effective alternatives to mere acceptance, it seems to me like teaching people to be satisfied with living on their knees, when they can in fact be helped to stand and live on their feet again.

In its method of creating change, CBT teaches the person to engage in something of a conflict with the thinking errors—to dispute and do

---

[6] The basis of claims of CBT's superiority are often "meta-analytic" studies which review and summarise all research reports of a particular topic. Where meta-analyses do suggest that CBT is superior in treating the most common psychological complaint, depression, research published in 2010 by Cuijpers and colleagues in the British Journal of Psychiatry clearly indicates the operation of a "publication bias" with CBT. That is, journals generally only report CBT research which shows a positive outcome and rarely publish the research which find negative outcomes. As such, it is of little value to only take into account the published research as this is biased towards only research with positive outcomes. When this factor is taken into account statistically, the benefits of CBT revert to being much the same as most other approaches to psychology.

[7] Hayes, Strosahl & Wilson (2003). *Acceptance and Commitment Therapy: An Experiential Approach to Behavior Change.*

battle with them. William James, viewed as one of the originators of depth-psychology, warned against this tendency as long ago as the late 1890s. He suggested that it often proves fruitless to attempt changing worries, anxieties, and self-doubts with the tool of conscious thought. In fact, such efforts may only add momentum to the problematic thoughts, allowing them to build in strength. James favored an approach whereby we learn to not rely on our forebrain (the seat of conscious thought) to solve all problems, but rather passively surrender to *what is* with a more relaxed attitude. In so doing, he suggested many answers to our compelling problems will simply emerge from within us (from "the greater Self") as "regenerative phenomena"— what I refer to as the self-corrective tendency. There are some overlaps here to more recent developments in psychology such as "Mindfulness" and the ACT approach (see Chapter 17).

As medicine has suffered from Cartesian dualism, focusing almost exclusively on physical phenomena, psychology has also suffered from this split with its own near-total focus on non-physical phenomenon. The distinction between the physical and the non-physical realms as proposed by Descartes has had far reaching consequences which still hamper our health practices many centuries later. Also, the mechanistic mind-set has dominated both psychology and medicine, with each reflecting a tendency to view their subject matter as elaborate machines rather than as growing, living organisms. The obvious reality is that the physical and the non-physical aspects of human functioning and experience are flip sides of the one organic coin—they go together, and in reality cannot be separated in anything but an arbitrary fashion. Where possible in this book I will use the terms mind/brain or mind/body to underscore this reality, as the brain can be viewed as the organ of the mind—or to put it another way, the mind is what the brain does.

"Holism" and health care

An awareness of the need to take into account both physical and psychological factors is referred to as "holism" in the health industry, and has unfortunately suffered poor credibility due to its association with many new-age health fads which have no evidential basis at all. The current interest in new-age holism owes much to the radical rise of interest in Eastern spiritual practices and religions which erupted during the counter-culture movement of the 1960s and 70s, especially after celebrities like the Beatles embraced Indian forms of meditation and spiritual philosophies. Despite the many blind alleys which this cultural trend has taken us down, the large scale interest in Eastern practices and philosophies has brought about something of a correction in the Western mindset. This was much needed, and in the last three decades notions of mind versus body being a false dichotomy have become an almost mainstream understanding.

As already stated, the West also has its own traditions of holism going as far back as the ancient Greeks, and the indigenous and Pagan cultures of ancient European as well. This was evident in the accepted medical wisdom up to the early 20th century. Depth-psychology is also a representative of this Western tradition of holism in that it evolved from a cultural understanding that mind and body are essentially different aspects of the same process.

Unfortunately, both medicine and psychology turned their backs on this tradition, and instead focused on either the body or the mind respectively.

Psychological studies of chronic pain

Research reported in the medical journal *Spine* examined the role of emotional distress from abuse in recovery from back pain and reveals some important findings.[8] One hundred people who were to undergo surgery for lumbar disc herniations were interviewed prior to the surgery in relation to the occurrence of specific life events. Each was asked if he/she had experienced any of the following in their childhood years:

- physical abuse
- sexual abuse
- emotional neglect/abandonment
- loss of one or both parents (divorce, death, etc.)
- drug abuse at home (alcohol, prescription drugs, etc.)

---

[8] Schofferman (1992). "Childhood Psychological Trauma Correlates with Unsuccessful Lumbar Spine Surgery." *Spine*.

On the basis of their responses, patients were then allocated to one of three groups:

- none of these experiences
- one or two of these experiences
- three or more of these experiences.

The success of the surgery (i.e. the elimination of pain) was then evaluated according to the above groupings. Ninety-five percent of those people who had experienced none of the above forms of abuse demonstrated "excellent improvement" post-operatively. Those people who had suffered one or two of these abuse experiences demonstrated 73% improvement. And finally, those who had three or more of the abuse experiences demonstrated only 15% improvement. These results strongly suggest that the success or failure of the surgery, and the existence of post-operative pain, actually had little to do with the surgery itself. They had all received the same surgical procedure, but with widely different outcomes. Clearly, the success or failure was related to the occurrence of multiple abuse experiences in childhood. Psychological factors related to these traumatic experiences appear to have been the most important issue in determining the surgical outcome. Follow-up research indicated that people in the abuse categories could achieve better post-operative improvements with the introduction of brief psychotherapy focused on the abuse/pain nexus.

Personality factors could also play an important role in the causation of chronic pain, especially when these interact with distressing experiences. Research shows that a large proportion of chronic pain sufferers share common experiences as well as personality traits.[9] Studies have found that many sufferers have a very strong work ethic, are overly self-reliant, relate strongly to caregiver roles, and idealize relationships.

A large proportion of the chronic pain sufferers studied also avoided conflict and tended to deny emotional problems. As many of them started work at young ages, the researchers concluded that the higher-than-average amount of chronic pain amongst this sample of people is the result of more opportunities to harm themselves at work as they had been doing it

---

[9]   Barsky (in Grant, 2009). *Change Your Brain, Change Your Pain.*

harder and for longer than others. This conclusion is perhaps yet another example of identifying significant psychological factors but failing to connect the dots, and instead resorting to a physical explanation for the pain. Hopefully, this book shows how the researchers failed to recognize the true significance of these personality factors. They are all significant psychological characteristics, suggesting "risk-factors" for chronic pain.

In other informative work, researchers conducted a large scale prospective study with 3,020 aircraft employees in an American Boeing factory.[10] The workers were assessed on a range of factors including both the existence and history of back pain events, other health measures, personality measures, and a survey that measured their level of job satisfaction. Four years later they were reassessed, and it was found that 279 workers reported to having back problems. When the researchers statistically analyzed the results, they discovered that apart from a recent experience of back pain, the factors which best predicted whether four years later a worker would be amongst those with back pain or not was 1) their level of work satisfaction; and 2) other psychosocial variables as measured on a personality test, the MMPI. Workers who reported four years earlier that they "hardly ever" enjoyed their job tasks were 2.5 times more likely to have wound up with back pain than workers who reported that they "almost always" enjoyed their job tasks.

As there are a range of tasks at an aircraft factory, it is possible that the least enjoyable jobs were also those which entailed the heaviest and most tiring tasks. This factor was also measured and taken into account in the statistical analysis four years later. No differences were found between those reporting back pain and those not reporting back pain in regards to the specific tasks which they had to perform in their jobs. That is, someone with a light/sedentary role was just as likely to report a back injury as was a person whose job entailed heavy lifting. The extent to which people enjoyed their jobs was not a simple function of which job they had—other personality factors were more important in determining job satisfaction than were the specific roles and tasks.

---

[10] Bigos and colleagues (1991). "A Prospective Study of Work Perceptions and Psychophysical Factors Affecting the Report of Back Injury". *Spine.*

When we look at what contemporary research is telling us about the role of psychological factors in the production of chronic back and neck pain, an article featured in the medical journal *Spine* is worthy of mention.[11] This meta-analysis detailed the results of a comprehensive literature review in which 913 research study articles from medical and psychological data bases were examined. From this overview, thirty-seven prospective studies that appeared in scientific journals were reviewed. Prospective studies are ones in which people who are assessed as being well at point A in time (in this case, free of back and neck pain). As well as being diagnosed as free of pain at that time, a range of psychological measures of such factors as stress, distress, anxiety, mood and emotions, cognitive functioning, pain behavior, personality factors and experience of abuse were taken. The researchers were asking the question as to whether people who displayed the most psychological distress would be more likely to be suffering from chronic back or neck pain at point B in time. When point B arrived (usually several years later than point A), they were reassessed and measures of their levels of back and neck pain were again taken. The article author reports that, "The prospective studies indicated that psychological variables were related to the onset of pain, and to acute, sub-acute, and chronic pain. Stress, distress, or anxiety as well as mood and emotions, cognitive functioning, and pain behavior all were found to be significant factors."

Personality factors were found to have mixed results, while abuse was found to be a potentially significant factor. The conclusion was that psychological factors have been found in the scientific research reviewed to play a significant role in chronic pain.

In the light of such research findings, why isn't psychotherapy offered as the first treatment of choice for people in chronic pain? As discussed in an earlier section, psychology as a discipline is relatively young. As a result, there are a range of highly differing views and opinions within psychology, and little agreement as to which is the best way to help people. In addition, psychological interventions are not as suited to the gold standard of research as are physical interventions, i.e. the double-blind controlled research study. This approach to studying the effectiveness of a particular intervention

---

[11] Linton (2000). "A Review of Psychological Risk Factors in Back and Neck Pain." http://www.ncbi.nlm.nih.gov/pubmed/10788861

requires that the therapy be compared to another intervention which is assumed to have no therapeutic value at all (a placebo treatment). Ideally, neither the subject in the study nor the researcher should be aware of which condition, genuine or placebo, is being applied to which subjects (thus the double-blind element). Where the legitimate treatment out performs the placebo treatment, it can be viewed as effective.

But psychological phenomena cannot usually be studied in this way, any more than they can be studied in a laboratory test tube, or viewed under a microscope. Obviously, physical therapies are going to be a lot more suited to this type of research approach than are psychological therapies. But just because a psychological approach is difficult to research does not mean that it can't be researched at all, or that the psychological therapy is not valuable.

John Sarno reports that in the twenty-five years between 1973-1998, he worked with around ten thousand patients in chronic pain.[12] This is a very large sample of patients indeed, and was added to by his subsequent work in the same capacity from 1998 until his retirement in 2012. His observation is that the vast majority of his patients overcame their chronic pain simply by processing accurate information about mind/body phenomena. Such an observation, based on a very large number of people, with consistent outcomes from a particular intervention also constitutes a scientific enterprise, albeit not a double blind controlled study approach.

Need we be limited to an experimental approach to science which does not suit the topic area being studied? Does it even make any sense to try to apply a model of science well suited to physical phenomenon to subjects which are literally in a different realm of experience, such as human emotions? Just because these realities cannot be studied in an experimental laboratory does not mean that they cannot be rigorously studied at all. Clearly, different approaches to the scientific study of human phenomenon are needed. A considerable amount of psychological research has been conducted in this area, albeit rarely of the double-blind controlled nature, but the results do indicate the value of bringing psychology to the table.

It is apparent that chronic pain is a multi-factorial and complicated equation taking in a range of important psychosocial and physiological

---

[12] Sarno (1998). *The Mindbody Prescription.*

factors. These psychological factors are the focus of this book, and a significant part of the treatment is in understanding their contributions to chronic pain. In essence, this subject speaks to what it means to be a human in our society, and chronic pain highlights our culture's failure to come to grips with fundamental issues of what it is to be a whole person—that is, both psychological and physical.

CHAPTER 4

Chronic Pain Misunderstood

Chronic pain does not equate with damage

S HORT-TERM ACUTE PAIN IS OFTEN the result of damage, however this is rarely the case with chronic pain. Some form of reoccurring or chronic pain is nearly universal in our society, and is rarely ever evidence of a medical illness. As already detailed, I experienced a long-term chronic pain in my groin, as well as two or three bouts of extreme back pain that lasted for days to weeks. I am in good company, as most people can relate to this experience.

Rather than being evidence of current or unhealed damage, The Hidden Psychology of Pain suggests that most chronic pain is psychogenic in nature, i.e. psychologically generated. As Professor David Cherry states "Healing has long since finished by the time a patient is diagnosed with chronic pain behavior."[1]

That such pain is psychogenic does not mean that it is imaginary, but simply that its origins are caused by the mind/brain. Most chronic pain results from an alteration of soft tissue (muscles, nerves, tendons, ligaments), and not from a problem of the spine or a vague collection of muscle conditions mis-attributed to overexertion, lack of exercise or poor posture, as is commonly suggested.[2]

---

[1]   Cherry (2009 p.6). "Managing Chronic Non-Malignant Pain." *Medicine Today.*
[2]   Sarno (1991). *Healing Back Pain: the Mind-body Connection*

John Sarno and his psychologist colleague, Dr. Stanley Coen suggest that the coexistence of other common psychosomatic complaints in 88% of patients with chronic back, neck or shoulder pain indicates the pain's true nature.[3] That a high proportion of chronic pain sufferers also experience a range of conditions which have a large emotional/psychological component suggests a relationship between these ailments. Further, the many examples of people resolving their chronic pain as a result of psycho-educational programs, with no other physical intervention, suggests that the problem is essentially a *psycho*-physiological one.

Theories of causality are extremely important as they inform treatment approaches. When Sarno began his work in rehabilitation medicine, he did what few other clinicians at the time were doing: he accepted that medicine actually knew very little about the causation and treatment of chronic pain. As a result, he began his observations of patients with few preconceived ideas. In addition, he reviewed the research literature pertaining to physical damage in the body and the experience of pain. In the days before the Internet, this was not such an easy undertaking.

In seeking research-based information, Sarno discovered that there was no neat one-to-one relationship between the existence of damage in the body and the experience of pain. There are plenty of people who report experiencing intense physical pain, but upon examination with sophisticated imaging technology, no structural abnormality in the spine, neck or shoulders can be found. In fact, research clearly demonstrates that when people who are free of pain participate in such research, a high percentage of them show evidence of structural pathology of the spine—however, they are *not* in pain. Despite this lack of correlation, the same structural pathologies when seen in people with chronic pain are generally assumed to be causing the pain.

It is a natural and understandable assumption to make that people in chronic back, neck or shoulder pain must be suffering from structural pathologies of the spine. The person is in pain in a particular part of their anatomy, and if they are a statistically normal person, X-rays or scans will reveal that they are likely to have structural pathologies in that area (e.g. disc pathologies)—the same type of structural pathologies that are assumed to

---

[3] Sarno & Coen (1989). "Psychosomatic Avoidance of Conflict in Back Pain." *Journal of the American Academy of Psychoanalysis,*

be the culprits when people are in chronic pain. Some research indicates that if over the age of forty, there is a greater-than-not chance that people will have *multiple* sites of disc pathology, but most of them will not experience chronic pain. If between the ages of twenty and forty, there is the same high chance that they will have at least one site of pathology in their spine, but not be in pain.[4]

Rather than providing evidence of a causal relationship between structural pathology and pain, the research clearly indicates that structural pathology of the spine is the *norm*. The same pattern also holds true for most other forms of chronic pain. For example, the structural problems that are assumed to be responsible for carpal tunnel syndrome (impaired median nerve conduction) are also seen in around 40% of people with no pain. Many people older than forty also have slow nerves, commonly viewed as evidence of carpal tunnel syndrome; however, they have no pain symptoms at all.[5]

As we age, the discs between vertebrae can lose their elasticity, shrink and weaken. If they rupture, the inner gel-like substance (similar in consistency to tooth paste) can herniate, causing a bulge, or escape through the fibrous outer part. As this is usually related to aging, it is often referred to as "grey hair of the spine"—an essentially benign condition which most people will experience if they live for long enough.

However, much of the pain industry blames such structural pathologies for chronic pain. This explanation may very well hold for acute pain (by definition, less than three months duration), however when it comes to chronic pain (over three months duration), it simply is not supported by the evidence. This is because our bodies are very good at healing damage—give or take a short time, most hard tissue injuries will be healed within three months, depending on other factors such as age, general state of health, etc. Most soft tissue injuries, such as strains and sprains, will heal within a matter of weeks.

As stated, structural abnormalities of the spine are so prevalent in the asymptomatic population (i.e. people with no pain symptoms) that one would have to wonder if it makes sense to continue calling them "abnormalities" at all. As Barnsley states, "Numerous studies have demonstrated a poor and

---

[4] Sarno (1991). *Healing Back Pain: The Mind-Body Connection*
[5] Lucire (2003). *Constructing RSI: Belief and Desire.*

unreliable relation between back pain and degenerative, osteoarthritic or spondyloytic changes in X-rays of the lumbar spine."[6]

Research has established no association between low back pain and spondylolysis, transitional vertebrae, spina bifida, spondylolisthesis, spondylosis or Scheuremann's disease. MRI studies have revealed a high rate of abnormalities such as annular tears, disc protrusions, endplate changes or zygapophyseal joint degeneration amongst forty-plus year olds that are *not* related to symptoms of pain.[7] The same findings can be seen reocurring in the medical research literature over the last forty years, each coming to the same conclusion, despite using increasingly accurate and sophisticated diagnostic tools from X-rays to CAT scans to MRI scans.

Personally, I have snapped two of the three biggest bones in my body in half (femur and tibia), fractured my fibula, and fractured both ankles as well as three vertebrae in my neck. All of these breaks were healed within three months of the injuries. I am certainly not statistically unusual to have this healing occur; it is normal, and essentially what our body is designed to do. Why is it, then, that most of the pain treatment industry seems to be proliferating the notion that structural pathology of the spine is responsible for chronic back, neck and shoulder pain?

When I first came across Sarno's claims, I decided to conduct my own literature search to ascertain if what he was saying could possibly be true. A sample of the research I found is presented in Appendix 7. These studies are only a small example of many that come to the same conclusions: *there is no necessary relationship between structural damage in the body and the experience of chronic pain.* It is clear that this statement is well-validated by the relevant research.

Imagine two forty-five year old men who are next door neighbors—call them Harry and Jack. Both are doing some back yard gardening on the weekend. Harry hurts his back, whereas Jack does not. Being a typical man, Harry may wait a week or so before seeking help, but if the pain is strong enough, eventually he will see his local GP. The GP orders X-rays and/or scans, and the results demonstrate that he has sites of disc pathology in the

---

[6] Barnsley (2010 p.20). "The Significance of Chronic Back Pain." *Medicine Today.*
[7] Ibid.

same part of his anatomy as he is experiencing pain, i.e. in his back. Due to the close proximity of the sites of damage to the site of pain, the logical conclusion to arrive at is that these phenomena are related. Specifically, it may be presumed that the disc damage is causing the pain. Everyone is satisfied that they have found the answer, and Harry is advised to seek physical manipulation via massage, chiropractic or physiotherapy. He may also be advised to avoid using his back, and then to only use it in particular ways. There is a small chance that surgery may also be suggested and explored. While the pain is still short-term, the diagnosis may be entirely accurate, as it may be originating from a new injury.

But what if the pain lasts for longer than three months? The confusing factor is that while the disc pathology may adequately explain the short-term pain associated with a recent injury, it cannot provide an adequate explanation for chronic pain. If Harry caused a disc herniation on the weekend that he was doing the physical work, it is quite likely that this would result in short-term pain. Three months later, if he is still in pain (which would now be termed as chronic pain), the disc pathology becomes increasingly irrelevant.

When I fractured three vertebrae in my neck during a surfing accident a few years ago and picked up a couple of disc bulges in the process, I was informed by a physician on my first night in hospital that they may need to operate due to the damaged discs. I managed to ward this suggestion off with the statement that "The majority of the population over the age of forty have multiple sites of disc pathology and no pain, and they don't need surgery, so why would I?" No answer to this question was given, and no surgery happened. This suggestion, albeit well intended, was a massive invitation to be highly anxious. Needing to take injuries seriously, the medical profession is very able to frighten patients. Fortunately for me, I was well enough informed to not accept the invitation to be any more frightened than I already was. Beyond the initial first few weeks of recovery, I have been pain-free ever since.

What doesn't happen in the scenario presented above is that Harry's next door neighbor, Jack, has not injured his back. As a result, he does not go to the GP and request scans because he is not in pain. If he did request such assessments, however, there is a very high chance that his results would also show multiple sites of disc pathology, just like Harry, as this is the statistical norm for people over forty.

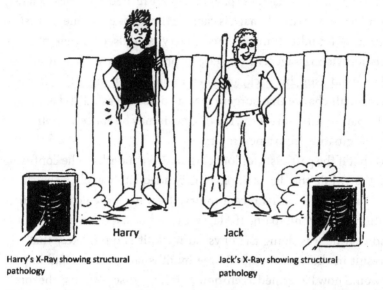

Harry   Jack

Harry's X-Ray showing structural   Jack's X-Ray showing structural
pathology   pathology

Neighbours, Harry and Jack doing some weekend gardening. There is a high probability that they both have a similar amount of structural pathology of their spines, but only Harry is in pain.

If it was the same GP seeing both of them (and if the GP was confronted by many cases of people like Jack—those not in pain), then s/he would have to question the assumption that structural pathology of the spine causes chronic back pain. However, GPs are rarely confronted by people who are not in pain; they are mostly confronted with people who, like Harry, are in intense pain. As such, the faulty notion of structural pathology causing chronic pain keeps being reinforced in medical practice as it appears to explain the pain of the patients who they do see, but not the lack of pain in the people who they do not see. This is one of the problems with clinicians arriving at conclusions only the basis of the patients they see, rather than on research studies.

Pointing the bone in a scientific culture

As a culture, we take our cues from the medical establishment in regards to health issues, and it appears that many health practitioners confuse their own personal ideas, perhaps based on their own experiences, with scientific facts. The recent CareTrack study, published in the *Medical Journal of Australia,* evaluated the medical interventions given to 1000 patients of a representative cross sample of physicians.[8] The medical interventions were gauged against the best practice guidelines suggested by scientific evidence. It was found that only around half of the medical interventions (57%) were in accordance with what the evidence suggests is best practice. This finding is in accord with ten year old American research which concluded that medical interventions there were conducted as per the evidence around 55% of the time. Whether health professionals use guidelines or not shows a remarkable consistency around the world in that guideline recommendations are only adopted 40% to 60% of the time. What physicians and other health professionals are doing the other 60% to 40% of the time remains anyone's guess. They are likely to be promoting their own 'pet' theories.

In addition to this problem, the pet theories promoted by many health practitioners in regards to chronic pain are likely to be inculcating sufferers in wrong notions of what is going on. Proust stated many decades ago, "For each illness that doctors cure with medicine, they provoke ten in healthy people by inculcating them with the virus that is a thousand times more powerful than any microbe: the idea that one is ill."[9] This concern is entirely applicable to the structural theory of chronic pain which most sufferers are likely to leave a health consultation with.

An interesting phenomenon of traditional Australian indigenous culture pertains to the practice of "pointing the bone." This was a form of condemning to death the recipient of the bone-pointing by a suitably qualified "magic man." Folklore, anecdotal and eyewitness accounts testify to the effects of such a practice usually being the rapid death of the recipient who was otherwise healthy and not expected to die.[10] This outcome is

---

8   Runciman (2012) "CareTrack: assessing the appropriateness of health care delivery in Australia". *Medical Journal of Australia*

9   Proust (1921). Cited in Lucire (2003), *Constructing RSI: Belief and Desire.*

10 Lockwood (1962). *I the Aboriginal.*

only possible within a cultural context wherein the predominant view is a subscription to certain magical beliefs. It is unlikely that a person not of that culture would respond in the same way.

But there also exists the possibility of a similar phenomenon in our "scientific culture," where predictions of health or illness that are presented from medical practitioners may demonstrate the same power of belief over biology.

A shocking example of this is presented by Jon Kabat-Zinn.[11] "Mrs. S" was in hospital receiving weekly treatment for a low-grade congestive heart failure that resulted in modest swelling of her ankles; however she was able to maintain her usual employment and household chores. A professor of cardiology conducted a weekly outpatient clinic at the hospital in which trainees would examine patients and then the professor would assess their findings. On the round in which he examined Mrs. S, the professor reported to the trainees that "this woman has TS" (referring to tricuspid stenosis), and then promptly departed. As soon as the professor left, Mrs. S became highly anxious and displayed all the physiological and psychological signs of panic. One of the trainees inquired with Mrs. S as to what the matter was. She responded by stating she knew that the "TS" statement by the professor referred to "terminal situation."

Her body began to show signs of catastrophic dysfunction in that her pulse raced to more than 150 beats per minute, and her lungs developed moist crackles at their bases due to excess fluid (unusual for her particular heart condition). The trainee cardiologist attempted to reassure Mrs. S as to the correct meaning of the professor's statement, however she remained panicked and her lung congestion worsened, which resulted shortly afterwards in a massive pulmonary edema. Mrs. S died later that day from intractable heart failure, despite all medical attempts to save her.

This case is a clear example of the power of words and ideas to create negative changes in the body. If this can occur to such an extent that traditional indigenous people can die, despite being entirely healthy, by having a bone pointed at them, and a woman in a modern and sophisticated medical context can die in much the same manner, then it is hardly fanciful

---

[11] Kabat-Zinn (2009). *Full Catastrophe Living: Using the Wisdom of Your Body and Mind to Face Stress, Pain, and Illness.*

to suggest that words and ideas can play a large role in the causation of chronic pain.

The fact that the medical idea of what causes the pain (structural pathology) is usually consistent with standard public idea only reinforces the physicality of the explanation. Most patients are as satisfied with the explanation as are most treating health professionals, and the erroneous ideas keep being reinforced over and again.

Theories used by patients to make sense of their own symptoms actually occur somewhat ahead of the medical explanations. Doctors learn how to treat particular conditions from a range of sources that include the patients themselves, as well as from popular literature, the media, and gossip and hearsay.[12] Medical and scientific sources may only be one competing source of guiding information, and with the rising strength of the Internet, perhaps not even the most powerful source of information.

Patients seeking arbitrary medical opinions are enabled in Australia where people have a great deal of choice about which GPs to seek treatment from. In the UK, patients are allocated to their local medical practice where they have to consult with the GP provided. If they don't like the views expressed by the GP, they are unable to "doctor-shop" until they find one who will support their notion of the problem.

RSI as a case example

An examination of the Australian RSI epidemic of the late 1980s provides a useful case study for developing an understanding of the causes of chronic pain. In many ways, this epidemic demonstrates the universal nature of chronic pain, and demonstrates many of the points made in this book. From extensive research, Lucire concluded that the phenomenon of doctor-shopping was a major social factor in the production of the epidemic.[13] She reports that most sufferers of RSI changed GPs, some up to four times, until they found a physical explanation that confirmed *their* view as to the cause of the problem.

---

[12] Lucire (2003). *Constructing RSI: Belief and Desire.*
[13] Ibid.

For most people afflicted with RSI, there was no suggestion that the pain was not real—only that the pain was not being caused by the physical tasks that were commonly viewed as the culprits. With hindsight, this can be clearly seen. The incident rates of RSI have fallen in recent years almost as dramatically as they rose at the beginning of the epidemic, with no real changes in work conditions that could explain this. During the epidemic, a range of causes were blamed for the radical increase in the incidences of pain, from chairs of the wrong height, to badly positioned monitors, faulty work stations, old typewriters, poorly designed furniture and/or equipment, inactivity, incorrect posture, etc. In fact, the epidemic required a constantly changing list of "causes," as each one failed to account for the pain experienced. The supposed causes were addressed with changes in work practices, none of which produced lasting changes to frequency of RSI.

People have been performing repetitive and straining actions ever since humans have been on the planet. Where a real physical injury occurs, the "natural history" of such injuries follows a predictable path in which rest usually resolves the problem. RSI did not conform with this natural history in that short-term rest would often appear to make the pain worse, not better. Many of the workplace actions that were viewed as culprits had been performed for generations before the rise of RSI. The same actions were being performed in both private enterprise organizations in Australia, and in organizations overseas, with nothing like the injury rate reported in Australian government agencies.

People will rarely suspect that their physical problems are being caused by their emotions in combination with their faulty beliefs about causality— it does not seem to be an understanding which spontaneously arises within us. Many GPs tried to suggest this possibility to people suffering from RSI, which resulted in the doctor-shopping until a physician was found that supported the notion of physical causes. The physical explanation of RSI shot to prominence despite the lack of any evidence (in fact, usually *in spite* of the scientific evidence), until it became the conventional wisdom of both the general public and the medical and treating professions alike.

With the lack of opportunity to doctor-shop, it is entirely unlikely that the RSI epidemic could ever have started in the UK where patients are stuck with the GP provided by the National Health Service. The erroneous ideas associated with RSI were eventually taken up in other parts of the world, including Britain, as the epidemic gained momentum. But these ideas could only *begin* in a country where people have the freedom to search for validation of their own causal theories of pain by looking for a doctor until they find one who agrees with their own diagnosis.

In regards to RSI and its presumed inflammation of tendons, Dr. Jill Cook, Professor of Physiotherapy at the Musculoskeletal Research Center of Melbourne's La Trobe University, states that tendinitis (meaning inflammation of the tendons) is itself a myth. RSI was popularly assumed to be an inflammatory problem of the tendons. While the pain is entirely real, research simply provides no evidence of inflammation for most people presenting with chronically painful tendons. When the painful tendons are thoroughly examined, they do appear abnormal, but with no white blood cells that are indicative of inflammation.[14] Tendonitis is a myth that has a long history, and was no doubt was partly responsible for fuelling the whole RSI epidemic.

Where painful tendons are the result of overuse, as with some professional athletes who spend most of their time practicing certain actions with a great degree of exertion (e.g. Olympic swimmers), the natural history of such conditions is apparent, i.e. rest from the repeated action will usually allow the tendon to recover with time.

As with the research that shows no association between structural abnormality and chronic back pain, Professor of Physiotherapy at the University of Queensland, Bill Vincenzino, states that when "the cells involved in making the collagen that goes into the tendon becomes dysfunctional, they become abnormal."[15] Pointing to a confounding contradiction, Cook states that tendons "... can be ragingly abnormal, *but they don't have pain.*"[16] (italics added). That is, having abnormal tendons is not necessarily related to having tendon pain. As such, the source of the pain is not the structural pathology of the tendon, as this often does not correspond with the experience of chronic pain. Again, like back pain, something else is clearly going on here, and it is not related to inflammation or to other structural abnormalities in the tendon.

---

[14] Cook (2002). Personal communication.
[15] Vincenzino (2010). *Corticosteroid Injections for Tendon Injuries.*
[16] Cook (2002 p.3). *The Tendinitis Myth.*

As can be seen, when it comes to RSI, and the associated chronic pain of nerves, muscles and tendons, the research clearly does not support the conclusion that structural disorders are responsible.

Rather than see normality and relative health in the structural pathologies of most patients, medical and other health practitioners are much more prone to see illness, which necessitates medical or other physical treatment. This makes perfectly good sense when we are talking about potentially serious health conditions such as heart disease or cancer, as a failure to do so could be catastrophic. However, the evidence suggests that this is rarely the case in regards to chronic pain, especially after more serious competing explanations have been eliminated.

The tendency to see illness where there isn't one is reinforced by a general public who often want to have this view endorsed. The attitudes of both the public and the treating professions can each reinforce a set of erroneous ideas. Lucire states that, "Epidemics of symptoms follow the circulation of ideas, as in education and prevention campaigns, and symptoms afflict the anxious and depressed."[17]

The transition from acute to chronic pain

As the distinguishing feature between acute and chronic pain is the length of time the person has suffered, there obviously must be a degree of overlap between the two. All chronic pain, by definition, is pain that has lasted for more than three months, and therefore must have started as a short-term acute pain. In Linton's meta-analytic study of chronic pain research, evidence was found that psychological factors can play a role in the transition from acute pain to chronic pain. This is a particularly important stage in that the pain which accompanies the acute injury can be so frightening to people that the distressed emotions can emerge, and with it the prospect of TMS pain arises as an "overlay" on top of the initial injury. Chronic pain can thereby take over from where the acute pain left off, generally some time before the three month mark, even when the whole process began with a physical injury.

---

[17] Lucire (2003, p.153) *Constructing RSI: Belief and Desire.*

Had my back pain lasted for more than three months, it would then have qualified as chronic pain; however it would have *firstly* qualified as acute pain. As such, it is apparent that the psychological explanation for chronic pain must also be partly true for some acute pain as well (as long as the pain is not resulting from a recent injury).

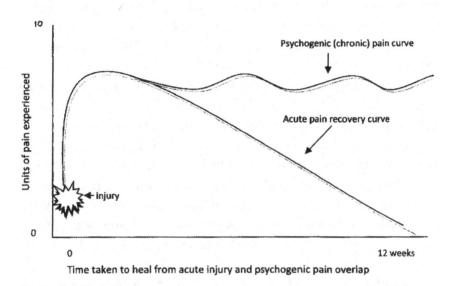

Time taken to heal from acute injury and psychogenic pain overlap

On one of the occasions that I have experienced back pain, it was clearly derived from emotional causes—I had done no injury to my back, but I was in a conflict situation that was getting worse before it got better. The transition from short-term psychologically created pain to longer-term chronic pain can be greatly assisted by the stress and anxiety relating to the pain; by worries about its increasing intensity; and by a decreasing ability to earn an income.

Such additional worries are extremely potent psychological factors that can then feed back into the emotional turmoil, adding to the intensity of the pain. This is referred to as *psychological overlay*—the collection of distressed emotions which may accumulate in addition to the distressed emotion which your mind/brain was trying to protect you from by creating the pain in the first place. Much of the psychological overlay will pertain to all the worries and anxieties associated with being in such terrible pain, and all the ramifications which this can have on your life.

Pain following an injury

As with Harry (in the example given at the beginning of this chapter), a person who has actually been injured (e.g. soft tissue disc injury) is likely to first present to their GP while their pain is still in the acute phase, i.e. within the first three months. In most cases, it is only within this time-frame that it makes sense to attribute the pain to the injury. A physical injury may very well have occurred, acute pain results, and the person is slowed down by it so as to allow the healing to occur within the next twelve or so weeks.

The problem is that an appropriate explanation for acute pain is then inappropriately applied to chronic pain, simply because the symptoms being described by the patient are very similar. If Harry internalized the notion of damaged discs being responsible for the pain, and misapplied this explanation to chronic pain (guided by his health professional), then he would become much more vulnerable to it becoming long lasting. Again, the importance of accurate information is obvious in this example. What explains short-term pain cannot explain most chronic pain, as most times the body is able to repair and recover from acute injuries before chronic pain is even diagnosed.

The situation can be further complicated, and the person even more convinced that the cause of the pain is structural, when people report to hearing or feeling a pop, crack or a snap when the pain begins. While a real sensation, no evidence of any structural derangement has been found that could account for this type of experience.[18] It may be similar to pops and snaps that people experience when cracking their knuckles or when receiving chiropractic treatment. However, being in a therapeutic context, people rarely associate the chiropractic experience with damage being done to their spine.

Explanations for such experiences include the escape of gases like nitrogen and carbon dioxide contained in the synovial fluid of joints. When a joint is "cracked," the gas is released and the pop sensation occurs. A snapping sound can also be felt/heard when a joint moves, with the tendon becoming slightly out of position and then returning to its original position. These are

---

[18] Sarno (1998). *The Mindbody Prescription.*

totally benign and normal events in the body which are not associated with any structural damage.

My groin pain of nearly two decades began with such a "popping" sensation in my lower back when I was bending and twisting whilst operating a ride-on lawn mower. It did not hurt in that moment, but when I came to stand up an hour later, the tearing pain in my groin, which lasted for the next eighteen years, began. I immediately associated it with the crack I felt in my back an hour earlier, and made sense of the entire experience in light of my spine being "out of whack" from the head-on car accident a year and half earlier.

When the groin pain did not resolve, both chiropractors and physiotherapists reinforced the view that it was resulting from some unspecified structural spinal abnormality caused by the car accident. All of the treating practitioners I saw over the next couple of years associated the crack I felt in my back with the existence of the pain in my groin, and this explanation seemed entirely logical to me at the time. The problem is that the treatments which followed from this explanation simply did not produce any lasting changes. Only the introduction of useful information did produce a change. This fact alone supports the contention that the pain was never being caused by a spinal pathology, as information is not able to correct a pathology in the structure of the spine.

The range of human experiences associated with chronic pain argues against a simple physicalist explanation, as many experiences just do not conform to the explanations offered. Other observations that demonstrate a lack of correspondence between standard explanations and pain are discussed next.

Chronic pain sufferers with no structural pathology

There are many chronic pain sufferers who are in very real physical pain, but with no observable structural pathology at all. Pain researchers Deyo & Weinstein state that as many as "eighty-five percent of patients with isolated low back pain cannot be given a precise pathoanatomological diagnosis."[19]

---

[19] Deyo & Weinstein (2001 p.363). "Low Back Pain." *New England Journal of Medicine.*

I have worked with many people whose lives have been irreparably turned upside down as a result of their pain. Some of them have even lost relationships and marriages, careers, their homes, and their families due to unrelenting pain and inadequate treatment. Of course, there are some people who will "put it on" for the sake of obtaining some kind of monetary pay-off or other secondary gain. But for the majority of people, the negative consequences of pain can be so extreme that it is hard to believe that they could possibly be putting it on for the sake of a little sympathy, or even an insurance pay-out. Very often they get neither, and in fact often lose everything important to them as a result of the pain which has become entrenched.

Lucire states that the medical profession in general fails to understand the concept of "psychogenic," or psychologically generated pain, which refers to conditions being caused by ideas and emotions.[20] This lack of understanding results in the awful situation which many patients complain of, in which a physician has told them that the pain condition is not real, it is imaginary or "all in your head."

Some physicians will also make the mistake of associating the concepts of psychogenic or psychosomatic pain with mental illness, which it is not. What is being described in *The Hidden Psychology of Pain* is *normal* psychology, not abnormal. Physicians are also often very concerned about offending their patients with mention of psychosomatics or psychogenesis of pain, as most people simply don't want to hear of this as an explanation. This is due, partly, to a fear of being viewed as somehow "crazy." So, it is not easy for either a physician or a psychologist to suggest that the chronic pain could be caused by psychological factors—this must be done skillfully and carefully.

When no pain results from injury

More interesting evidence of the lack of causal relationship between structural pathology and pain are war-time observations. Combat veterans often report to having sustained injuries during battle, but having been unaware of it

---

[20] Lucire (2003). *Constructing RSI: Belief and Desire.*

until sometime later. Sapolsky, in discussing this "stress induced analgesia," states that approximately 80% of civilians request morphine, while only a third of soldiers request the pain killer for injuries of similar severity.[21]

It appears that as long as a soldier's attention is focused on doing what is required to stay alive, their mind/brain doesn't notice an injury unless it interferes with activities necessary for survival, e.g. running or fighting.

The meaning of the injury, especially in a war context, is very important. An observation of the WWI trenches was that significant injury was often a soldier's "ticket" away from the front line and towards survival. This meaning of the injury could have such a positive effect on wounded soldiers that some were seen to be in a celebratory mood after an injury, rather than in pain.

Neurologists such as Norman Doidge suggest that rather than pain being a necessary consequence of certain physical injuries, it occurs from the mind/brain's assessment of what *should* result from the injury.[22] As such, he is suggesting that pain is more an "opinion" that the mind/brain arrives at rather than a necessary response. It would seem that the mind/brains of soldiers who are injured in battle are otherwise so engaged in simply staying alive that they don't arrive at the opinion that they should be in pain, until it is safe to do so.

A similar incident was recently reported in which a man recalled celebrating New Year's Eve five years earlier when he received a "blow to the head," but didn't seek medical attention at the time due to the festivities. Five years later, he became aware of a lump on the back of his head, and on seeking medical assistance, was amazed to discover he had a .22 caliber bullet lodged beneath his scalp.[23]

Had he felt the blow at another time, it is very likely that he would have been aware enough to investigate it, would have discovered blood and a wound, and would subsequently have experienced pain. As he was too preoccupied at the time to allow his mind/brain to make sense of the blow, his mind/brain failed to form the opinion that he should be in pain. He had been fooled to not arrive at the opinion that pain should follow the blow, as he had barely perceived it. It is unimaginable that this could have occurred

---

[21] Sapolsky (2004). *Why Zebras Don't Get Ulcers*

[22] Doidge (2007). *The Brain That Changes Itself.*

[23] http://news.ninemsn.com.au/world/7950481/man-shot-but-only-notices-years-after

without pain had he been able to accurately interpret what had happened to him.

I recently had an experience which demonstrates the role which the mind/brain has in deciding whether to "do" pain or not. In a dream, I brushed a spider's web with my hand, and found it impossible to remove the web despite my frantic attempts. Whilst struggling, I discovered that there were several small dangerous red-back spiders still in the web, now stuck on my hand. To my horror they began biting me. As I was waking up from the fright, what struck me was how real the pain felt. It was an actual *physical* experience which stayed with me for a moment or two after I awoke from the dream. I could feel the pain of being bitten, even though I know it didn't actually happen. Obviously, my mind/brain had decided that being bitten by a bunch of spiders was going to hurt, and it accordingly gave me the appropriate dose of pain.

Another example is the use of a "mirror box" for treating phantom limb pain, devised by Vilayanur S. Ramachandran.[24] A significant amount of people who have lost a limb, particularly in traumatic circumstances, experience chronic pain in their missing limb. It appears that if the mind/brain's last experience of the arm or leg was a painful one, then this is the last "impression" of the limb which can remain with the person. Thus, the pain or discomfort can continue for many years afterwards. It is not unusual for amputees to complain of an itch that can't be scratched, or a cold absent limb that can't be warmed, or a pain that can't be soothed.

When the remaining limb is placed on the outside of a box with a mirror on its side, and the stump is placed in an opening of the box, such that to the person the reflection makes it look like the absent limb is again present, the mind/brain is given a "newer" experience of the limb. The sensory data from the eyes to the mind/brain is that of the limb again being present. It can then be seen to be scratched or warmed (via the visual experience of the remaining limb being scratched or warmed), or the person can simply have a visual experience of the missing limb which is not a traumatic and painful one. With this new experience, the mind/brain is able to change its opinion about what the ongoing experience of the missing limb should be. Often, it

---

[24] Doidge (2007). *The Brain That Changes Itself*

decides that pain is no longer the appropriate experience as a more recent, non-painful experience has been had.

What determines the mind/brain's opinion of whether the person should be in pain or not? We see spiritual devotees in Hindu cultures piercing and punishing their bodies, but apparently experiencing no pain. As such, it is reasonable to conclude that our culture's notions of pain, and the meaning of particular behaviors and social contexts, are highly relevant. There aren't too many examples of Hindu sadhus in Western culture, however we see similar experiences every weekend in both professional and amateur participants playing high-impact sports.

The most popular form of football in my country is Australian Rules Football, a unique contact sport characterized by heavy tackling, no off-side rule, moving the ball with long kicks, and, at the professional level, as much running per game as a half-marathon. It was first played over 150 years ago, and is thought to have evolved as an amalgam of an Aboriginal game and European ball games. To the uninitiated, it looks something like a cross between a rough version of Irish Gaelic football, rugby, and Greco-Roman wrestling at high speed, with no padding or helmets used for protection. Critics sometimes refer to it as Australian "No-Rules" Football due to the apparent on-field mayhem which thirty six players can make on the huge oval.

Professional Australian Rules footballers have completed games with broken ribs, noses, collarbones and legs, and similar feats are known in the rugby codes as well. The mind/brains of these footballers have not settled on the opinion that pain should always follow a hit because heavy tackling is a part of the game, an expected element of the sporting contest. As such, the meaning of the hit in this game is significant. A normal Australian Rules Football tackle to a soccer player is likely to result in more pain, as such rough treatment is not a part of the soccer player's expectations of what happens on the field.

There are also many reports of surgery being conducted without anesthetics while the person is under hypnosis.[25] It would seem that with some highly hypnotizable subjects, the hypnotic suggestion is able to convince the mind/brain that no pain need to occur, thus changing its

---

[25] Milne (2007) *Hypnosis and the Art of Self-Therapy.*

"opinion." Unfortunately, many people are not adequately hypnotizable, otherwise this would be a viable treatment approach for chronic pain in the general population.

When the prevailing culture promotes the relationship between structural pathology of the spine and pain, then we are vulnerable to this view and consequently to chronic pain. The idea itself constitutes a metaphoric "disease," as it can cause pain when internalized. Powerful messages and meanings have been transmitted to the individual via our culture, which help the mind/brain to arrive at the opinion that pain is the inevitable outcome. These messages keep being reinforced by health authorities, who confuse the reasons for acute pain with the reasons for chronic pain.

To summarize the research evidence: on the one hand, there are the majority of people in the pain-free population with demonstrable structural pathologies of their spine, but no pain. And on the other hand, there are people with no structural pathology, but who are in real pain. And there is every possible combination in between.

The only rational conclusion to draw from this evidence is that in most cases, there is *no necessary one-to-one relationship between structural pathology and chronic pain.* Most people in chronic pain are not suffering from a medical disorder, even though it feels like they are as the symptoms manifested are all-too physical. The medical profession is reluctant to consider emotional causes for physical pain for many of the reasons stated above, even where the evidence is clearly in its favor.

This reluctance results in medicine's "wholesale failure" to correctly diagnose the cause of the problem, and instead to focus on physical factors which are for most part irrelevant, or merely coincidental to the causation of chronic pain. This failure is a not so much the isolated failure of the medical profession, but more broadly the product of a cultural notion of the human organism as an elaborate machine, and is no more the physician's fault than it is all of ours. The difference, of course, is that physicians and other physical therapists are viewed as credible authorities on such issues, so their views simply reinforce this basic cultural error.

The only sensible conclusion to settle on is that most chronic pain is not caused by structural abnormalities at all. Amongst the exceptions to this are undetected cancers and spinal infections. The experience of fever, along with no relief from lying down may indicate a spinal infection.[26] And cancer could be a possible cause of chronic back pain when accompanied by a similar lack of relief from lying down, along with frequent and/or painful urination, unexplained weight loss, neurological deficits and a history of cancer.[27]

As stated previously, it is worth having a thorough medical check-up before concluding that your pain is psychologically generated, as self-diagnoses can lead to dangerous mistakes. There are tragic stories of people having received psychotherapy for chronic headaches over many years, only to later die of a brain tumor that was causing the pain all along. This is a mistake that should be avoided with all forms of chronic pain.

Multiple factors

Any health professional will tell you that it is common for one set of symptoms to have a range of possible contributing factors. Depression may be experienced in an adult as a result of haunting memories of childhood abuse, by unfavorable current life circumstances, by recent traumatic experiences, by thyroid problems, by unhealthy diets, by overloads of stress, or by various illicit or pharmaceutical substances. It is faulty to assess that depression is resulting from overloads of stress when the person is actually suffering from thyroid disease, or from the adverse side effects of medications or other drugs. The wrong problem will be treated, and the person is not likely to recover.

Of course it is possible, and even probable for there to be multiple causes or contributors to any health problem. Such a depressed person may have had an abusive childhood, a bad marriage, financial problems, a recent car accident, substance abuse problems, adverse side effects of medications, *and* thyroid disease. Any combination of the above factors is more than possible in the reality of people's lives, and in any one individual, these various factors may be contributing different amounts to the problem. Clearly, we are both physical and psychological beings.

---

[26] Deyo & Weistein (2001) Low Back Pain. *New England Journal of Medicine.*
[27] Ibid.

Peptic ulcers are perhaps the classic example of this interaction between physical and psychological factors. Until the relevant bacterium was found in the early 1980s, the general consensus was that peptic ulcers resulted purely from psychological factors such as stress. With the discovery of *Helicobacter pylori*, the consensus of opinion swung to the notion that peptic ulcers were a purely physical condition, with no psychological input at all. However, current research makes it clear that such ulcers are the product of both bacterium *and* psychological factors like sustained emotional stress. The emotional stress is also more likely to result in poor life-style choices such as excessive alcohol and cigarette consumption, missing meals, and also an overreliance on such medications as aspirin. Excessive secretions of stress hormones are also likely to play a role. Most health conditions are likely to result from a combination of relevant factors, both physical and psychological.

With chronic pain, it is possible for the syndrome to begin with structural damage of the spine from an injury resulting in acute pain. At some time over the ensuing few months, as the injury is naturally resolving, a psychological overlay can begin to take over where the pain associated with the acute injury naturally diminishes. It is not possible to definitively assess what the exact cause of such pain is, or the relative contribution of physical and psychological factors. If rest and time has not resolved it, nor have a range of physical interventions, and if serious physical causes have been eliminated, then the chances of there being a psychological factor rises.

As stated above, treating the wrong problem is not likely to result in a cure. Where health professionals remain unaware of the research data relating to acute and chronic pain vis-a-vis structural pathology, they will continue to misdiagnose the problem, resulting in the wrong treatments, and the person is likely to remain in pain.

As there are likely to be both physical and psychological contributions to chronic pain, the task is to work out the relative contribution of each, and to address these appropriately. The closer to the time of a physical injury, the more relevant are physical factors likely to be in the ensuing pain. The further away from the moment of a physical injury, the less likely are physical factors to be of primary causal relevance to the chronic pain.

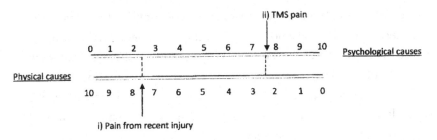

The continuum of relative contributors to pain due to i) a recent injury, and pain due to ii) emotional factors (TMS). You will see that each type of pain will also contain an element of the other. There is no physical injury without psychological consequences, and no psychogenic pain without physical factors involved. The contribution from each source can move up and down the continuum.

People typically become more and more distressed as one physical treatment after another fails to provide lasting relief. As mentioned earlier, it is not at all unusual for such people to then become depressed about the pain, and the worsening prospect of ever being free from it. These upset emotions become yet another rich layer of psychological burden for the person to carry, in addition to the already existing emotional problems, creating a negative feedback loop. As long as the focus remains on treating the wrong problem, then no circuit breaker to this feedback loop can be in place. As with all negative feedback loops, the problem just intensifies and the emotional and physical pain continues to worsen.

The difficulty in the early stages of an acute pain is to establish if it is resulting from purely physical causes, and/or from distressed emotion. The best guide in answering this is whether you have been injured or not. Sometimes, people can pick up a physical injury and barely be aware of it, but this tends to be under extreme conditions that are unusual. More often than not, if you have injured yourself through an accident or inappropriate movement, you will know it.

If you are not sure whether the pain you are experiencing is in accord with the injury itself, get a medical opinion. People have different thresholds of pain—what is excruciating for one person may be quite manageable for another, so there are no objective standards or measures of this. However, if a physician tells you that it is quite reasonable to expect pain from what you have undergone, then this is a useful guide.

If you have had no accident of any kind, then it is unlikely (although not impossible) that you have had an injury. If that is the case, you may then consider emotional factors that may be contributing to the pain. Begin considering your level of emotional distress at the time when the pain began. These distressed emotions are not always the most obvious ones, such as stress. Look for deeper implications of the stressful situation. Often, the culprits will be painful emotional dilemmas, or extremely negative views of yourself which can come about because of a stressful situation. This will be explored further in later chapters.

If you have been injured, then resting the injured area of your body and allowing the natural healing process to occur makes sense. If you conclude that the pain is likely to be resulting from psychological causes, you have several options available. You will find out early that to exert yourself when in extreme pain is likely to exacerbate the pain, even if the pain is being caused by psychological factors. As such, it would be wise to refrain from a *normal* level of exertion; however, you need to avoid the opposite mistake of resting too much. Try to strike the right balance of physical activity while you undergo the psychological process of addressing the pain, as per the strategies in this book. Most physicians and physical therapists are aware these days of the need to keep moving, for both injury-caused pain and psychologically induced pain. Be guided by their opinions on what is a sensible level of activity.

Thinking psychologically is your main tool to overcoming a pain that is not likely to have resulted from a recent physical injury. Without the correct psychological understanding of what is causing the pain, you will limit your chances of getting better and put yourself at risk of the pain becoming chronic. If your pain is resulting from a large stressor in your life that is not "solvable," then the pain may last until the stressful situation itself changes. In the meantime, it is likely that you will be able to have a positive impact on the pain by thinking psychologically about it. However, it is also possible that you may remain in pain until the circumstance itself has changed.

Most life circumstances, even bad ones, change with time—if not the entire situation itself, then at least aspects of it are likely to change over days or weeks. These changes may take the pressure off in some important ways, resulting in less distress and less chronic pain. Thinking psychologically about the pain may help you to prevent it from becoming chronic and debilitating.

You can also learn how to manage the associated stress in specific ways, such as by problem solving, relaxation exercises, meditation, prayer, gaining social support, etc. Counseling can help with problem solving strategies and clarifying the issues for you. Again, this can take some of the psychological pressure off the difficult situation, and allow things to settle down again.

The physicality of pain

A problem with thinking psychologically about chronic pain is its very physicality. I recently had an episode of acute low-back pain which lasted for around three to four days, the first such attack I have had in around thirteen years. The last time I suffered in this way was prior to my knowledge of The Hidden Psychology of Pain. As such, the episode eighteen years earlier lasted for several weeks, during which time I underwent a range of chiropractic and massage interventions, all to no avail. In hindsight, I can easily see that during the pain episode years earlier, I was under enormous emotional pressure from relationship difficulties which were simply compounded by additional life stressors. In my recent episode of low-back pain, I was aware that the physical pain was closely related to an emotionally painful conflict situation that I was experiencing. Several important points became apparent to me.

Firstly, my experience of pain was entirely *real* and in no way imaginary. If I did not know better, I could have sworn that something was actually broken in my lower back. Having fractured three vertebrae in my neck, I am in a reasonable position to compare the degrees of pain. This episode of back pain was as painful as my neck injury, however it was nowhere near as serious in cause or consequence.

Secondly, despite being fully aware of the role of distressed emotion in the causation of pain, I experienced it anyway. This is the human condition, and very few humans are exempt. I knew that I had done nothing physical to my spine at all that could explain the pain. In fact, I was resting on a four day holiday when the pain began. I might have thought that I would be exempt from such pain because I have an understanding of the role of emotions. Unfortunately for me, I was still vulnerable to it just by virtue of being human. More than likely, my knowledge of The Hidden Psychology of

Pain helped me to only experience the recent back pain for a few days, rather than it becoming deeply entrenched as a chronic condition.

Thirdly, I realized that if I worked physically for a living, my ability to earn an income would have been severely compromised by the back pain. I found it difficult to just stand up and move freely, not to mention bend, twist, carry weight, or even tie my shoe laces. Were I dependent upon my ability to move to provide for my family, I would have become highly anxious even after just a few days.

This is an extremely important consideration for people who do work physically. Once the pain kicks in you are often rendered disabled, and any attempts to use your body when the pain is at its worse will just increase its intensity. Each effort to "push through" the pain will increase your level of disability until you are almost unable to move at all. Even though the pain is coming from what is a terrible but essentially benign condition, it is still best to not overly exert yourself and aggravate it. Where possible, you may need to cease engaging in your normal levels of exertion, and this may mean not doing your normal work for a few days to a couple of weeks.

It is not always easy or realistic to just not work due to pain, especially if self-employed, or if your employment is casual and therefore not secure. This means a lot of people, as an increasing proportion of Westerners now find themselves casually employed. However, trying to push through the pain, and thereby risking making it worse, is likely to increase your fear and anxiety about it, which feeds into the psychological overlay, which then feeds back into the production of the pain.

You need to find a balance between not aggravating the pain from trying to push through it, and not completely giving into it through becoming immobilized. Modifying your work duties in the short run may help, rather than staying away from work and seeking total rest. If you have a supportive employer, you may be able to negotiate some alternate duties so that you can still be a productive employee, just not in your normal capacity for a relatively short time.

If you feel the need to persevere despite the pain so as to keep earning an income, an awful double bind can become more and more established. With the increase in pain and levels of disability comes an increase in anxiety and fear of where it is all heading. When the pain is at its worst, most people will be extremely worried about ever being able to earn a living again. It is little wonder, then, that most chronic back pain is experienced by people who are smack in the middle of these "years of responsibility" with families and mortgages, rather than in younger people with no financial obligations, or older people who have fulfilled their financial obligations.

The longer people go in this pattern of suffering, the more intense the pain and distressed emotions become. This is the path to chronic pain, which is viewed as largely untreatable from within the standard physical paradigm. With better information about the true nature of pain, this vicious cycle can be broken.

Chronic pain myths

As you have read, faulty ideas can play a very large role in exacerbating and maintaining pain as well as creating a high level of disability. If you are able to *manage* the incorrect ideas, beliefs and myths, then you have an excellent chance of gradually emerging from pain when the stressful situation has sufficiently changed either by its own accord, or as a result of your problem solving. Pain cognitions, or your beliefs about the pain, are extremely important and powerful. Some beliefs have the power to help you overcome pain, and some beliefs will only make the pain worse by deeply entrenching it.

The following are common myths about chronic pain which are adhered to and promoted by both clinicians and sufferers alike. None of them are an accurate reflection of the current state of knowledge.

1. *Chronic pain is the result of damage*

The reality is that highly sophisticated imaging studies are generally unable to locate specific forms of structural damage which is responsible for chronic pain. This is further demonstrated by the regular finding that structural abnormalities which are often believed to be causing the chronic pain are usually found in high proportions amongst the *pain-free* population. Most people have structural pathology but no chronic pain.

2. ***Chronic pain is evidence of spinal/body weakness & vulnerability***
    Your spine is your body's core strength. It is rarely seriously damaged, even by those who participate in highly physical contact sports. The fact that superbly fit and strong athletes can also experience chronic pain is evidence against the notion of vulnerability via weakness.

3. ***Chronic pain is only likely to get worse with time***
    With the right type of information and recovery program, there is no reason for most cases of chronic pain to get worse with time. In fact, given the right intervention, most will actually improve with time. The rates of chronic pain in the population decrease as age increases. This suggests a connection between the "years of responsibility" and chronic pain, and not a relationship between increasing years and increasing chronic pain.

4. ***Chronic pain is ultimately crippling***
    While many people experiencing bouts of chronic pain can be somewhat "crippled" by it, there is nothing inevitable about this. The fact that many sufferers are able to overcome the pain and decrease their level of disability, suggests that ultimately others can overcome it too. Professor Alan House in the UK has demonstrated that when similar factors produce "hysterical" paralysis, people are still able to overcome the condition and learn how to walk again.

5. ***Chronic pain precludes independence or the ability to earn***
    Many people who have suffered from serious chronic pain, to the extent that they have lost their jobs as well as their independence, have managed to rebound from this to lead full and happy lives again. Such people have returned to pre-pain employment and recreational activities. I regularly see this happening in my work, and this observation is echoed by other like-minded therapists.

Psychology Professor Keith Petrie has extensively researched the role which people's perceptions of their health conditions can play in determining the health outcomes of a wide range of conditions.[28] He and his research colleagues have studied the influence that beliefs about such factors as causal theories of illnesses, "catastrophizing," and the diminished sense of control over the condition can have. In a recent review of the research literature they demonstrated that how a person views their illness can actually play a *larger* role in determining the outcome than the actual severity of the condition itself. That is, what people believe about their pain is a leading factor in producing either a recovery from, or a worsening of the condition.

Petrie and his colleague's research has found that people who believe that their pain is the result of damage, believe that there is nothing they nor treating professionals can do to help, have a poor understanding of the condition, tend towards an emotional catastrophizing about their pain and/or are hyper-vigilant to pain are more likely to be highly disabled by it and less likely to recover. Their research demonstrates that when a psychological pain intervention is able to counter these beliefs, pain and disability levels decrease. This shows the importance of obtaining accurate and useful information about chronic pain, making sense of why the pain is happening, and using this information to aid in your recovery.

If you are able to train yourself to think psychologically about your pain, you are likely to avoid adding to it by believing chronic pain myths. It is likely that the type of understandings presented in this book will help to heal you of the condition. At the very least, having a correct understanding of the relationship between your emotional and physical experiences will equip you to *not* add unnecessary layers of psychological overlay on your pain.

Many people who progress from acute pain to long term chronic pain have succumbed to these damaging ideas and myths. As a result, the layers of psychological overlay become so solidly and deeply entrenched that it takes considerable effort and time to overcome them. These are the people who are most adversely affected by chronic pain. However, as seen with Max in Chapter 1, even people with extreme pain and solid psychological overlay are able to overcome the syndrome with the right information.

---

[28] Moss-Morris, et al (2007). "Patients' Perceptions of their Pain Condition across a Multidisciplinary Pain Management Program." *Clinical Journal of Pain.*

CHAPTER 5

The Physiology of Chronic Pain

Two PROPOSITIONS HAVE BEEN PRESENTED in this book: 1) chronic pain is real; and 2) structural abnormalities are not responsible most of the time (as suggested by voluminous research evidence). If we accept these propositions, then in terms of making sense of chronic pain, limited possibilities arise. Either the sufferer is malingering, perhaps seeking to manipulate a situation or others, imagining the pain; or alternatively, something else must be causing it.

As already stated, while it must be considered possible, it is actually quite rare in my experience for people to consciously be seeking to manipulate situations with their chronic pain. Gains to them hardly ever eventuate as a result, but plenty of misfortune often accompanies the disabling pain, and these usually outweigh any potential benefit. In addition, it is almost incomprehensible that people could be imagining the pain—while perhaps not an absolute impossibility, it must be considered a somewhat fanciful explanation with little credence and no evidence. As such, something other than structural pathologies of the body must be causing chronic pain. From a physiological perspective, mild blood and oxygen deprivations are the likely candidates.

The role of oxygen and ischemia

In addition to locating research evidence essential for putting together the chronic pain jigsaw puzzle, Sarno made an important observation early in his rehabilitation medicine career. He noticed that most of his patients reported that at least one of three things helped to alleviate the pain. These actions did not allow the sufferer to become pain-free, but at least took the "edge" off the pain temporarily.

Most people report that a decrease in pain can result from:

i)   the effects of heat pack (or an ice pack, which paradoxically, can increase the muscle temperature), or

ii) physical manipulation in the form of massage, or

iii) movement or activity.

The only thing that these three interventions have in common is that they all bring blood, and with it oxygen back into the affected area as a result of the increased muscle temperature which ensues.

Our entire body is an organic electro-chemical system. The food we eat and the oxygen we breathe combine in our body cells to produce the electricity that our system runs on.[1] Things just don't work the way they are meant to without sufficient supplies of electricity derived from food and oxygen. These essential ingredients are utilized in the part of body cells known as the mitochondria, where they are converted into a molecule called adenosine triphosphate, or ATP. These ATP molecules are the principal type of food that cells burn and can be thought of as tiny batteries that travel throughout the cell providing the energy required for cellular processes.

Metabolic stress occurs when the cells can't produce enough ATP as a result of not enough glucose entering or being available for the cell. A typical cell requires around one *billion* new ATP molecules each two minutes, after which they empty of energy and are readily replaced by another billion ATP molecules. This process is what keeps our system ticking over. Without it operating properly, we would be simply unable to function, and even basic requirements such as keeping our bodies warm on a cold day would not be possible.

A lot of blood is required to keep the cells freshly oxygenated. When at rest, our hearts are pumping around 343 liters of blood an hour, or around 8,000 liters per day. The cellular demand for oxygen increases when a person

---

[1]   Arden (2010). *Rewire Your Brain: Think Your Way to a Better Life.*

engages in vigorous activity, as this increases the workload on the muscles involved.

The observation that interventions that increase muscle temperature also alleviate pain, suggests a biological cause of the pain. Chronic pain is often related to a blood deficiency, and subsequently to a mild oxygen deficiency in the pain affected parts of the body. Such an oxygen deficiency is technically referred to as ischemia, and is experienced as a painful cramp or spasm. When the blood and oxygen supply has been decreased, a deficiency in ATP ensues and the cells can experience metabolic stress. All muscles, nerves, tendons and ligaments require a sufficient supply of oxygen in order to function as they are meant to in a pain-free manner. When the oxygen supply is deficient, pain ensues.

Muscles and nerves obtain their oxygen supply via the blood which carries it through the body. When the blood supply decreases by even a small amount (not enough to cause any cellular damage), ischemia of muscles and nerves can result, and you will wind up in pain if it is affecting muscles; or pain, numbness, tingling, and maybe weakness if the nerve is affected. Many people will experience both odd nerve sensations and muscular cramp simultaneously.

Most of us have experienced cramps that resolve fairly quickly, usually by stretching and/or massaging the pained area. However, the pain can last long after the spasm has come and gone, possibly due to the decrease in blood supply which results a buildup of lactic acid in the muscles. Sarno's experience over many decades suggests that the vast majority of chronic pain cases are essentially a problem of mild but persistent ischemia, and the associated build-up of lactic acid.

Rather than occurring in someone's head, it appears that this is the biological pathway relevant in the production of chronic pain—and it *is* happening in the body, where the pain is felt. However, the picture is a little more complicated than this as the mind/brain is entirely involved in all experiences of physical pain, including the pain of stepping on a nail (see Appendix 2). That is, pain is never an experience purely of the injured part of the body, but the mind/brain is always central to the perception of pain sensations. Chronic pain is not resulting from "imagination," but actually reflects a biological process occurring in the body which the mind/brain is very active in making sense of by producing a perception of pain.

The problem can be extreme, even disabling, when the cramp occurs in the postural muscles of the neck, back and buttocks. These are the muscles with an almost constant workload on them as long as we are upright. As such, they are nearly always in demand and therefore requiring new supplies of oxygen in order to replenish ATP. This type of pain can also extend to the shoulders, usually in conjunction with neck pain. As long as we are in an upright position (most of our waking hours) the postural muscles are always requiring more blood, and with it oxygen, in order to replace the ATP molecules which are expended through the constant exertion of being upright.

Researchers have demonstrated experimentally what happens to body parts when they are deprived of blood and ischemia results. You can perform your own experiment now—just raise your hand above your head and see how many seconds it takes for nerves to be affected, giving you odd tingling sensations. How long would you need to keep your hand elevated in order to experience pain? Probably not much longer.

The literature relating to hypnosis is full of accounts of people being able to raise or lower the temperature of their hands whilst under the influence of hypnotic suggestion.[2] A thermometer in one hand will show the temperature falling, while a thermometer in the other hand will show the temperature rising. On the next hypnotic suggestion, the hands can be instructed to swap temperatures, and the thermometers will be seen to fall in one hand and rise in the other. These changes of temperature are being governed by changes in the flow of blood. The hypnotic suggestions go straight to the "control center" that is the mind/brain, changing the flow of blood from one hand to another—one hand becomes somewhat drained of blood, while the other hand becomes engorged in comparison.

There are also reports of the control of pain during surgery whilst under hypnosis, and other reports of hypnotic suggestions to keep blood away from the surgical site until after the operation; then allowing a flow of blood in order to wash away impurities, followed by an adequate supply of blood to the area to allow healing to occur. Again, this is brought under control by the mind/brain, particularly the autonomic nervous system, which controls involuntary functions such as digestion and blood circulation.

---

[2] Milne (2007). *Hypnosis and the Art of Self-Therapy.*

A more common example of changes in blood flow may be when driving your car after having a meal, a dog runs out on the road and you need to take evasive action to avoid an accident. Immediately, your mind/brain will change the flow of blood supply. The circulation of blood around our body is under the control of the autonomic nervous system, which is a subsystem of the central nervous system. As digestion is not a priority during an emergency, the blood supply to your stomach will be restricted, while blood needed to respond to the situation will be sent rapidly to your arms and legs. This allows you to apply the brakes and move the steering wheel with the force required to exert control over the vehicle. All this occurs in a nanosecond, and none of it occurs under your conscious control. We don't need to think about altering our blood supply; it just happens automatically. As such, the mind/brain is constantly controlling the flow of blood to the various parts of our body, usually without any awareness on our behalf.

All blood vessels are surrounded by connective tissue, around which is a layer of vascular smooth muscle, more highly developed in arteries than in veins (arteries take the blood away from the heart and to body organs, whereas veins bring blood back to the heart). Surrounding the vascular smooth muscle is another layer of connective tissue that contains the nerves and capillaries that supply these muscles. Changes in the blood flow to downstream locations can be created by a contraction of the layer of muscles surrounding the arteries, thereby constricting their inner dimensions.

Vasodilation (resulting in an increase in the cross-sectional area of the artery) and vasoconstriction (resulting in a decrease in the cross-sectional area of the artery) are used to automatically regulate body temperature. In a very cold environment, through simultaneous vasoconstriction and vasodilation, blood will be directed away from the extremities and to the body core to ensure that the torso is able to remain as warm as possible. In a freezing situation, this change of blood supply, protecting the essential organs, will increase the chance of survival.

This is the opposite to what happens with the blood supply in a near accident as described above, whereby the blood is sent to the extremities to increase the chance of survival. The constriction of blood vessels is achieved by the action of vasoconstrictors, which include a range of hormones and neurotransmitters that are part of the functioning of the nervous system. As such, it is apparent that our brains are altering blood flow as a normal aspect of biological functioning.

It is clear that the postural muscles in the neck/shoulders, back and buttocks are especially vulnerable to ischemia. The gluteal muscles in the buttocks are susceptible to ischemic pain due to their ongoing role of keeping the body upright on the legs without tipping forwards or sideways. The lumbar muscles, just above the buttocks in the small of the back, are very often affected by ischemic pain, usually in association with pain in the glutes. Muscle pain in the neck and the top of the shoulders is also very common, and again can result from ischemia. Such muscles can be expected to suffer ischemia when there is an almost constant workload on them, and the blood supply has been reduced by only a small amount. With more exertion, the gap between the amount of oxygen the muscle needs and the amount that it gets continues to increase, and with it so does the pain—the deficiency in oxygen simply gets larger with more exertion. As a result, using muscles already suffering from ischemia makes them become even more painful.

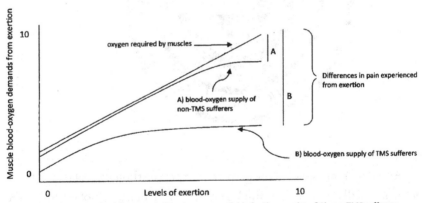

This table shows the differences in blood-oxygen available for the muscles of A) non-TMS sufferers during exertion compared to B) sufferers of TMS during exertion. This difference results in more pain for the TMS sufferers due to the larger deficit in available blood-oxygen from ischemia.

The pain pattern & psychological overlay

The longer the pain lasts, the more the pattern of thoughts, feelings, behaviors relating to the pain and subsequent social interactions become deeply embedded within the person. This begins to constitute an ever growing pain pattern which grows stronger and stronger as time goes on. As this continues, the pain, as well as a range of debilitating emotions such as fear and anxiety (about the pain getting worse) become more deeply entrenched. Grief develops about a lost rosy future, as well as lost sense of self, and lost life opportunities. Frustration also grows with the failure of treatments to eliminate the pain. Anger develops with one's own body and with life in general. Ultimately, despair and depression are often the consequence of the accumulation of these feelings, and a prevailing sense of helplessness becomes normal for chronic pain sufferers.

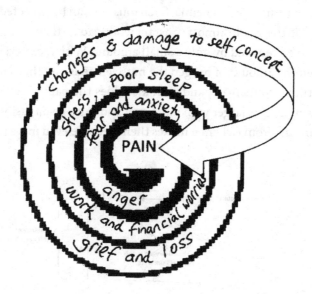

An important aspect of the pain pattern are the thoughts related to these feelings: "I will always be in pain; I'll be an invalid for the rest of my life; there is nothing I can do about the pain—I am powerless; my spine is vulnerable and easily damaged; my life is a wreck; I will be financially destitute; I am useless, etc." It can be seen how this intensifies already negative beliefs. Extreme worry about the pain only increases anxiety and hyper-vigilance, and this will consequently aggravate the pain and nerve symptoms. This may be known by the sufferer, but it is very difficult to *not* worry when you are in severe pain.

Certain patterns of bodily movements and muscular tension also become part of the pain pattern, as does a shrinking social and vocational world. This is compounded even more when people experience some of the physical consequences of decreased blood supply, such as easily torn muscles, which can then be mistakenly viewed as evidence of serious damage.

As you would expect, the feelings, thoughts, behaviors and interactions that constitute the pain pattern can themselves become deeply embedded forms of psychological distress which the mind/brain can then try to protect the suffering person from with even more intense pain. A vicious negative feedback loop can be created with additional layers of psychological burden on top of the original distress and few apparent avenues out.

Just the thought of it is enough to generate pain and make you depressed. However, the strategy of the mind/brain has worked well. Whatever the original problem was has taken such a back seat (kept in the unconscious) that as long as the physical pain lasts, there is little chance of worrying about the original upset. All that distressing material has safely receded back into the unconscious where our mind/brain figures it belongs, as we now have more immediate pain concerns to worry about.

Physical pain is entirely compelling. We are more able to ignore emotional pain, with a range of defense mechanisms, than we are able to ignore physical pain. As we are not designed to ignore physical pain, it is amongst the most effective defense mechanisms in that it commands our attention.

Additional muscle problems

In addition to ischemia, a painful problem can occur when muscles that are already suffering from an insufficient supply of oxygen become more vulnerable to tears in the muscle fiber due to exertion. The pain that results may be due to a muscle tear *on top* of ischemic pain which has resulted from a decrease in blood supply. As such, an acute pain (from a muscle strain or tear) can occur in addition to a longer term chronic pain (caused by psychologically induced ischemia).

People often report that the offending action, such as lifting a particular weight, is something that they have always been able to do without a problem—the fact that pain has resulted from the lift is viewed as being unusual. Perhaps the weight itself was not the problem. Instead, the pain was the result of a muscle strain due to putting an increased workload on a muscle already compromised by ischemia. This is often confused with the idea that, for example lifting, will produce more pain because it aggravates the structural pathology. However, as stated earlier the structural pathology is likely to be normal, even amongst people who are not in pain. The increased pain with increased activity is more likely to result from the increase in oxygen deficiency of the muscle, as described above, and may unfortunately result in a muscle tear on top of the already painful ischemia.

This can happen when people try to push through their pain for work reasons. A sharp increase in the pain can result and remain for a substantial period of time as the muscles can stay in this combined state of ischemic and muscle strain pain, resulting in a spasm that maintains the ischemia. If this occurs in the postural muscles of the back, many normal activities, such as putting on socks or tying shoelaces, can be excruciating and almost impossible. The idea that you have a *serious* spinal injury is an easy conclusion to arrive at, even though most of the time it will be wrong.

A muscle tear can be either partial or complete, and depending on how much of the muscle is affected, can take varying times to heal. Mild tears, affecting less than 5% of the muscle fiber are experienced as "pulled" muscles and are referred to as first-degree strains. This will produce only mild pain and little loss of strength. A second-degree strain affects more than 5% of the muscle fibers, but is less than a complete rupture. People with second-degree strains are likely to feel considerable pain and will be able to only partially contract the muscle. Standing or walking without a limp may be difficult. Third degree ruptures are the most serious and entail a complete tear across the width of the muscle, often rendering it unusable. This can be so serious that much internal bleeding occurs and surgery may be necessary in extreme cases to ensure proper healing.

Around 90% of people fully recover from muscle strain or sprain within a month, as most are not of the third-degree level of seriousness. Like bones, muscles also have a great capacity for self-healing. Like most muscle tears, mild ischemia itself is not generally a serious physical problem. The most sensitive nerve fibers will be affected by a lack of oxygen first. With higher levels of oxygen deprivation, muscles can become debilitated. Clinical observations indicate that mild ischemia (as seen in TMS) is usually reversible and results in no permanent damage to muscles.

The painful effects of muscle strains and tears on top of ischemic pain is similar to the causal factors relating to peptic ulcers. Both psychological and physical factors are relevant, and this reality prevents a simplistic assumption of the condition being either purely psychological or physical. We are both physical and psychological organisms. Rather than arguing for a single cause of psychological factors, chronic pain must be viewed as both physical and psychological realities. None of it is "all in your head," as though your psyche could exist without a body. Likewise, none of it is all in your body, as though your body could exist (in any meaningful way) without a mind/brain.

In *The Hidden Psychology of Pain*, there is an assumption that all of the painful conditions have biological pathways that produce changes in the body resulting in pain. This approach is arguing for a consideration of psychological factors, which work in tandem with biological pathways to produce pain. The conventional treatment approaches to chronic pain and health conditions, for the most part, ignore these psychological factors.

A confusing factor in deciding if you are suffering from ischemic muscle or nerve pain is the fact that our backs or necks are not sensitive enough for us to clearly determine if our pain is originating from a particular vertebra or damaged disc, or from the muscles, nerves or tendons in the immediate vicinity of the structural pathology. Surrounding our spine are layers of ligament and muscles, referred to as paraspinal muscles. Our backs are not sensitive enough for us to know if we are in pain due to the spine itself, or the paraspinal muscles. We just know that there is an intense pain in our buttocks, back, neck or shoulders without being able to accurately pinpoint the source of the pain.

Many physical therapists are familiar with "trigger points" that exist in various parts of the body. These are spots of extreme sensitivity which can be easily hurt with a little pressure applied. They appear to be the central zones of oxygen deprivation, and will usually persist in being tender even after the person has resolved their chronic pain or health condition. This tenderness generally points to a role for the mind/brain in the production of the pain, and not a specific location of structural abnormality.

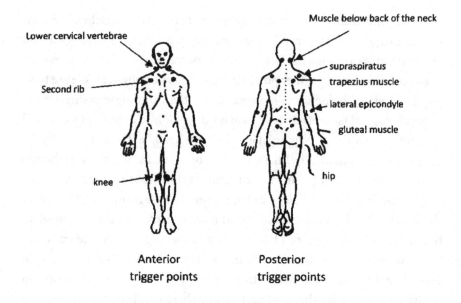

Anterior
trigger points

Posterior
trigger points

Most people suffering from emotionally generated chronic pain will be highly sensitive in these trigger points. For example, even when the main pain is in the right lower back, pain may be felt with pressing trigger points on the top of both shoulders, on the small of the back or on the outer part of both buttocks. Sarno states that pain on pressing the tendons around the knees, and the long tendon that covers the entire length of the lateral thigh and passes beyond the body outcrop of the hip is found in around 80% of people with TMS, irrespective of the site of their main pain. Further, in around 99% of people with TMS, pain on both sides of the lateral upper buttock, deep in the lumbar region of paraspinal muscles, and on the top of the shoulders (trapezius) is experienced on pressing.[3]

A high level of sensitivity in trigger points (in the absence of competing explanations such as cancer, infection or recent injury) generally indicate that the chronic pain you are suffering from may be a product of chronic blood and oxygen deprivation to key muscles, nerves or tendons/ligaments. If you are not sure whether you are suffering from chronic ischemia and build up lactic acid, it could be worth being assessed by a physician or physical

---

[3]   See Sarno (1998) under heading of "Physical Examination for Patients with Low Back and Leg Pain" (p.66), *The Mindbody Prescription*.

therapist to see how sensitive your trigger points are. Sarno provides a brief guide to assessment that medical doctors and physical therapists may find very useful in helping them to accurately diagnose the true nature of the problem[4]. You may also have sites of structural pathology on which the physical therapist may want to focus, however remember that most people who are not in pain will also have the same type of structural pathologies.

Whenever a physician assesses your pain condition, rules out serious medical conditions, and suggests "conservative treatment," *The Hidden Psychology of Pain* can be considered a viable option.

Nerve pain

Nerves are cords which are made up of equal measures of neurons and ligament. As such, they are generally quite strong, but both the neuronal and ligament parts do contain danger sensors, and can therefore send alarm messages up to the brain (see Appendix 2). Nerves can be injured by a range of assaults, including cutting, banging, squeezing, and pulling. They can also suffer from irritating chemicals around them, and by reductions in blood and therefore oxygen supply. It is possible for nerves to undergo damage, but not generate any danger messages or subsequent pain for days or weeks. In fact, some bodies donated to science show damage in the dorsal root ganglion (a nodule that contains neuronal cell bodies) without the person ever having experienced nerve pain. Many other people are found to have damaged, compressed or somehow otherwise altered nerves, but no pain.[5]

Psychologically generated pain usually presents as a *regional* process, meaning that general areas are affected by ischemia rather than just specific structures. As such, both muscles and nerves of a particular area in the body are likely to be affected at the same time as all the tissues in that area are suffering from ischemia.

Nerves are more sensitive than muscles, so ischemic pain of nerves can be more extreme as is the case with muscles. Less of an oxygen deficit is required to produce nerve pain compared to muscle pain, and nerves can

---

[4]   Ibid.
[5]   Butler & Moseley (2003) *Explain Pain.*

be more damaged than muscles from continued ischemia. Damaged nerves are also more sensitive to stress chemicals, which can create something of a vicious circle. In the absence of a viable explanation for a pain (none is usually given by health professionals), the brain can conclude that you are under some kind of threat. This sense of threat will generate the release of more stress hormones, which activates 'danger' messages from sensors, which then tell the brain that you are under threat, etc.[6]

Sarno & Coen state that, "Ischemia of nerve roots or peripheral nerves are additional sources of pain and may produce other sensory, and occasionally motor changes."[7] Symptoms often associated with nerve pain include pins and needles, burning, itchiness of the skin, and odd sensations such as prickly, pulling.

Nerve compression from a disc abnormality, like a herniation, is often viewed as the cause of a referred or nerve pain—the proposition is that the disc is impacting on the sciatic nerve to produce pain. However, Sarno states that, "Neurophysiologic logic suggests that although continued compression of a nerve might be painful for a short time, it would soon result in a total loss of feeling because the nerve could not continue to function in the face of persistent compression."[8]

Most people in chronic pain do not complain of a loss of feeling, but do complain of debilitating pain—that is, *too much* feeling rather than not enough of it. Again, the observation of many pain sufferers becoming pain-free, simply by using these ideas supports the notion that the pain was being caused by the mind/brain. If pain in the sciatic nerves was being produced by protruding disc matter, the simple introduction of information could not create a change in that structural abnormality and result in a decrease in pain. That this relief is regularly seen in people who work with *The Hidden Psychology of Pain* suggests that the physical abnormality of disc compression was not producing the pain to begin with.

The nerves that seem to be most affected by ischemia—the sciatic nerve, lumbar spinal nerves and brachial plexus nerves—are all located within muscle structures—the gluteal, lumbar and upper trapezius muscles

---

[6]   Butler & Moseley (2003) *Explain Pain.*
[7]   Sarno & Coen (1989 p. 360). "Psychosomatic Avoidance of Conflict in Back Pain." *Journal of the American Academy of Psychoanalysis.*
[8]   Sarno (1998). *The Mindbody Prescription.*

respectively. Ischemia in the sciatic nerve can produce pain in a range of leg locations such as down the entire back of the leg, only a part of a leg or foot, the front or back of calf, or the top/bottom of the foot. When the lumbar nerve is affected, pain may exist in the upper thigh or groin, or the lower abdomen. Lower sacral spine nerves may produce pain in the genital region, and this can also result from involvement of the upper lumbar spinal nerves.[9]

Most nerves have a mixed function in that they will transmit information to the brain (as sensory nerves), and bring messages back from the brain to direct muscle action (as motor nerves). As a result, pain and other sensations, as well as retarded motor function (e.g. weakness in the muscles), can be observed in many people who suffer chronic pain. Muscle pain, as well as nerve pain or odd sensations, often occur at the same time. Other nerve sensations can include pins and needles, tingling or numbness, or maybe even weakness in the legs or arms, which is demonstrable and measurable in electromyographic (EMG) studies.[10]

It is no wonder that people become frightened, especially when these symptoms are accompanied by pain. It can take some convincing that where serious medical conditions have been ruled out, the pain is resulting from an essentially benign condition.

Nerve weakness found in EMG studies are usually viewed as evidence of structural compression of nerves, however the structural abnormalities are usually unable to explain the broad extent of nerve weakness observed. This all supports the notion that chronic pain is a genuine physical condition, albeit one generated by the mind/brain.

My own personal experience dovetailed remarkably with a client's experience of pain and emphasized to me how nerves can be adversely affected by the brain. Within a month of fracturing three vertebrae in my neck (from a surfing accident in which I landed head-first on a sand bar), I returned to work. On one of my first days back, I took a big stretch while having morning tea. As I stretched and my neck flexed backwards, I felt a very sharp stabbing pain in the middle of my chest. It was of such intensity

---

[9] Sarno (1991). *Healing Back Pain: The Mind-Body Connection.*
[10] Ibid.

that it took my breath away and left me gasping before subsiding a few minutes later.

I knew that nothing was actually wrong with my chest, as it had not been injured in the accident. But the pain was reminiscent of the sensation of several thousand volts which I felt surging down my left shoulder and arm at the moment of fracturing my vertebrae. As soon it happened, I knew the pain was the result of nerve damage. My shoulder and arm were not actually injured but they were still in intense pain. A month later, while stretching at work I felt the same type of pain in my chest. I knew that it must be coming from the vertebrae impacting on my recently damaged nerves. The fact that part of my left hand was still numb from the nerve damage also gave me a fair indication. From prior reading, I knew that the vertebrae that had been damaged were in the same vicinity as the nerves that are responsible for sensations in both the arms and the chest, where I now felt the pain.

After recovering from this burst of pain while stretching, I proceeded to meet with my next client. As fate would have it, he was a man suffering from an intense persistent pain in his middle chest—the same location where I had minutes earlier experienced extreme nerve pain.

Ronald told me that he had been in chronic pain for the last three years and that it was so intense that he had stopped working. He revealed that he had been born with a deformity in his chest bones—a large concave in his chest that had been assumed to cause the intense pain. Interestingly, although he was in his fifties by the time I met him, and he had never lived a day *without* the chest deformity, he had never experienced any pain prior to the previous three years. As the deformity was so apparent, and it was located in the part of his anatomy where he felt the pain, it was logical to conclude that the deformity must be causing the pain. Various explanations for the pain had been offered to Ronald. He reported that there was one surgeon in the world who was able to perform corrective surgery. This surgeon was located overseas, and Ronald was desperate to receive the surgery, despite the enormous cost of many tens of thousands of dollars.

Having just experienced my own intense chest pain resulting from nerve damage, my mind immediately leapt to the possibility that his pain may also be nerve related. Knowing that nerves, like muscles and tendons, require a sufficient supply of oxygen, The Hidden Psychology of Pain seemed like a reasonable line of inquiry.

I asked him what had been going on in his life at the time when the pain had started. Ronald told me that it was during the time of the build-up to the invasion of Iraq in 2003. He had been at the forefront of the anti-war movement that was quickly gaining momentum as the invasion became more inevitable. Ronald had serious misgivings about the morality of invading another country, with the predictable deaths of many thousands of innocent civilians in the absence of any demonstrable justification. As no weapons of mass destruction had been found in Iraq, he believed that the whole plan for invasion had more to do with protecting oil and military interests than with liberating the Iraqi people from a cruel dictator. As such, he was a passionate opponent to military intervention.

However, at the same time Ronald had a much-loved son who was a serving member of the Australian Army. This sincere young man, like most other servicemen and women, was equally committed to a set of high ideals of service to one's country and notions of freedom from tyranny. His unit was due to leave Australia to participate in the invasion of Iraq when Ronald experienced his first attack of extreme chest pain. He told me that, "The attack was so intense that I was immediately hospitalized in a cardiac unit in what we all thought was a critical condition. My son was given compassionate leave from the army as everyone thought I was dying from a heart attack. As a result, his unit left without him and he missed out on participating in the invasion." Ronald's son went to his father's bedside in hospital and remained with him. After a week or so of undergoing a battery of heart assessments, Ronald was released from hospital as no evidence of cardiac disease had been established. It was still believed that he may in a serious condition, although no real problem with his heart could actually be found.

In varying degrees, the pain stayed with him over the next three years, sometimes requiring emergency admissions to hospital again. The ultimate medical conclusion was that due to the chest deformity, his heart did not have enough space to function without being in pain. As with other types of persistent pain, it was important that Ronald be medically checked for a more serious condition such as heart disease. Had he not already done so, I would have insisted that he obtain such a medical assessment of his heart before proceeding with psychological possibilities.

Clearly, he was experiencing a terrible dilemma when the pain began. As a father myself, I can easily imagine the anguish which he must have been in, having a sincere and decent young son getting caught up in a historical event which he viewed as being morally dubious. Worse, the invasion of Iraq could take his son's life. The prospect that his son may either be killed, or participate in the killing of other people without what Ronald viewed as being a morally sufficient reason, was highly distressing. The more he looked into it, the more the reasons for invading Iraq appeared to be morally suspect. But, his son had sworn to serve and obey, and had every intention to do just that. Seeing the potential role which this dilemma could play in his pain, I decided to bring Ronald's attention to this issue. I wondered out loud with him whether this awful dilemma, which had no apparent answers, could be more relevant to his chest pain that the bone deformity? We then spent some time discussing The Hidden Psychology of Pain.

When I saw Ronald two weeks later, he reported that the chest pain had radically diminished. As such, he was very interested in the prospect which I had proposed to him and we discussed it further. Two weeks later again, he reported that the pain had gone away. At my last contact with him, several months later, the pain had not returned. A year later, I learned from Ronald that he went back to his former employment and decided that he had no need for the expensive corrective surgery of his chest. Without being in pain, he felt he could easily live with the benign deformity.

This was a clear case of the relevance of hidden psychology to nerve pain. It is likely that his mind/brain had decreased the blood and oxygen supply to his chest nerve, a part of his anatomy that he would never question had a genuine physical condition. The ensuing physical pain guaranteed that he was no longer focused on the emotional dilemma, as he and everyone around him believed that he may be dying. The pain performed its role beautifully as a distractor from the emotional dilemmas. This was never a conscious ploy to keep his son from participating in the invasion, and he would have been morally repulsed by such a deliberate strategy. However, a deeper part of his being took the only action available to it by monopolizing his attention with a physical pain that he could not ignore.

The title of Gabor Maté's book, *When the Body Says No* sounds very relevant to this case. Cardiologist Binh An P. Phan refers to such heart pain that Ronald experienced as "broken heart syndrome," also referred to as stress cardiomyopathy.[11] It can result from extremely emotionally stressful experiences such as the breakup of relationships, the death of a loved one, the loss of an important job, or even extreme anger. The symptoms are very similar to a heart attack and can include difficulty breathing and chest pain. Dr. Phan suggests that following extremely stressful events, the heart can be overwhelmed by a surge of stress hormones including adrenalin (referred to epinephrine in America). This can result in a narrowing of the arteries which supply the heart with blood, resulting in very real physical pain. As seen with Ronald, stress cardiomyopathy is reversible and results in no lasting damage to the heart.

With his son missing the invasion, Ronald's awful emotional dilemma had diminished. However, with the prospect of his son's involvement in the ongoing war, the pain never went away until Ronald learnt about its real cause. At that point, the pain no longer served its purpose, and he was free of it. His pain had served the function of helping him to avoid consciously dealing with the seemingly unsolvable dilemma that he was in. He chose to become aware of and confront the emotional dilemma instead.

Tendon/ligament pain

Almost any tendon or ligament can be in chronic pain, however those in the knees, shoulders, feet and elbows are especially susceptible. While Sarno suggests that chronically pained tendons are also suffering from an oxygen deprivation, Professor of Physiotherapy Jill Cook refers to studies that suggest a different possible biochemical source of tendon pain. In a personal communication, she referred to Swedish research that suggests that the activated cells in the tendons are themselves responsible for producing substances that can cause pain.[12]

Contrary to Sarno's proposition, Cook informed me that there is no evidence of oxygen deprivation being the problem with chronically pained tendons. The question then becomes whether emotional/psychological

---

[11] Phan (2012). "As Valentine's Day Approaches, Cardiologist Describes Broken Heart Syndrome." *Science Daily.*

[12] Cook (2010). Personal communication.

factors are able to produce the observed cellular level changes in tendons through processes other than ischemia. A large amount of research in psychoneuroimmunology would suggest this to be the case. Cook reported that the current research "suggests that acetylcholine [a neurotransmitter], noradrenalin/norepinephrine [a stress hormone and neurotransmitter] and glutamate [a nerve transmitter] have increased expression for the substance and the receptor in activated cells." In response to my next question, she reported that "There is certainly potential for sympathetic activation," indicating the involvement of the mind/brain via the functions of the autonomic nervous system (which can generate arousal of sympathetic nervous system as seen in the fight/flight/freeze response).

The role of distressed emotion is generally involved whenever a biochemical process entails a role for stress hormones such as noradrenalin/norepinephrine. Based on current research, the role of stress hormones in the process of biochemical changes in tendons provides support for Sarno's *general* contention, if not a specific role for oxygen deprivation in tendon pain. Over a decade ago, he stated, "If research were to demonstrate some other autonomically induced pain pathology, I would not be disturbed. What's important is not the method the brain uses to produce symptoms; it is the fact that the brain *is* inducing symptoms."[13] Cook's comments, based on current research evidence, suggest that Sarno was correct in proffering that the mind/brain, via distressed emotions, is highly involved in tendon/ligament pain.

The type of structural diagnoses that are usually offered to explain such tendon-ligament pain include chondromalacia and unstable kneecap and trauma for knee pain; neuroma, bone spur, plantar fasciitis, flat feet and trauma due to overuse for foot pain; bursitis or rotator cuff disorder for shoulder pain; carpal tunnel syndrome or RSI for wrist pain; and trochanteric bursitis for hip pain.

The evidence, which demonstrates the possibility of a psychogenic cause of the tendon pain, is in the sufferers who become pain free as a result of learning of the role of distressed emotion. (see Rebecca's story in Appendix 10). This appears to be the case, even if the biological processes responsible for chronically pained tendons ultimately prove not to be changes in oxygen,

---

[13] Sarno (1998, p.50). *The Mindbody Prescription.*

but the type to which Cook refers. The mind/brain, via powerful emotions, appears to play a vital role in the causation of chronic pain in tendons. If the introduction of ideas alone can change a person's experience of pain, then the pain *must* have originated in the mind/brain to begin with.

The same impressive results are found even in the less common circumstance when knees show swelling. Again, viable competing explanations such as acute injuries must be eliminated first via a medical examination. Various biological pathways are required to create physical changes resulting in pain and swelling, but the process begins with emotional distress at a very deep level, and our mind/brain's efforts to protect us from the full conscious awareness of this distress.

CHAPTER 6

Conscious & Unconscious Factors

Conscious stressors

We ARE ALL GENERALLY AWARE of the role which stress can play in producing certain bodily sensations and experiences. It is not unusual for our shoulders to slowly rise over the course of a busy day, and for this to produce some stiffness in our neck. We are also familiar with the experience of blushing when embarrassed, or of stressful situations resulting in headaches. These experiences are widespread and easily recognized by most people. As such, they tend to be about the stressful situations of which we are *consciously* aware. We know when we are having a bad day at work, or when there is strain in our relationship, or that we don't want to have that meeting with our boss. If such stressors are sustained over a long period of time, they can lead to health-damaging consequences.

Chronic stress makes us more vulnerable to common complaints such as colds, flus and other opportunistic infections. Many researchers and clinicians also believe that the damaging effects are so powerful that chronic stress can make us more vulnerable to serious conditions such as cancer and heart disease. The health conditions that can follow chronic psychological stress clearly demonstrate the true nature of the human organism, being both mind and body.

The body reacts to psychological stress in typical ways, including a range of hormonal and physiological changes. Adrenal fatigue, as an example, can have a broad range of health consequences, and psychology is highly relevant via the effects of sustained emotional stress on the body. This syndrome occurs when psychological stress has become so prolonged that the adrenal glands, which respond to stress with raised secretions of adrenaline/epinephrine and cortisol, have become exhausted from almost constant arousal. As a result, the secretions of these stress hormones become diminished, and a range of health problems can follow.

Although too high levels of cortisol are responsible for many health problems, via its immune dampening effects, it is still needed at adequate levels to "turn off" the immune response at the appropriate time when the danger has passed. When the adrenal glands have become exhausted, they may be unable to produce even enough cortisol to allow this to happen. The results of this can be associated with inflammatory problems and many other serious health conditions.

Other lifestyle factors such as diet, exposure to toxins, substance use patterns and exercise all play an important role, along with psychological factors, in producing adrenal fatigue. Dietary changes and a range of herbal, mineral and vitamin supplements are often required to overcome this condition. And naturally, it is important to become aware of the psychological stressors which feed into the whole condition; and to use psychological coping strategies to decrease the negative impact of these factors. It makes a lot of sense to do what we can with problem solving strategies, given the opportunities and restrictions inherent in the situation. Relaxation exercises, meditation and prayer are excellent options for such times. They can help us to slowly take the tension out of our minds and bodies by focusing on progressive muscle relaxation and peaceful guided imagery.

The above discussion refers to psychological stressors of which we are aware. But what about the psychological stressors of which we are either not at all, or just barely aware? It appears that in cases of chronic pain, the mind/brain has diverted a small proportion of blood away from nerves and muscles, thereby producing the intense pain via an oxygen deprivation. *But why would the brain choose to do this?*

The unconscious purpose of chronic pain

If we want to make sense of the various quandaries that chronic pain poses, we need to leave behind purely physical explanations—there simply *are* no physical explanations for most of these phenomenon. Unlike acute pain, there is no adaptive value to chronic pain. It doesn't help us to slow down for healing purposes, to do anything well, or to improve the quality of our lives in any apparent manner. As such, the only other way of making sense of chronic pain is from a psychological perspective. But keep in mind, this is not to say that the pain is "all in your head,". Despite a high level of involvement from your mind/brain, as is the case in all pain, it is clearly in your body where you feel it. There are psychological reasons for your mind/brain to use real biological pathways to produce real physical pain in your body. These reasons are the essence of *The Hidden Psychology of Pain*. What could these psychological reasons be?

Remember the depth-psychology notion of there being a conscious mind and an unconscious or subconscious mind? Like the ice-berg, most of the psyche appears to be below the waterline, or below the level of consciousness. It contains material that we are simply not aware of, but it is there regardless. The unconscious mind can also be thought of as a storehouse, or a warehouse for all of the experiences that we've had over the course of our lives from childhood through to teenage years, through to early adulthood and up to the present moment.

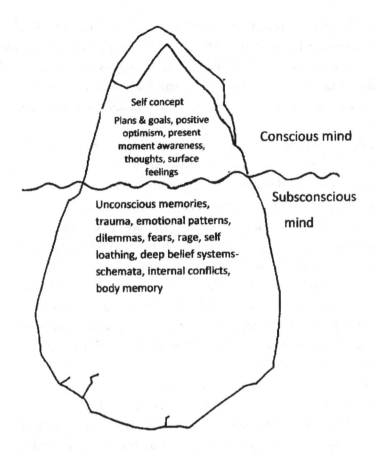

Iceberg/depth-psychology model of the psyche

Neuropsychologist John Arden, referring to experiences from infancy that we are no longer able to remember, states that these memories are neither forgotten nor suppressed.[1] Most memories are encoded in various brain areas via the hippocampus. However, when the experience is terrifying, it appears that the amygdala, the part of the limbic system that generates fear, is able to store the memory rather than have it stored in the normal manner. This is because the stress hormones which flood the brain during the traumatic event make the amygdala more excitable, and can inhibit the functioning of the hippocampus, preventing the normal memory consolidation process.

---

[1]   Arden (2010). *Rewire Your Brain.*

This will lead to fragmentary memories, as the thinking parts of the brain were overridden by the limbic system during the ordeal (see Appendix 2). Such memories are often referred to as unconscious memories, or 'covert recollections' by neuroscientists. Unlike normal memoires, they can remain hidden for many years, and are often only available in fragmented flash-backs.

These "lost" memories are only available to our consciousness as emotional patterns—they present themselves to our awareness in the form of habitual emotional reactions to situations, but not in the recollection of specific events. Often, these responses will seem to be out of proportion to the situation. However, the size and patterned nature of the emotional response indicates upsetting experiences which have been lost to our conscious awareness. Despite this, they tend to permeate everything we do.

Many of the experiences which our mind/brain will store away are positive. The memories and associated feelings that go into our unconscious can be happy ones reflecting the good experiences in life. Many others will be negative and unpleasant ones. All of us have *some* kind of distressing experiences from childhood, teenage years, and early adulthood, not to mention possibly now in our current lives.

The unconscious mind (being the processes of the sub-cortical brain areas in the limbic system—including the amygdala—and the brainstem) has stored up all those experiences along with the associated thoughts and feelings. It is also taking in things on a daily basis now, things that we are not quite aware of. For example, research has demonstrated an increase in heart rate when forms of frightening stimuli, such as large spiders, are presented in a person's peripheral vision. Surprisingly, this increased heart rate occurs even when the person has no conscious awareness of seeing the spider, as they are focused on the stimuli ahead of them. At some unconscious level, a moving object with eight hairy legs is perceived and the person's body can demonstrate a fear response in their physiology, even without the person knowing why. This is referred to as "blind-sight."

Other experiences in our normal daily life can "wind us up" without us being entirely aware of them, as they are so common. Buses or trains running late again; people pushing in front of us in a queue, or being rude to us in shops; relationships not going the way we want them to; our jobs not being so good, or chronic unemployment being even worse—all the normal things in daily life that people get upset about. The emotional content of all these experiences are also going into the storehouse of the unconscious, joining the other experiences that have been filed away.

You can think of the contents of your unconscious as being like pots of water on a gas stove, which are being kept on a constantly low simmer. The contents of the unconscious, like the water are not cold or inert. Rather, there is still a small amount of life in them—the water is still lukewarm.

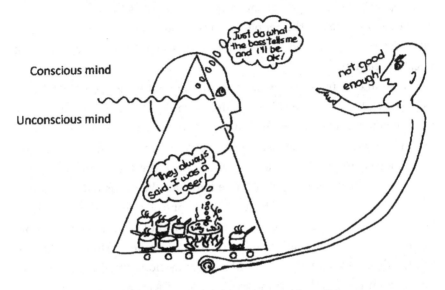

Turning up the heat on unconscious distress

As with Max (introduced in Chapter 1), the distress related to his brother's sexual abuse of him never ended, died or went away—rather, it remained 'warm' and somewhat alive within him. For his development and progress in life, it may have been important for Max to put the associated hurt behind him and just "get on with life." In an ideal world, he would have been able to tell his parents when the abuse first happened, but perhaps due to his young age, the lack of social power of children at the time, and the shame that most perpetrators manage to instill in their victims, he was unable to disclose the abuse.

This was even more so during the 1960s and 70s when the abuse was happening to Max. At that time, there was no public discussion of child sexual assault as there is now and as a result, most young victims were simply not in a position to raise what was clearly a taboo topic. Consequently, Max had to make a decision as a young person—to be a victim and live under the shadow of what had been done to him for his entire life; or try to "get over it and move on."

Our culture encourages the latter option. Most of us try to come to grips with what has happened to us, put it aside and refocus on the tasks ahead. People who suffer from psychogenic pain tend to be the "copers," i.e. those who appear to hold it together and keep on persevering despite the odds. By and large, they are not the people who just tend to give up and wallow in a pit of despair. To succeed at this will require some degree of repression of negative feelings.

Max, like many people who have suffered, put his energies into living as normal a life as possible. He socialized, had girlfriends, maintained his involvement with his family (including his brother), got a job, married, and began his own family. The distress was never far from the surface however, as evidenced by his "wild" adolescence and more-than-normal alcohol consumption with socially disruptive behavior. With his defenses down while drunk, he did confront his brother on one occasion about the abuse; however his brother retreated in distress and Max never raised the topic again. As long as he was able to focus on the tasks required for a productive life, the distress that dwelt within Max's unconscious remained lukewarm, on a low simmer. It didn't die and go cold, nor did it erupt and boil over. This was the equilibrium that he managed to find. Once he had matured out of his adolescent excesses, his life was relatively stable and normal—at least on the surface level.

Max's equilibrium was radically disturbed when two events happened. Firstly, he became a father for the first time. All of a sudden, he felt responsible for a child whom he knew was vulnerable, just due to his age. The second event, his brother getting a job at the same workplace, was more disturbing. The "lie" that Max had chosen at some level to live, that he and his brother had a normal and healthy relationship, became unsustainable at a very deep level. On the surface, he joined in with other people's pleasure at two brothers now working together. However, at a more unconscious level, he was in a terrible dilemma. Did he confront the brother again, this time as a sober adult, telling him to leave the job and get out of his life? How would he explain this to his employer, workmates or to his mother? His brother was content to leave the history between them alone and never revisit it, as evidenced by his response when Max did confront him years earlier. What would the impact be of revealing to his mother what his brother had done to him? Their father had since died, so the brother was now living with his mother, ostensibly to look after her. Would his mother throw the brother out and be left on her own? Would she suffer a heart attack or a stroke on learning of what one son had done to the other?

As you can see, these were terrible issues for Max to grapple with, and none of them had easy answers. The material which had been on a low simmer in his unconscious for many years now had the gas turned up. Even though he had always known that the abuse had happened, the full enormity of the emotional distress (perhaps including a murderous rage) was still largely unconscious, and had remained relatively dormant since the abuse stopped. He was barely aware of the building pressure of these emotions threatening to emerge from his unconscious, as he was still focused on coping with the tasks required for life, i.e. working, looking after his family, maintaining relationships. This was the psychological context in which his back pain first emerged.

As is so often the case with sufferers of chronic pain, some part of the mind/brain realizes the need to protect the person from the deeply distressing feelings that are bubbling away at an unconscious level.[2] The mind/brain does this by creating a compelling diversion: chronic pain.

Most people state that they would prefer to consciously deal with the distressing feelings rather than have their mind/brain create physical pain as a distraction, and this would be a rational response. However, the unconscious does not use the same rules of logic or rationality as does our conscious mind. Rather, the unconscious often uses a childlike irrationality in its normal functioning, and reason may not play too much of a role. There

---

[2] Sarno obtained the understanding that pain was operating as a defense mechanism from his psychologist colleague, Dr. Stanley Coen, who had been influenced by psychoanalyst Franz Alexander. Until that time, Sarno had assumed that chronic pain was simply a physical manifestation of anxiety or other emotional distress. Coen helped Sarno understand that the pain, or other equivalent symptoms, are being created in order to help the person *avoid* having to consciously deal with difficult unconscious feelings that are usually repressed.

is, however, often a rationality of sorts to the avoidance strategy developed by the mind/brain, but it is generally not what people would choose consciously for themselves.

Unacceptable feelings

Just what could this unconscious material be that we apparently need protection from? It will often relate to feelings that are embarrassing to us, are painful or hurtful, or in some way unpleasant or "unacceptable" by society's standards. The associated feelings that then need to be repressed include anxiety, anger/rage, and feelings of inferiority. Some part of the mind/brain does not want us to be in touch with them at all due to their threatening nature, and certainly does not want them to be apparent to others.

The existence of unconscious conflicts, and their role in generating conscious anxiety, has recently been demonstrated in an experiment conducted at the University of Michigan. Researchers gathered a list of words that were viewed as being related to the unconscious conflicts of eleven subjects who had undergone some sessions of psychoanalytic therapy. The words, relevant for each individual, were then played back to them at a subliminal rate which the conscious mind is unable to detect—at one thousandth of a second. Subjects were connected to scalp electrodes which measured their brain's reactions to the words. Their brains were seen to react to the unconscious conflict words only, and not to unrelated words; and only when they were presented subliminally. Through variations in the study methodology, the researchers were able to demonstrate that the words relating to unconscious conflicts were responsible for the conscious experience of anxiety. Clearly, we are only aware of limited features of our mind/brain functioning.[3] Some of the cornerstones of psychoanalytic psychology continue to receive evidence based support through research using sophisticated brain imaging technology.

---

[3] University of Michigan Health System (2012, June 16). Freud's Theory of Unconscious Conflict Linked to Anxiety Symptoms. *Science Daily*.

Martin, a musician client of mine, had been somewhat crippled by arm and shoulder pain that prevented him from playing his instrument and performing. He was highly skilled, but due to his childhood experiences of being asthmatic in a sports-mad culture, he grew up feeling never quite good enough. As an important indicator of the motives of his unconscious, he revealed to me that the pain had prevented him from having to deal with his lack of confidence in publicly performing music, so he was effectively "off the hook." The pain had been quite debilitating to him, such that he would never have consciously chosen to experience it. However, his unconscious was using a childlike logic in preventing him from having to confront his own feelings of inadequacy by giving him the pain. Like repressed prisoners in jail, these feelings of inadequacy were wanting to escape—to burst into his conscious awareness. As such, there is a need to distract attention away from them in order to avoid having to confront these difficult feelings should they succeed in becoming conscious. Speaking of this around one hundred years ago, Freud wrote, "The unconscious itself has no other endeavor than to break through the pressure weighing down on it and force its way either to consciousness or to a discharge through some real action."[4]

Ronald's mystery chest pain was also a very good example of the unacceptability of certain feelings. My guess was that at a very deep level he felt horror with his son's potential involvement in the invasion of Iraq. Part of this may have involved a disappointment in his son; part would have involved despair at the chance of his son killing or being killed; and part may also have involved a sense of failure in himself as a parent for having raised a boy who was willing to participate in such an activity. As he also loved and respected his son, these feelings would have been very threatening to him and therefore had to remain at a deep unconscious level.

Martin the musician was not traumatized by his childhood experiences; however, it is apparent that he felt somewhat humiliated by his asthmatic condition (my assumption would also be that his asthma may have resulted from distress in his childhood that he no longer has any awareness of).

A certain amount of unconscious anger or rage is inevitable for most children, regardless of how diligent and caring their parents are. All young children will experience frustrations at being smaller, younger and weaker

---

4   Freud, Sigmund (1961). *Beyond the Pleasure Principle.*

than older siblings and adults. They will all be frustrated by their parents as the socialization of society's expectations is a necessary component of child raising, and this entails plenty of *no's*—some of which are reasonable, and others less so.

When children are abused by dysfunctional or malicious adults, then the addition to their reservoir of distress is larger. Some parents, with all the best intentions, will fail to raise their children in a healthy manner because of their own burdens of distress. The quality of bonding between the primary caregiver and a baby will create flow-on effects later in life.

In Max's case, it would make sense that the deeper feelings, from which he needed protection, would have included both a revulsion and shame in himself (unwarranted, but not unusual for people who have been sexually abused), as well as an intense anger and hatred towards his brother. None of these feelings were straightforward. The adult part of Max knew that he was not responsible for the abuse. He didn't invite nor did he want the abuse, and his brother was older and stronger than him. However, the child part of him suspected that he may be in trouble and feared being blamed if he disclosed to his parents. He felt ashamed of his involvement as well as forever dirty and unworthy.

In regards to his feelings about his brother, he was also ambivalent. He could see the better sides of his character as an adult (the brother hadn't hurt him since) and recognized that his brother was also young when he perpetrated the abuse. On the other hand, Max was so angry with his brother that at times he wanted to kill him. There is no easy answer to or reconciliation between these competing feelings. In addition, for a child to endure years of sexual abuse at the hands of a sibling suggests that his parents were not at all "tuned-in" to his needs or distress. This implies that an insecure form of attachment may have characterized Max's relationship with his parents, setting him up to feel anxious and unworthy even before his brother's abuse started.

In the years beyond adolescence, Max had developed a self-concept which included being a gentle and decent man—certainly not a potential murderer. His sense of self, while damaged by the abuse, still included being a reasonable human being. As such, his murderous urges were entirely threatening to his sense of who he was.

As is typical for people suffering from psychogenic pain, the clients discussed so far overcame the urge to indulge in their misfortunes and attempted to get on with life in as positive a manner as they could. As such, there was a level of self-imposed positivity as a preferred option to shriveling up and dying. It is not as though they ever actually succeeded in this attempt at being positive, as it remained an uphill battle for them to remain positive enough to just keep on living. Undoubtedly, this positivity is the preferred option; however, such a rational decision (to be positive) does not mean that the deep emotional distress just goes away. It may simply drive the distress deeper into the unconscious and thereby make it even more powerful as it threatens to erupt into awareness. This could increase vulnerability to chronic pain.

The people who appear to be most susceptible to this scenario are those who make the most concerted efforts to get on with life in the best way they can—again, the "copers." This response is not to be discouraged, but it can come at a cost. Personally, while still recovering from my car accident as an eighteen-year-old, I went for my first "jog" down the street while still using a walking stick after six months on crutches. Two weeks later, on the day I came off the walking stick, I jogged 20 laps of an Australian Rules Football field (the size of a large cricket oval). I was not going to let the damage control my life, either physically or psychologically. But I spent most of my adult life with chronic groin pain, being thirty eight years old before it went away— this is what self-imposed positivity did for me. Of course, there was an upside to this positivity, but the downside was nearly twenty years of ongoing pain. Those who give in to their distress may be crippled with emotional problems, but they tend not to suffer from as much chronic pain.

Richard Davidson, a neuropsychologist who has been at the forefront of brain research regarding emotions over the last thirty years, provides an important piece to the jig-saw puzzle of chronic pain. His research has demonstrated that people's typical emotional style, either positive or more negative, is reflected in certain types of brain activity. Providing another piece to the puzzle, research by Baliki and colleagues have recently demonstrated that these same brain areas are also important for chronic pain. Specifically, Davidson notes that people who can be characterized as more emotionally positive display a higher level of neural activity between their pre-frontal cortex and their nucleus accumbens.

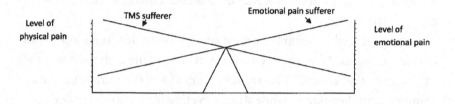

The 'see-saw' effect of experiencing either psychological/emotional pain, or psychogenic physical pain. Typically, if people allow themselves to feel the emotional pain, they tend not to feel so much psychologically caused physical (TMS) pain. Alternately, if they repress their emotional pain, they tend to feel more physical (TMS) pain.

From reading Appendix 2, you will recall that the largest neuroscience predictor of chronic pain following an injury is the high level of communication between two brain regions, the pre-frontal cortex and the nucleus accumbens (NAcc).[5] The more communication people have between these two brain areas, the higher is the chance that they will suffer from chronic pain; the less communication between these two areas, the more likely are people to recover after an injury, and the pain resolve before it becomes chronic. Is it merely a coincidence that neuroscientists now report that people who are the most able to sustain positive moods (the least depressive) are the people who also have a *high* level of communication between the pre-frontal cortex and the NAcc, just like the chronic pain

---

[5] Baliki et al (2012)"Corticostriatal functional connectivity predicts transition to chronic back pain". *Nature Neuroscience*.

sufferers?[6] Conversely, those who are more negative (i.e. emotionally pained) have *less* communication between their pre-frontal cortex and their NAcc, and are less likely to experience chronic pain. The above diagram, showing a see-saw effect between chronic physical pain and emotional pain, appears to be supported by cutting edge neuroscience.

Level of communication between pre-frontal cortex and NAcc	**Low** communication	**High** communication
Emotional experience	More **negative**	More **positive**
Physical experience	**Low** chronic pain	**High** chronic pain

The above table shows the inverse relationship between emotional pain and chronic physical pain. Those who give in to their distress may feel overwhelmed with emotional problems, but they tend not to suffer from as much chronic pain as do people who attempt to remain positive. Distressed feelings tend to make their impact felt either directly as debilitating emotions, or indirectly as the avoidant strategy which is chronic pain.

What would have happened had Max's distress and the related dilemmas reached such a temperature that they finally erupted and burst into his conscious awareness? He could have experienced something of a psychological episode, or "nervous breakdown" as it is commonly called. That is, he may have become so psychologically distressed so as to become immobilized, or he may have become homicidally angry. He may have actually hurt or even killed his brother if he gave full vent to the feelings that were erupting from within his storehouse of distress. However, this did not happen, as his awareness became monopolized by the new physical pain, which he began to experience not long after his brother turned up at his workplace. As anyone in serious pain knows, once the pain starts, it demands your full attention and little else seems important.

As Max was required to engage in heavy lifting for his job, the first twinges of back pain caused him a great deal of concern. He had to modify and restrict aspects of his work. As the pain got worse rather than better with

---

6   Davidson & Begley (2012) *The Emotional Life of Your Brain*. Hudson Street Press, New York.

time, he became more worried. When the days turned into weeks with no improvement, this worry became even more intense. A month or so later, the pain was pretty much all Max could think or talk about. He reluctantly had to take time off work. As his X-rays showed structural pathologies in his spine (disc bulges), his treating GP signed him off as unfit for work, concluding that these bulges were producing the pain. (This may have been an accurate diagnosis if the disc bulges were recent, meaning that he was suffering from an acute pain due to a recent injury; however, he recalled no recent event which would suggest a new injury).

As the financial implications of his pain became even more evident, the pressures on his young family escalated. Within a few months, the pain could no longer be called acute but was now chronic. Just over a year later, he and his wife had their second baby and the difficulties just mounted. Max never got to hold either of his babies while standing, as his back pain would allow him to carry no weight. As his babies grew into toddlers, he was never able to get on the floor and play, nor run or kick a ball with them. The emotional pain just mounted as he came to view himself as a worthless husband and father.

By the time I met Max, five years after the onset of his pain, he was still in physical agony as well as feeling suicidally depressed. He and his wife had the barest of relationships. He was totally disengaged from his children, living on a disability pension, and spent his time moving between his living-room couch and his bed. He was obsessed with his pain, as it curtailed and limited every aspect of his life.

What had happened to his dilemmas and feelings in regards to his brother? They had receded back into the recesses of his unconscious mind/brain. In my analogy, the gas had been turned down again and the deep emotional hurt simmered back down again to the level where it had been before. This happened as his conscious attention was well and truly focused on his pain and all of its consequences in his life—and these were substantial. As such, there was no threat of the unconscious distress erupting into his awareness and causing a psychological overwhelm as long as the pain dominated his conscious attention.

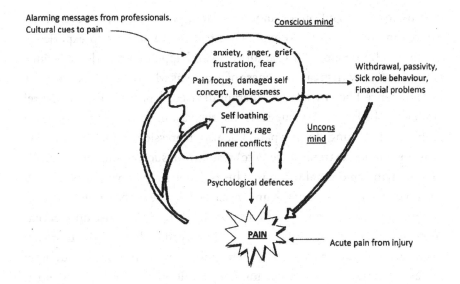

Vicious pain cycle and pattern

The Hidden Psychology of Pain suggests that agony, such as that experienced by Max, serves a psychological purpose. The purpose is to take the person's attention away from the emerging awareness of emotional material (eg. hurts, dilemmas, feelings of inadequacy, guilt, anger, etc) at the time when they are threatening to erupt into conscious awareness. An unconscious part of the mind/brain, being aware of the deep emotional issue, uses biological pathways to create real physical pain as an attempted 'solution' to the problem of these issues bursting into conscious awareness. Instead of this occurring, perhaps resulting in a 'psychological break-down', a focus on physical pain develops. In my own case, chronic groin pain was unconsciously created for eighteen years in order to protect me from a conscious focus on psychological trauma. As such, the pain operates as something of a 'solution', and to the unconscious emotional part of the mind/brain creating it, is more important to have than not to have.

It seems odd, especially in this age with a focus in psychology on our conscious thoughts, that an unconscious part of us can experience an underlying emotional problem (often relating to some kind of wound we have undergone); can construct pain as an attempted solution to the problem associated with that wound, whether the problem be the threat of conscious recognition, or another related problem; can believe that it is more important for us to experience this 'solution' than to experience the original problem; and that all this can happen with little conscious awareness, but with great awareness of problems which the pain creates for us. Coherence Therapy, a psychotherapy devised by Bruce Ecker and Laurel Hulley[7] in the late 1980's, suggests that the vast majority of psychological problems (including chronic pain, but also depression, anxiety and panic, substance abuse, extreme anger, etc) result from such attempted solutions to underlying emotional wounds. This psychotherapy involves assisting a person to become aware of the unconscious purpose of the symptom vis-à-vis an emotional wound, as the symptom tends to make sense only in that context. Coherence Therapy is entirely in accord with the TMS approach to chronic pain, and represents a therapeutic method that allows sufferers to learn of the underlying reason for their condition. I highly recommend it.

Depth-psychologists use the term "defense mechanisms" to describe psychological strategies that prevent us from becoming aware of problematic material in the unconscious. Chronic pain operates as such a defense mechanism. It appears that our mind/brain decides that we can better cope with physical pain rather than with intense emotional pain. The fruitless search for the alleviation of the bodily pain with physical therapies can monopolize our lives for many years, and keep obscuring the real need to address distressed emotion.

As research has demonstrated, traumas experienced by children are highly related to the experience of chronic pain as adults.[8] But some people will be confused by their symptoms of chronic pain, as they cannot relate to the stories which others tell of terrible childhood abuse experiences, horrible war experiences as adults, or even car accidents. Obviously, the psychological culprits are not always overt traumas. Additional forms of psychological distress will be explored in the next chapter.

---

[7] Ecker & Hulley (1996) *Depth Oriented Brief Therapy.* Jossey-Bass Publishers, San Francisco.

[8] Schofferman (1992). "Childhood Psychological Trauma Correlates with Unsuccessful Lumbar Spine Surgery." *Spine.*

CHAPTER 7

The Depths of the Unconscious

As discussed throughout this book, just because we lack an awareness of relevant psychological factors does not mean that they are not present or affecting our lives in ways which we do not realize.

Childhood attachment patterns

One of the primary sources of unacceptable thoughts and feelings is the quality of our relationships with primary caregivers as infants. In varying degrees, we are all grappling with the realities of our early lives. Most of us suffered in some ways as children. Sometimes, this suffering has been through overt abuse or severe neglect, and sometimes it resulted only because we were smaller and had less social power than those bigger than us. Powerlessness, lack of control and frustration is the norm for young children, and can leave psychological scars on all of us in varying degrees.

Unless we were repeatedly abused as children, or experienced some other extreme situations, very few of us will have any memory of the quality of the relationships we had with our primary caregivers as babies and toddlers. For little people, life is an often scary and potentially difficult proposition. How we psychologically attach to the adults in our lives is crucial in terms of whether we become anxious or calm children.

Attachment style is the way in which children come to connect with their primary caregiver (mostly, but not always mothers). The attachment style of primary caregivers has crucial lasting effects, not only for children's emotional functioning, but also for our later emotional patterns as adults. From many years of research, four main attachment styles have been identified:[1] [2]

- *Secure* attachment styles occur when caregivers tend to respond quickly and consistently to the infant's needs. As a result, the child is likely to feel worthy of love, and experience feelings of closeness in their relationships. As adults, people who experienced secure attachment are more likely to have high self-esteem, and to be more emotionally resilient. Secure attachment styles occur between caregivers and their infants around two thirds of the time. The remaining attachment styles are all referred to as "insecure."

- *Avoidant* attachments are where caregivers tend to be somewhat unresponsive to their infant's distress, discourage crying and promote separation. As adults, people who experienced this style are likely to be described by their peers as aloof, unlikable and highly controlling. They find it difficult to trust their partner, are anxious in relationships, feel unworthy, worry about abandonment, are clingy and jealous, and are prone to addictions. This attachment style occurs around 20% of the time.

- *Ambivalent* attachments are formed when caregivers tend to behave in an inconsistent manner, with sometimes being indifferent to the infant's distress, and other times being attentive. This tends to result in adults who are anxious and insecure, and occurs around 10-15% of the time.

- *Disorganized* attachment styles are where the caregivers tend towards being impulsive and depressed, as well as abusive toward their children. Such parents show an extreme lack of

[1] Arden (2010). *Rewire Your Brain.*
[2] Siegel (2010). *Mindsight: The New Science of Personal Transformation.*

attunement with the child's emotional needs, and are often frightening to them. Adults who experienced this style as infants tend to have difficulties relating to others and regulating their negative emotions. This style occurs around 10% of the time in the general population, but around 80% of the time in certain subgroups, such as with drug abusing parents.

Adults who fell into one of the three insecure attachment types as children are more likely to be mistrustful and defensive, prone to pessimism and have poor self-esteem. In addition, they are more likely to be anxious, and to experience mood problems. In contrast, adults who had secure attachment styles with their primary caregivers as children are more likely to have achieved their intellectual potential, be respected by their peers, have positive relationships with others, and are more able to regulate their emotions. Guess which people are more likely to suffer from chronic pain?

As these emotional problems relate to a pattern of very early life experiences, it is possible for people to have few conscious memories of specific experiences that reflect these attachment styles. The part of the brain most responsible for long-term memory, the hippocampus, is not mature until around three years of age. Rather than clear memories of upset relating to specific events of insecure attachment style, there is simply a feeling within of distress and unworthiness, which can easily be triggered by current experiences.

These early distressing experiences occurred before the brain had developed the capacity to retain them as memories. However, the part of the brain that becomes highly active during times of distress, the amygdala, is thought to be fully functioning when the baby is born. It is likely that the distress associated with insecure attachment styles becomes stored in the amygdala, the brain area that registers fear.[3] An emotional pattern of fear, insecurity and unworthiness can be established at an early age, and result in a lifetime of distressed emotion. It is possible to have no memories which relate to these feelings, but an *emotional* memory remains, as discussed in relation to cover recollections. Emotions are products of body and brain processes that occur at much deeper levels than thinking cortex. As such, it

---

[3]   Carter (2010). *Mapping the Mind.*

is fair to say that most emotions are somewhat unconscious, at least in their origins. Freud was right when he suggested that consciousness is merely the tip of the iceberg.

It is likely that the emotional patterns of distress stemming from insecure attachment styles are amongst the types of feelings which our mind/brain is trying to protect us from by creating chronic pain. It is from positive as well as distressing experiences that children arrive at conclusions about their value as human beings (worthy or not), about the world in general (safe or dangerous), and about other people (benign or threatening). Unfortunately, when they have bad experiences, children will use the only type of logic available to them, which is little kid's logic.

It is not unusual for small children to blame themselves for bad things happening in their lives, such as parental conflict, or even abuse they experience at the hands of their parents. The fantasy of parental "goodness" serves them better psychologically by decreasing anxiety, than does the reality that they are vulnerable to the whims of people who may be little more mature than they are. As such, some extremely unfortunate conclusions can be drawn by children from the ages of three or four until around ten.

It is typical for children that have been sexually abused, for instance, to blame themselves and conclude that they are bad and dirty people. In the absence of caring adults who will listen to them and take appropriate action, this type of faulty conclusion may *feel* safer to the abused child than the realization that they are at the mercy of an abusive parent or other adult. As adults, they may rationally believe that this is not true—they were not responsible for the abuse. However, the distressed emotions can still remain, coming from a much deeper level than the rational mind.

This conclusion of blame, leading to a lack of self-worth ("I am bad and dirty") will often be carried by the person into their adulthood. We are all attempting to make sense of our experiences, and we use such conclusions to assist us in making sense of a potentially confusing world. These conclusions (e.g. "I am worthless," or "the world and people in it are dangerous") then become templates for our understanding, a frame of reference to help us make sense of potentially confusing experiences.

We take these templates, or "cognitive schemas," with us into the next chapters of our life such as school. They allow us to make ready sense of why, for example, the teacher might mean to us—"Because I am a worthless person." The fact that the teacher is having a bad day, or doesn't like his job, is an adult understanding and may not occur to the child. However, a self-deprecating explanation is already available and has worked in the past to decrease anxiety. It allows the child to retain some sense of control, with the notion being that they can impact the situation by behaving differently—"They will treat me better if only I can behave better." A sense of control can be restored by the child, even if illusory.

Although most children's experiences of life will include both positive and negative responses, we have a tendency to only pay attention to those responses from others that conform to our template of who we are. Those who have internalized a template of "I am unworthy" will tend to focus on the responses which confirm this template, as this provides some level of predictability. We may not *like* what this entails, but at least we are able to predict what is likely to happen as a result of being "unworthy." People may disregard our feelings and needs, and preparing for this can help restore a sense of control—"I just won't expect them to care about me."

Over time, and with a succession of life experiences, these conclusions become solidified through repetition and reinforcement, until they appear to be self-evident basic "truths" about the self. Thus, the template can become a well-entrenched psychological pattern governing emotions, thoughts, behaviors and interactions with others. It is normal for these patterns to be operating largely outside of our conscious awareness.

It is these patterns of distress that can make us vulnerable to The Hidden Psychology of Pain. The manager at work looks at us in a critical manner, and at a very deep level this triggers feelings of unworthiness that our scornful parent used to instill in us. The deep-set feelings of unworthiness can be so painful that our mind/brain would prefer us to experience a bout of extreme physical pain than the associated emotional pain.

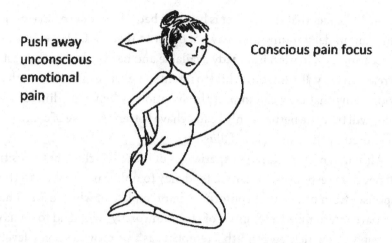

Push away
unconscious
emotional
pain

Conscious pain focus

Chronic pain as a psychological defense mechanism

Thoughts, feelings & the body

While not endorsing the simplistic CBT notion that thoughts cause feelings, it is clear that such a relationship between thoughts and feelings does exist. However, there is considerable evidence that emotional states can play a large role in determining the nature of thoughts (rather than thoughts necessarily producing feelings). Thoughts are able to have a reciprocal influence on emotions in that they can reinforce and help to entrench the distressed feelings. Many feelings are also much more powerful than thoughts. The neural pathways from the emotional systems to the thinking systems in the brain are stronger than the pathways that run the other way. More neural traffic comes up from the limbic system than goes down from the neo-cortex. It makes most sense to view thoughts and feelings as merely different but highly related aspects of psychological and physiological experience rather than assigning an overriding importance to the role of thoughts.

Neuroscientists distinguish between emotions (which they regard as primarily a physiological state characterized by identifiable bodily changes), and feelings (which they regard as an internal subjective state, such joy or sadness). Many of the same physiological states, such as increased heart rate, can be associated with widely different feelings. Your body may react to winning the lotto in the same way it does to a home invasion, however the associated feelings are extremely different. It is the emotional limbic system, in conjunction with the thinking cortex, that takes in all the cues relating to the particular circumstance, reviews past messages learnt about such circumstances, and then constructs the feeling state which is appropriate to the situation, e.g. fear or exhilaration.

How the body instinctively reacts to a situation is extremely important in this process. This is determined largely by the actions of the brainstem that are constantly scanning the environment for danger. The mind/brain takes this information from the limbic system/brainstem and combines it with past learning experiences as well as cues in the situation to arrive at a particular feeling. As such, the eventual subjective feeling is constructed by the combined efforts of the body, the thinking cortex and the emotional limbic system/brainstem. The sequence of arriving at an awareness of a feeling state is as follows: a physiological reaction in the body to danger cues in the environment → "I think I should feel scared" → "Yes! I seem to be feeling something" → "It must be fear." As you can see, it is a bit more complicated than thoughts causing feelings. However, in making sense of the situation itself, and reviewing messages learnt from similar situations, the thinking brain does have a role to play.

As such, it is important to look at distressed feelings as well as the types of thoughts that are more likely to be associated with them. Such distressed thoughts/feelings are more examples of psychological "packages" that have an unacceptable quality to them, and which the mind/brain is likely to try and protect us from via the creation of chronic pain.

Psychologist Jeffrey Young has identified four main types of belief systems, or what he refers to as schemata, which are related to emotional distress.[4] This is a way of formalizing and grouping the types of negative emotional patterns, described previously, usually developed during childhood. These belief systems contain thinking and emotional styles typical of people in psychological distress. They are:

1. *Disconnection and rejection,* wherein the person doubts that their needs for safety and security, as well as respect and acceptance

---

[4] Young (1999). *Cognitive Therapy for Personality Disorders.*

are able to be met. They have underlying beliefs in their own unworthiness and/or lack of confidence in the world at large.

2. *Impaired autonomy and performance,* in which the person doubts their ability to function successfully or independently in the world.

3. *Other directedness,* when the person is overly focused on the needs and desires of others, and under-focused on their own needs and desires.

4. *Over-vigilance and inhibition,* wherein the person's approach to life entails an extreme amount of worry about things going wrong, and suppressing their own impulses and needs. People with this as a dominant schema tend to live their lives according to rigid rules and expectations, which they apply to themselves and all others, with predictable deleterious effects on their well-being, health and happiness.

Most of life's negative emotional experiences can be interpreted in relation to these schemata. There is an obvious relationship between insecure attachment styles and subsequent distress-schemata as adults—the less favourable attachment styles have "trained" the child in these thinking styles. Like many other psychological patterns, we are rarely aware of any of them until they are pointed out. As a result, with each new negative experience, the schema's strength can be constantly added to over the years of life until they have an all-encompassing nature. It is easy to see how the negative conclusions that children can arrive at about themselves from bad experiences are related to the schemas described above.

These belief systems are a useful way of categorizing the types of self-limiting beliefs that are likely to give rise to chronic pain via ischemia. With such beliefs often comes the need to keep them at a relatively unconscious level, as it would be extremely disturbing to have a conscious awareness of them.

In regards to our adult experiences of life, even if not highly traumatic, relationships are often not as rewarding as we want them to be. A rejection schema may be triggered by this reality. Most children will disappoint us in some way, even if simply by growing up and moving away from us in a successful manner—we may view this as evidence of our unworthiness that the kids no longer want to be with us. Many jobs can be unfulfilling in various ways. This may trigger our impaired autonomy and performance schema, as it can be seen as evidence of our inability to function well in the world. Many people are disappointed with life and how things have turned out for them, even if just by virtue of aging and losing good looks or valued physical capacities and attributes. This may reflect a focus on what use we can be to others, rather than focusing on our own needs, and can therefore reflect an other-directedness schema.

Our mind/brain will often employ a range of defense mechanisms to prevent us becoming fully aware of these schemata, and chronic pain is an excellent option as it will compel our conscious attention.

The hidden side of success

Chronic pain can also be triggered by *positive* success experiences in our lives, and this can be extremely puzzling. On a conscious level, we may be pleased with ourselves or with a particular outcome; however, at a deeper unconscious level something quite different may be happening.

Anna, a young woman who consulted with me over her low-back pain, revealed that she had been in pain since the day she was married three years earlier. She reported that she and her boyfriend had lived together for several years before deciding to get married—they had what she considered a perfect relationship. "The first day I experienced extreme back pain was on the day of my wedding. I thought it must have had something to do with wearing high-heeled shoes all day, as I usually avoid them. But I became really worried when the pain just kept on happening to me throughout the entire honeymoon."

Her pain was so intense that she spent most of their exotic-location honeymoon in bed, barely able to move, despite wearing no high-heeled shoes beyond her wedding day. Due to the pain she had to take two months off work on her return (an office job that entailed no heavy lifting), and since returning to work, it was in a part-time capacity only.

Anna reported that she loved her husband both before and since their marriage, and that there were no apparent problems in their relationship apart from the limitations which her pain placed on both of them, and these did entail significant stressors. But if The Hidden Psychology of Pain is relevant to this case, what unconscious emotions could have triggered her pain on the day of her marriage? Anna had experienced no traumas in her childhood or adolescence, and had never been abused or troubled by negative events before the onset of chronic pain.

Everyone has heard stories of the "perfect" couple who got along beautifully until they ruined it all by getting married. Even though rare, the notion of this happening is part of our cultural psyche—call it "Murphy's Law of Relationships." At a level deeper than her conscious awareness, Anna was terrified of this happening to her—her perfect relationship being destroyed by getting married. This fear was internally generated and not triggered by any negative event between Anna and her partner.

When this possibility surfaced through our conversation, Anna was somewhat relieved. This fear, which had lurked deep within her, had intensified on the day of her wedding as the "gas" got turned up. What would have happened had this thought and the associated fear erupted into her awareness on the day she was to marry? Would she have had cold feet and pulled out? How could she do that to the perfect man with whom she had the perfect relationship? Rather than have to confront these feelings in her awareness, the protective part of Anna's mind/brain chose to prevent conscious knowledge of them, and instead created intense back pain for her to focus on. In the weeks that followed, she was not wondering if the marriage had been a mistake. Her awareness was now monopolized by the pain she was experiencing and the associated unhappiness that ensued. And that was its purpose—to ensure that she did not indulge in this emotionally painful question and the associated fear.

Daniel was a similar case, although in very different circumstances. His intense knee pain commenced at the time when he obtained his dream job as a teacher at a prominent school. Rather than follow the normal academic path to becoming a teacher, he had decided to remain at university and continue studying after the basic four-year training. He obtained a Doctorate in Education after many years of additional hard work. On the strength of this higher qualification, he landed what was for him the dream job. In the same week, his knee became painful to such an extent that he could barely walk. Surely getting the dream job was such a positive experience that it would be a big stretch to associate this with his pain?

The flip side of the positive always needs to be considered. What if, after so many years of additional study, the dream job turned out to not be so good? Or what if he turned out to be a lousy teacher? As with Anna, the stakes were extremely high, and the fear of failure was lurking at a deeper-than-conscious level.

Classical conditioning

An additional component of chronic pain can be classically conditioned physiological responses. As with all the other factors discussed in this chapter, we are rarely, if ever, aware of having been classically conditioned by either our experiences or our environment. The reality of classical conditioning is usually unconscious.

Although not suffering from pain, Jerome suffered from chronic rhinitis: year-round hay fever. He'd been almost constantly sneezing for around ten years, and until learning about the role of psychology, had never suspected the unconscious factors underlying it. He reported that the sneezing had begun when he and his new wife and infant son went away for a summer holiday. As their dog spent time in the house, fleas had spread to the extent that they decided to set off a flea-bomb. Upon returning to their home a couple of weeks later, fleas were no longer biting but Jerome began sneezing profusely. Immediately, he concluded that it must be related to the toxins from the flea insecticide.

As the weeks turned into months, the sneezing didn't stop and instead got worse. He reached a point where it was not unusual to have fits of up to 50 sneezes at a time up to five or six times a day. The associated post-nasal drip meant that he could barely talk during the day, which was a problem as his work involved considerable talking with customers. By the end of the day, he was exhausted and his voice was hoarse from the strain of so much sneezing.

Jerome consulted with a GP who prescribed antibiotics. Knowing that he did not have an upper respiratory infection he chose not to use the script, but instead sought help from a naturopath as a second option. The naturopath's view was that he was suffering from a range of food allergies, in particular to wheat, sugar and dairy. As a result Jerome did the best he could to avoid bread and other wheat products, began drinking soy milk and eliminated most foods with sugars. Yet the sneezing continued unabated for many years. He ended up on such a restricted diet that just eating enough was becoming more and more challenging. The list of acceptable foods diminished, but unfortunately his symptoms did not.

After around ten years of this torment, Jerome came across The Hidden Psychology of Pain (or sneezing, in his case) which detailed the range of non-pain symptoms that the mind/brain could inflict on a person. Looking back to what was happening when the sneezing started, he could see that he was newly married, had a new baby and his wife was pregnant with their second. He maintained that he had always loved his wife and baby. However, it is plausible that at a more unconscious level, he was actually reeling from the rapid increase of responsibility that he had accrued to him so suddenly. Only a couple of years earlier, he was a young man in his mid-twenties with very few responsibilities or cares in the world. Now, he was entirely loaded up with responsibilities—life had become a serious business all of a sudden. He confessed to having been quite immature when he became a husband, and then a father shortly afterwards.

On a conscious level, Jerome was confident in his ability to cope, and deliberately maintained a positive outlook. This was difficult, as he and his wife argued and fought quite a lot in their first few years of marriage. However, he was as optimistic and as resilient as he could manage. If asked at the time, he would never have admitted to himself, much less to anyone else, that lurking deep within was a part of him that wanted out. Rather than become aware of this aspect of himself, as it was clearly "unacceptable" by every standard he held, Jerome's mind/brain gave him the symptom of sneezing. He sneezed all day and much of each night. As the years rolled on, he continued sneezing despite having finally matured into the role of being a husband and father.

Ten years later, he began to see that the unacceptable emotions were more responsible for the symptoms than were either the flea bomb or wheat, sugar or dairy foods. He could see that the sneezing had effectively monopolized his conscious attention for around a decade as he had become quite obsessed with the symptoms and offending foods. It had worked beautifully to keep him from thinking about the deeper problems in his life. After becoming aware of unacceptable emotions, the problem was that his sneezing did not quickly dissipate. He had learned that the symptoms could be kept alive, no longer by the original cause but by virtue of classical conditioning. Research in the field of psychoneuroimmunology (a field of science looking at the connection between psychology, neurology and immunology) demonstrates that the immune response, like many other bodily responses, can also be trained to respond in a certain way via a classical conditioning process.[5]

If you learn to associate particular stimuli (such as sugar) with a particular immune response (such as sneezing), then the stimuli on its own can eventually elicit the same immune response just by virtue of having learnt the association, whether it is a 'real' association or not. This is referred to as a classically conditioned response. As an example, people who sneeze in response to flower pollen can be triggered to have a sneezing fit on the presentation of life-like plastic flowers which obviously have no pollen at all. It is even reported that some people can also sneeze just on the presentation of *photos* of the offending flowers.

Jerome came to the conclusion that with the help of the naturopath's suggestions of food allergies, he had learned to associate wheat, sugar and dairy with sneezing, whereas, in fact, there may have been little physical basis to this belief. In the absence of knowing that the sneezing was keeping him from becoming aware of his deeper anguish, the naturopath's advice seemed plausible. Taking this information on board over time, he classically conditioned himself to sneeze whenever he slipped up and consumed some of the forbidden foods (finding that it was quite difficult to totally eliminate all these food types).

In the end, there was not a lot of difference between what he was doing, and what had happened to Pavlov's dogs that were salivating just because a

---

[5] Classical conditioning is a process of learning first articulated by Russian physiologist, Ivan Pavlov. He managed to teach dogs to salivate upon the presentation of certain forms of stimuli that would not inherently cause salivation. If he paired these two things together often enough, the dogs would end up salivating simply when a bell was rung, even in the absence of any food.

bell went off when food was presented. This conditioned response remained for years after the emotional causes of his symptoms had resolved.

The process of recovery for Jerome was to embark on a journey of inquiry as to what role the symptoms had played for him. He learned about the relevance of the mind/body syndrome, even though the biological pathways involved in causing the chronic rhinitis are not the same pathways involved in causing back pain, i.e. no ischemia is involved. Rather, his histamine response had been stimulated into over-reacting.

The next step was to slowly re-condition himself over a period of time by gradually increasing his exposure to the offending foods. In order to do this he needed to become conscious of the classical conditioning which had occurred over many years, and to counter-condition himself. In a sense, he needed to become aware of the conditioning factors of which he had been unaware for the previous ten or so years, and a big part of this process was the very *belief* that certain food types would cause the sneezing.

Even though he continued to sneeze upon consuming the forbidden foods he worked hard at breaking the connection in his mind/brain between the foods and the symptoms. Much of this entailed repeatedly reminding himself that he was sneezing because of a classically conditioned response, and that there was no essential reason for these foods to produce these responses.

As with most human ailments, it is likely that Jerome's symptoms were caused by a combination of both psychological *and* physical factors. Just because we are introducing an awareness of psychology does not mean that we can ignore physiology. If there is a role for food intolerances in such cases, it can be thought of as similar to the role of physical factors in stomach ulcers. The helicobacter virus is a necessary pre-condition for stomach ulcers, but without psychological stress, it is not sufficient in it's own right to produce symptoms.

A genuine physical basis, such as a virus, food intolerance or a gut disorder, may play a role in the *beginning* of the process. The mind/brain is aware of the intolerance and can build a full syndrome, such as chronic rhinitis, around the initial physical condition in the same way that the mind/brain can create a chronic pain syndrome around an acute injury. In a way, the mind/brain is doing this in an opportunistic fashion, exploiting the physical basis to the complaint for a psychological purpose, and in the process making it more extreme and protracted, i.e. chronic.

The initial physical basis for the complaint may play only a relatively small role in the overall syndrome that eventually develops. The chronic pain, or the chronic rhinitis, is a much larger problem than the original physical issue, and represents a high degree of psychological overlay which has developed on top of the initial symptoms. In this case, it is the intensity of the symptoms that serves the psychological purpose, and the initial physical basis has become a relatively minor contributor to the overall syndrome which eventuates. With conditions that are often referred to as food allergies, the initial food intolerance has been added to by a classical conditioning process which ensures that more serious symptoms ensue until a full syndrome is experienced.

Another possible physical basis to Jerome's rhinitis could have been an allergic reaction to dust mites. Although this may be considered a purely physiological reaction, it is also worth noting that not all people respond to dust mites in the environment in the same way, or to the same degree. In these individual differences, it is somewhat like the differing responses people have to various pollens. Most of the allergens which people have a reaction to should actually be tolerable to our immune systems. It is the nature and the intensity of the response of the immune system that creates the associated symptoms of sinus congestion and inflammation, watery eyes, and sneezing.

There is a similarity here with the observation that structural pathology of the spine is normal in the pain-free population. Most people who do *not* suffer chronic rhinitis also have dust mites in their environment. Why the highly differing responses? It may be psychological issues which take a reaction to dust mites from a mild response to an extreme and ongoing chronic rhinitis. The fact that Jerome's sneezing ultimately stopped as a result of his learning of its hidden psychology would suggest that suppressed emotions and classical conditioning were important factors in his symptoms. Perhaps, he would also have benefited from eliminating dust mites.

After several months, Jeremy succeeded in reconditioning his response and the sneezing greatly diminished to the point where he only sneezed at times when he was under unusually high levels of emotional pressure, or when it was appropriate to sneeze in order to clear his sinuses of aggravating matter. He considered this to be a vast improvement over sneezing all day, every day. He was still exposed to dust mites, but the sneezing lost its intensity.

Classical conditioning can play a similar role in many seemingly inexplicable symptoms, including chronic pain. Luke, a plumber I treated, had to cease working due to his back pain, but oddly he could continue surfing. For some reason, he had not learned to associate surfing with being in pain despite a strain to his back muscles. He had, however, learned to associate leaning forward while cleaning his teeth with being in pain. As such, he would experience intense pain every time he came to clean his teeth, but not when surfing. As with all of my clients presented here, Luke was not making up the symptoms.

Many sufferers of RSI believed that a particular physical action at work, or a piece of equipment would result in pain.[6] As such, they had classically conditioned themselves into experiencing pain with actions or equipment that had not resulted in pain for many years prior to the epidemic. The pain was real, but as with Jerome, the belief about what caused the condition was misleading or simply false. The belief can end up having the power to generate the symptoms if it suits the mind/brain's desire to obscure emotional difficulties at an unconscious level.

The "why there?" of pain

What determines whether a person's mind/brain chooses to locate pain in the back, neck or shoulder; or decides upon other chronic health symptoms such as asthma, hay fever, or skin rashes; or even goes to the extreme of creating paralysis in parts of the body? Unconscious factors also play a role in determining the nature and location of symptoms.

As described earlier with Martin, the musician who experienced intense pain in his shoulders and arms that prevented him from performing, symptoms can sometimes have an inherent logic to their location. His shoulders and arms were the obvious place to locate a pain in order to help

---

[6] Lucire (2003). *Constructing RSI: Belief and Desire.*

him avoid playing his instrument, and thereby prevent him from having to confront the feelings of inadequacy that he carried within himself.

Similarly, Sarah suffered from extreme pain in both her hands and wrists, which was put down to carpal tunnel syndrome. The pain was so intense that she was advised to have surgery on both wrists. She had already gone under the knife on one wrist when we met, but was reluctant to have surgery on the other due to the poor outcome. The first time I saw Sarah, she was in extreme pain, had a high level of disability, had been forced to quit her job, was highly medicated, and had both wrists in supportive braces. Within a few weeks of meeting, it came out in our discussion that a few years earlier, Sarah had spent hours with her mother practicing for a job interview which she had the next day. In particular, she was nervous about her hand-shaking technique, so spent the night practicing handshakes with her mother until she got it right.

Sadly, her mother died unexpectedly the next day. Sarah's symptoms did not arise until around two years later, when the shock of her mother's death had begun to wear off. At this point, an extreme grief threatened to overwhelm Sarah, and it appears that her mind/brain chose to locate pain in her hands and wrists rather than have her emotionally collapse. The "penny dropped" for Sarah when we realized the connection between plenty of hand-shaking the night before her mother's death and the location of her symptoms. The pain, which she had been told would be with her for life and could perhaps at best only be controlled with surgery, subsequently went away.

At the time of the hand/wrist pain arising, Sarah was doing hard physical work that entailed lifting heavy loads with her hands. The logical culprit was the work demands, and the possibility of the physical pain being related to emotional pain was way below the radar until we discussed this several years after the pain began.

In other cases, the location of the pain may seem less logical. Why had Daniel's mind/brain chosen to locate pain in his knee when he landed his dream teaching job? He had not injured it in any serious manner and the treating physiotherapist told me that there was no degree of damage that could possibly explain the extent of pain he was in. Although very painful, his sore knee was not going to stop him working as a teacher, nor was there any logical connection between knee pain and other aspects of his life.

However, on further investigation, Daniel revealed that his grandfather had sustained a serious injury in the same knee as a combatant during World War II. It appears that his mind/brain chose to locate the pain in his knee as this location would succeed in monopolizing his attention. He had grown up knowing the physical difficulties his grandfather had with his knee.

Part of Daniel's pain pattern was disgust with himself for experiencing the same level of disability without having had a serious injury. As such, the pain could not fail to monopolize his attention. He was appalled with himself for having the same pain as his grandfather but without having the brave war service or the injury. The resulting pain ensured that he didn't consciously question whether the dream job was actually worth it after all those years of additional study. He was so focused on the physicality of the pain, as well as his self-loathing for having the pain at all, that the fear of failing in his job never consciously arose.

A key factor in the location of pain or type of symptom is the extent to which the person is unlikely to recognize it as being emotionally induced. The fact that Sarah's work involved heavy and repeated lifting with her hands made her physical workload the obvious "cause." If it was obvious that the pain was stemming from emotional causes, then it would not be serving its purpose as a distractor. Anna's back pain followed her wedding in high heeled shoes. She had never worn them regularly before as she was aware that they were bad for her body. Jeremy was dubious about the safety of setting off a flea-bomb in his house, but he needed to do something to eliminate the fleas. The fears regarding high heeled shoes and toxic chemicals were pre-disposing factors which allowed these people's minds to seek relevant symptoms, and explain them in relation to their posed dangers. With these fears already in place, a sensible location for symptoms was already available—only the distressing emotional issue was needed to produce the chronic pain or health problem.

It is also not unusual for sufferers to have pain at the site of an old injury. The mind/brain knows that you probably won't associate the pain with emotional tension if it occurs in a place that has been injured. The injury will be blamed, even if it was only a minor injury that occurred years earlier.

My left foot was somewhat crushed, although probably not broken, in the car accident which snapped my leg bones as an eighteen year old. Around twelve years later I developed an intense pain in the foot for the first time since my recovery. As this was prior to my knowledge of the Hidden Psychology of Pain, I immediately "knew" that it related to the injury I had sustained in the car accident. The pain increased to such a level that on some days I couldn't walk without a limp. Within a few weeks, I had the foot X-rayed, although there had been no recent injury. The results showed no damage whatsoever and the pain promptly disappeared. Years later I played seven seasons of Australian Rules Football which involves plenty of running and ball kicking with both feet. Despite this, I never experienced the foot pain ever again.

The foot X-ray had blown the smokescreen of the pain, and once I learned there really was nothing wrong with my foot, my mind/brain had to find yet another place to locate pain as the foot pain wouldn't work anymore. In hindsight, I can see that the pain was helping me avoid the emotional impact of having moved my young family two thousand kilometers away from our home city on a risky "tree-change" adventure to live in the bush. At the time, I was aware of the challenges of this huge lifestyle change, but on a conscious level, I was focused on making the change work by being as positive as possible. At a deeper level, fears and anxieties were bubbling away, hence the need for the foot pain as a distraction.

We are constantly looking for reasons for our pain and our mind/brain, supported by the prevailing culture prefers us to look for reasons that are purely physical. If our mind/brain were to locate pain in a part of our anatomy that had never been injured, we would be more unimpressed with the pain and therefore more likely to simply ignore it, or suspect that it was psychogenic. The pain would go the same way as my foot pain after I knew the X-ray results. But this is not what the mind/brain wants. Rather, the mind/brain's goal is *not* to have us ignore the pain, so it will be in places where we are more likely to accept the logic of its location.

In addition, chronic pain can be located in a part of our anatomy which has just undergone a genuine acute injury. Our mind/brain is aware of every aspect of our biological functioning at all times, including sites of meniscus tears in knee joints or of the rotator cuffs in shoulders, or of herniated discs. At the time of injury, these structural abnormalities may be either severe and thereby cause acute pain, or they may be minor and subsequently cause either no or minimal pain. Regardless of the amount of pain necessitated by the injury, if our mind/brain is looking for a place to locate a distracting physical pain it is likely to locate it at a place of either an old or current injury. This structural pathology may then show up in an X-ray or scan and be blamed for the ongoing pain. As time proceeds from the point of injury to three months and over, in most cases this explanation for the pain becomes more and more inadequate.

Often, people with chronic pain will find it shifting from one of the conditions described earlier to another, since each performs the same function of distracting the person's from their emotions. When the "jig is up" and the person is suspecting the true cause of their pain, the mind/brain will often desperately try a different pain or another symptom in order to maintain their focus on the physicality of their experience. This can lead to a confusing array of seemingly unrelated symptoms with many different specialists each addressing their own area of expertise, but not seeing the unified cause underlying each of them.

Most health professionals will unwittingly reinforce the notion that chronic pain is arising as a result of injuries incurred years earlier. With this endorsement, the strategy which the mind/brain has created is strengthened, as we will usually take such opinions at face value. In this way, many genuinely caring professionals can further entrench the entire pain pattern without being aware of what they are doing. As stated earlier, this is a problem in our cultural understanding of the human organism, and such health professionals are merely treating us according to these cultural understandings.

Simon was a successful young computer programmer, having landed the perfect job for a recent university IT graduate. Living primarily for the enjoyment of computers, he loved his work until problems began to emerge with RSI symptoms in his wrists. Medical and physiotherapy advice suggested that he was overusing his arms in computer work and therefore suggested the need to take breaks from keying in order to rest his "inflamed" tendons. The prevailing cultural "knowledge" of what causes RSI (i.e. overuse) was lurking in Simon's mind. This was given a great boost by health professionals endorsing the view with an RSI diagnosis and relating it to overuse of computers.

Naturally, the development of this pain was a huge cause of concern for Simon. He began to feel threatened by the pain and worried about what it could mean for his work if it continued. Unfortunately, despite ergonomic changes in his work-station and taking more regular breaks (more reinforcement of the supposed physical causes), his pain simply got worse. As a result, he had to drop down to part-time hours, which resulted in excessive worry as well as financial hardship. The additional rest, which part-time hours allowed, did not reduce his pain, but rather, it continued to escalate.

Within a matter of months, he had to resign from his much loved job altogether as he was unable to use a keyboard. At least he still had his recreational computer use at home to fall back on as his only source of joy. Of course, his ability to engage in the recreational computer use was also highly restricted and before too long he was unable to use his hands for even this purpose. Now, not just his wrists hurt but his entire arms, shoulders, neck and upper back had also become extremely sore.

In desperation, Simon began using his *feet* to do the keying so that he could maintain some recreational computer use. But within a couple of weeks, the "RSI" had spread to his legs and feet and he was unable to continue with this adaptive strategy. His next option was to obtain a voice-activated program for his computer. This worked for a week or two until he began to experience *laryngitis* for the first time in his life. Like his wrists, arms, back, neck, shoulders, legs and feet, his voice also "gave out." Now he was unable to use his computer in any way.

The diagnosis given to him was fibromyalgia, a catch-all term for a syndrome of body wide intense aches and pains. There is no medical understanding of such conditions as fibromyalgia, and it is viewed largely as a medical mystery when considered without an awareness of unconscious psychological factors.

It was at the time when his larynx had failed him that I first met Simon. He presented as highly distressed, depressed, and anxious with a waxy quality to his skin. Despite being only in his early 20s, he seemed a young man well and truly "beaten" by life. The healing process for him began with an exploration of his background experiences. Simon did not have highly traumatic events in his earlier years. He was, however, a classic computer enthusiast. Throughout his teenage years, he was relatively shy and quiet, studious and serious—he was an intelligent and sensitive young man, viewed by many of his peers as a computer "geek." Most of his high school friends seemed to be the opposite. They were confident and outgoing, loud and boisterous, and did not put great value on academic skills. As a consequence, Simon felt grossly inadequate because he was simply different to the group. This was the emotional burden he was carrying, despite having succeeded in his chosen field. As a young man, he also wanted involvement with girls but his sense of personal inadequacy largely precluded this throughout all of his high school years, and now into his early adulthood as well.

Like other clients presented in this book, Simon was open to The Hidden Psychology of Pain and could see how his emotional/social difficulties had led to his pain symptoms. Over several weeks, during which time he was working with the ideas presented in this book, Simon gradually improved to the point where he was able to start swimming. Six months after I last saw him, I received an email from Simon stating that he now had a girlfriend, had resumed some part-time computer work, and was about to take his first sky-diving jump. Had I not seen this type of improvement on a regular basis, I would have questioned whether this could possibly be the same sickly looking young man I had first seen only six months earlier.

His case demonstrated the ability of chronic pain to "travel" between different bodily locations in the form of various pains, and also to jump to a seemingly unrelated symptom—in his case, laryngitis. Such movement between different types of mind/body symptoms is common. If a treating practitioner were to focus just on the supposed pathophysiology of each symptom they would be perplexed. If they took the structural pathology seriously, they would have to conclude that this poor young man was afflicted by a huge array of abnormalities, each of which would have required individual treatment by various specialists, and limited chance of healing would have emerged.

Cultural influences

Being the sea we swim in, our social environment or culture is yet another contributing factor to chronic pain of which we are largely unaware, in the same way that a fish is unaware that it spends its life in water. Many of the smaller hurts and disappointments which we pick up through our infancy and childhood will seem irrational or unreasonable to the conscious mind. We will often not be willing to own up to them, even to ourselves.

Simon found it difficult to admit that he had spent his adolescence feeling inadequate until I raised this possibility with him.

For most of us, the emotional pains don't end with the completion of adolescence. It is this "unacceptable" quality of the thoughts and feelings that causes the inner tension. The intense anger or rage that dwells deep within you may be quite disruptive to your sense of who you are, were you to become aware of it. Or even feeling very sorry for oneself may be considered unacceptable within a culture which is busily promoting a "can-do" and optimistic attitude towards life.

In getting a sense of what difficult emotions are likely to be "driven underground" in any particular culture, it is worth considering the virtues which are highly valued. Where some nationalities may emphasize exactness and precision, it makes sense that inner tendencies which violate those virtues will be less "owned" by its members, and will therefore be somewhat unconscious. We will have problems accepting those parts of ourselves that feel like failures if we live in a culture that only values success. Where some cultures are inherently more blunt and straightforward, then perhaps its people have less trouble in accepting their inner anger or rage, but will struggle with other disowned feelings such as vulnerability. As such, the hidden parts of ourselves which may be causing problems at an unconscious level are often an inverse reflection of what qualities are highly valued in a society. This varies from culture to culture, and from family to family.

John Sarno emphasizes the role which unconscious rage can play in causing such pain. Amongst other qualities, mainstream American culture seems to promote a certain "niceness" in social relations. While other countries may have learned to copy it, only America came up with the farewell of "Have a nice day." In Australia, we are more naturally inclined to wish people a *"good"* day, which may or may not be nice. To the extent that a culture creates a sugar-coating, then its inhabitants may be seething with an unexpressed rage below the surface, as anger is viewed as unacceptable.

Where cultures do not foster such a focus on niceness then unacceptable emotions other than rage may be more troublesome. For example, where liberty is the prevailing American ethos, the main Australian cultural ethos is egalitarianism. Australians who excel run the risk of being cut down by their peers as "tall poppies". As we are meant to be equal in all things, their success can undermine the ethic of equality. With a cultural bias working against individual success, feelings of unworthiness may be at least as prominent in Australian's unconscious as are feelings of rage—it is almost a cultural obligation to not get too big for your boots. The Australian "tall poppy syndrome" indicates a widespread cultural tendency towards a lack of sense of worth, such that anyone defying this is at risk of being resented and "cut down to size".

As countries like Australia, New Zealand, Britain, Ireland, South Africa, Canada and America are now so multicultural, it is more likely that in any of these countries, a wide range of cultural influences are operating. Variations of these cultural themes are therefore likely to be widespread and less confined to national borders.

Many of us would like to think of ourselves as good husbands or wives, a good son or daughter, a good mother or father, intelligent, successful, independent, strong, likeable, attractive, invincible, immortal, patient, loyal, loving, etc. But at the same time, we have all had experiences of unpleasant and distressing emotions such as fear, anger, guilt, anxiety, shame, sexual conflicts, and identity problems. We will all fail at times in trying to measure up to these high ideals.

As most of our life experiences aren't that intense, our mind/brain will usually succeed in keeping many of these distressing emotions at an unconscious level. The larger the threat to our self-concept is, the larger the need to keep these feelings suppressed. People who suffer from psychogenic pain often have a lot of the internal tension created by certain personality characteristics such as perfectionism, "goodism," the need to always please others, and being highly self-critical (as seen in Young's schemata). This creates enormous problems when we fail to live up to the unrealistically high standards which our culture sets for us, and which we internalize.

On the one hand, we have such high standards; and on the other hand we have experiences and feelings which are not in accord with these standards. For example, we may have internalized the notion that we should always feel love for our children or parents, but when conflicts arise, feelings other than these can emerge. Such feelings of dislike, disapproval or resentment may clash with our self-concept if it includes us always loving and respecting those who are closest. Internally generated and severe challenges to our self-concept can create the type of inner tension which a part of our mind/brain feels the need to keep from our conscious awareness.

What happens to stress that we don't express? When an alarm response is activated by a negative event, if we act on the feelings that arise, we will be propelled to some kind of action. When we are unable to run or fight because it is considered socially unacceptable, then we are left with more dilemmas. Our body has prepared us to escape from or to fight our boss or a police officer, but instead we may need to bury those feelings deep within ourselves.

Internalizing those feelings allows us to inhibit the outward signs of arousal and pretend that all is normal. Without the running away or fighting that our body is prepared for, we don't get the opportunity to expend the energy and reach a point of resolution when our heart rate can return to normal. Robert Sapolsky observes that when animals of prey have survived an attack from a predator, they will gently shake and quiver for a time before resuming their normal grazing in an undisturbed state. This shaking is allowing the release of stress hormones and prevents the animal from becoming overly traumatized or unwell because of the stress. Although there are some trauma therapies focused on it, we humans don't tend to actively embrace shaking when something stressful has happened to us. The inner stress remains internal and simply mounts with each new experience. As it has been driven deep within the psyche, it becomes one of the many types of unconscious emotions which our mind/brain may try to prevent from coming into full consciousness.

Why is it that non-Western cultures seem to be largely exempt from the current epidemic of chronic pain that is crippling so many in the West? This is despite the fact that in most of these countries people are regularly engaging in heavy-lifting (from a very young age onwards) with little or no awareness of the "right" way to lift or any other Occupational Health &Safety principles, and people continue exerting their bodies well into old age.

Could it be that they have no notion of the human organism being a complex "machine"? That they are more willing to experience their emotions than try to suppress them, as is the cultural ideal in the West? That they have well integrated communities and extended families with abundant family and community support? And that they have few helpful professionals constantly telling them how weak and vulnerable their spines are, with warnings against injury? I fear what will happen to non-Western cultures to the extent that they embrace our ways of being.

The cultural harm from "helpful" health professionals reached a ridiculous level for me several years ago when I heard a chiropractor on the radio news warning people against the damage that can accrue to their spines by sitting with a wallet in their back pockets. As the RSI epidemic gained momentum during the 1980s, new causal theories for RSI had to be found as many afflicted workers had none of the repetition or strain which keyboard work supposedly entailed.[7]

We are surrounded by health and OH&S warnings, all suggesting that the spine is a very fragile and easily damaged part of our body. While spines certainly can be injured, this does not happen easily. Our spine is our core body strength, and beyond the normal level of structural pathology (usually referred to as 'degenerative changes' that occur with aging), most of us will never experience a serious spinal injury, almost regardless of what we put it through. Look at the high physical impact football codes as an example. It is very rare, even under those bone jarring circumstances, for a serious spinal injury to occur. It can and does happen occasionally, but if you consider the number of amateur and professional footballers playing these impact codes each weekend, such injuries are tragic but really quite unusual.

Chronic pain is a benign condition that can hurt intensely, however it will usually not lead to further degeneration of the spine or any other serious condition as there is usually no cellular damage associated with it. Muscles, nerves and tendons are likely to hurt, but this is rarely the result (nor an indicator) of damaged cells. No one has become literally crippled as a result of chronic pain, nor has anyone died from it. The most important implication of the information in this book is that for most people, chronic pain is reversible. People can and do get better. Full recovery is possible and is regularly seen by practitioners who work with these ideas.

In arguing the importance of the unconscious mind/brain, *The Hidden Psychology of Pain* is swimming against the tide of contemporary thought. However, it is the contemporary mindset which is a significant part of the problem. Viewing the human organism as a machine, focusing exclusively on the nuts and bolts of physical functioning or maintaining a focus only on

---

[7] Lucire (2003). *Constructing RSI: Belief and Desire.*

stressors that we are consciously aware of, are each exacerbating the modern epidemic of chronic pain by obscuring the real causes. For most people to get better, accurate information is the key.

Depth-psychology has given us the notion that emotional factors hidden in our unconscious mind/brain are usually responsible for persistent pain. This is a cultural gem which we need to reclaim if we are wanting to overcome chronic pain.

CHAPTER 8
Getting Better

IN ORDER TO HEAL FROM chronic pain, you need to address the root cause, and not get sidetracked by merely treating the symptoms.

The root cause of much chronic pain is a combination of both erroneous ideas about pain, and distressed emotion operating at a less-than-conscious level. It is not necessary to eliminate every stressful situation or upset emotion in your life, although it does make sense to address the situations that you can. It is more important to become *aware* of the deeply held emotional causes of the pain, and how these interact with misinformation to protect us in some way- this is the hidden purpose of chronic pain, and it can continue until "the jig is up", and you realize what psychological harm the pain is protecting you from.

A very important implication of The Hidden Psychology of Pain is that our bodies are resilient, and not as fragile as the pain industry has led us to believe. Sarno states,

> It is totally without logic to propose that after millions of years of evolution, during which time we have become the dominant species on this planet, our bodies have become structurally incompetent, or that we have become so fragile that we must be careful how we move, use our bodies, or engage in repetitive activities. This is unadulterated nonsense. We are not papier-mâché; we are tough and resilient, adaptable and quick to heal.[1]

---

[1] Sarno (1998 p.96). *The Mindbody Prescription.*

As a result of this new awareness, I returned to playing amateur Australian Rules Football at the age of thirty-eight. I had not played since I was seriously injured in the car accident twenty years earlier. For the intervening two decades, I bought the notion that my body remained damaged and vulnerable from the injuries I had sustained, and that I needed to be exceedingly careful due to its supposed fragility. This fear remained for twenty years in spite of the fact that my body completed the healing required around nineteen and half years earlier. The persistent groin pain reinforced the belief in my physical vulnerability, especially in a presumed weakness of my spine

While I never set the amateur football world on fire, I did manage to play seven highly enjoyable seasons, usually against opponents roughly half my age. In addition, midway into this less-than-stunning return to football, I fractured three vertebrae in my neck whilst surfing. My neck injury happened in early January, and by April I was playing football again after having missed just the first game of the season. On only one occasion, after landing heavily and bracing my neck to stop my head from hitting the hard ground, did my neck hurt as a result of playing football. As any of my former teammates would testify, I am no iron man, nor am I particularly tough. It sometimes hurt when I was being hit by a burly twenty-year-old, and after each game I usually had trouble walking for a few days due to muscle stiffness. But I learned that my body was indeed resilient, and not as fragile as I had been led to believe for my entire adulthood.

Football allowed me to test this new possibility, as fear was no longer dominating my life. Was I just lucky to achieve this outcome? The observation of the few psychologists, psychiatrists and medical practitioners using this and similar approaches suggest that far from being unusual, my experience was actually quite common and typical for people who have learned and internalized the correct information.

I often have clients asking me, "Well, if it is as simple as this, why have I never heard of this approach before? Why isn't everyone receiving this treatment?" Firstly, most of the illness cues in our society which relate to chronic pain very clearly favor physical explanations. The problem is that while these make sense for acute pain, they have little relevance for chronic pain.

The medical and physical professions are largely unable to make accurate diagnoses of emotional or psychological factors which result in chronic pain, simply due to a lack of understanding (and often a lack of willingness). Of course, this problem is much wider than the physical therapy professions as it relates to psychologists as well, not to mention the general population. Very few of us naturally make psychological sense of physical pain. Instead, we generally focus on our physical experience and resort to physical explanations that seem to make sense.

A popular notion in the pain industry is that we have become such a sedentary civilization that our bodies are simply not used to hard work. When we do hard work, they suggest, we suffer the painful damage due to a habitual lack of exertion. But, there has always been a "leisurely" class in society who never did hard physical work—most of these people did not experience chronic pain as a result of the occasions when they did exert themselves by such recreational activities as rugby, tennis or polo. There is no evidence that strong muscles prevent back pain, as demonstrated by extremely fit and strong professional athletes who also experience this type of pain.[2] In addition, many people who suffer chronic pain these days have simply not exerted themselves in any fashion that *could* have produced pain. Low back pain is as common over a lifetime amongst white collar workers as amongst blue collar workers.[3] Chronic pain also affects both men and women equally, despite differences in the amount of heavy lifting undertaken over their lifetimes, or on any particular day.

Sociologist Ivan Illich coined the term "iatragenic" to describe conditions which medicine appears to make worse rather than better. The term "social iatregenesis" refers to health policies which reinforce illness and dependency in the population. Within the social factors that can reinforce chronic pain are the cultural beliefs which emphasize the causal role of structural pathology at the expense of psychosocial factors. The large scale social iatragenesis relating to chronic pain results in massive health expenditure, including invasive and surgical procedures, usually to no avail.

Many people in our culture fear that without a physical diagnostic label, their experience of pain will not be viewed as legitimate, and instead, they will be viewed as either a malingerer, or worse, as crazy. Despite many attempts to "de-stigmatize" mental health problems, such a stigma is still

---

[2]   Ibid.
[3]   Ibid.

well established in our culture. People who are viewed as mentally unwell are just not viewed in the same way as a person with a broken leg, despite regular urgings that they should be. Going crazy, or even being seen as crazy, is one of the biggest personal fears which people have in our society. This will remain the case as long as what are essentially human problems in living are viewed from within a medical perspective as stigmatizing "illnesses," rather than from a social perspective.

Psychogenic theories of chronic pain are too readily misunderstood by both the medical and general populations alike. As such, it is little wonder that many people are reluctant to take these ideas on board. The fact that you are even reading this book and entertaining the possibilities suggested here indicates a level of courage which is above the norm. Many people are simply too frightened by such ideas, and will just react defensively to these suggestions. You will discover this when you tell others about *The Hidden Psychology of Pain*, even if you report the benefits which you experience.

Another reason why these ideas are not more widespread is that just because we can make sense of what is responsible for chronic pain does not mean that it is necessarily simple to either find the relevant emotions, or to eliminate the symptoms. Even though most people are able to reduce or eliminate their chronic pain with these strategies does not make it automatically easy. Generally, a serious process of enquiry needs to be embarked upon with much reflection on one's own experiences in life and the emotional consequences. Not everyone is equally willing or equipped to do this.

Sometimes, the assistance of a skilled psychotherapist (who may or may not be a psychologist, clinical social worker or a psychiatrist) will be necessary to help us become more aware of what is operating at a less than conscious level within us. The unconscious is willing to reveal its secrets, but this can require the work of a psychotherapist who is firstly aware of the need to go down this path, and secondly has the skills to make this feel safe. Our mind can employ a range of defense mechanisms to prevent this material from emerging into our conscious awareness if this feels in any way risky. As such, we can easily fool ourselves that either the deep emotional hurts aren't there (another unconscious defense mechanism); or that we have found the "right" hurts, when in fact we have merely settled for something less significant or threatening. A skilled psychotherapist, experienced in such matters and having a more objective perspective than what you can have of yourself, could help you in this journey of discovery. But for many people, this will not be necessary, as the power of information can effect a positive change in its own right.

Thinking psychologically

For most people, the main treatment needed in order to overcome chronic pain is information about its hidden psychology. During the time needed for healing, correct information about what is going on is essential so that you do not panic, and internalize a wrong association between structural abnormalities and the experience of chronic pain. Remember that hidden psychological factors may also make your oxygen deprived muscles more vulnerable to strains and tears. The muscle strain can also be viewed as a symptom of a larger problem, namely, the emotional factors which your mind/brain has created the pain as an attempted 'solution' to. The solution may be in the form of protection or a distraction from psychological wounds, related emotional themes and overall schemas, or other purposes which may become revealed through investigation. Chronic pain also may be a 'stance' which the mind/body takes, a statement of 'no', where the person is unable to verbalise such a position.

Urging people to "think psychologically" about their pain is not to say that physical considerations are unimportant or irrelevant. It does mean, however, having a *primary* focus on the psychological factors which may be involved, and a *secondary* focus on the biological pathways and physical consequences of the mind/brain's strategy. It does not mean ignoring the importance of biology or physiology. For the most part, the pain industry's primary focus is on the physical, with a secondary focus on the psychological, if at all.

In his illuminating book, *When the Body Says No*, Gabor Maté urges people to consider "the power of negative thinking." Rather than advocating that pain sufferers wallow in their misery, Maté is arguing for the healing potential of delving into the negative aspects of our lives. Although it has become something of a cultural anathema, having the courage to explore such negativity as hurt feelings, unhealthy relationships and damaging experiences is one of the keys to improving health. Whether we want to acknowledge the reality of the negative or not, it remains a reality in everyone's lives. As suggested in this book, if we choose to deny and suppress strong negative emotions, there is little chance of them actually going away. They tend to just go underground, deep into our unconscious, where they will manifest in one way or another. These repressed feelings may seep out in inappropriate responses which are out of proportion to a particular situation. Or they may manifest in extremely disturbing or violent dreams. They may also find expression in various health problems. And if the unconscious mind/brain is fearful of them bursting into our conscious awareness, they may trigger chronic pain.

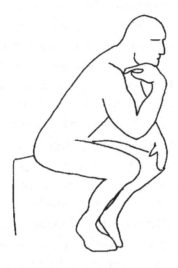

Thinking psychologically to overcome chronic pain

The other option to denial and repression is to allow for the reality of negative feelings, experiences, thoughts and perceptions. As stated in Chapter 6, studies in neuroscience confirm that allowing space for negativity is associated with decreased neural traffic between the pre-frontal cortex and the nucleus accumbens, and with less chronic pain. Richard Davidson suggests that if we are wanting to create space for a more negative outlook, a deliberate focus on negative aspects of life and possibilities is likely to result in less activity in the pre-frontal cortex and the nucleus accumbens, and weaken the connections between them. Research conducted by Baliki and colleagues demonstrates that less neural traffic between these two brain areas is associated with less chronic pain.

Is the suggestion here that we should be deliberately cultivating negativity in order to lessen the risk of chronic pain? No. The suggestion is that we would be well served by consciously *acknowledging* the negative aspects of our reality (not generating them), rather than attempting to force a cultivated positivity. Activities which deliberately cultivate positivity, such as writing down your positive traits, regularly expressing gratitude and complimenting others, are likely to improve your mood via strengthening the neural connections between your pre-frontal cortex and nucleus accumbens. And these neural changes are also more likely to make you vulnerable to chronic pain (as seen in the TMS-emotional pain see-saw diagram in Chapter 6).

Rather than leaping into defense mechanisms as default positions, we are able to explore the negative aspects of our experience further. Creating space for the negative raises certain constructive possibilities. We may be able to address unsatisfactory relationships; we may be able to confront our fears and anxieties; we may be able to look at and heal trauma from our past; we may be able to work out how to manage bad situations; we may be able to seek and gain emotional support in facing our challenges. All of these actions are the opposite to suppressing emotional distress, and relying on defense mechanisms such as denial to help us avoid having to do the needed psychological work. The very act of acknowledging the negative can be healing in itself, even if we choose to do nothing about them. Maté suggests that this focus on the negative is powerful, and the many clients who I have seen recover from pain when they overcome their denial would support this contention. The very act of allowing the negative, of no longer attempting to force positivity in the face of bad circumstances or a traumatic past, is likely to create the brain changes which Baliki and colleagues have demonstrated are related to a *decreased* risk of chronic pain.

Where this process of exploring the negative is simply too painful, a level of trauma may be evident. The less extreme end of the trauma spectrum may be successfully treated with self-help strategies as detailed later in this book. However, more severe traumas may very well require professional assistance.

The resolution of deeply unconscious conflicts is not necessary for most people to alleviate their pain. My client Max chose to do nothing about his experience of childhood sexual abuse. Had he chosen to, he would have been less vulnerable to such relapses as he experienced when his favorite aunt died. However, learning and accepting that his back pain was primarily due to his repressed emotions was sufficient to make a radical difference in his experience of pain. The same was true for all other case studies presented so far, and for countless other clients I have worked with over the years. Awareness of the psychosomatic process, knowledge that this condition is generally reversible, and a willingness to look into the negative is all that is required for most people to overcome chronic pain. However, it does require a consistent effort in processing these ideas and applying them to oneself.

The basic healing process begins with bringing sensible explanations and reason to the issue of chronic pain. This needs to be followed with a developing awareness and understanding of the underlying, largely unconscious causes, which will differ from person to person. The psychological wounds, associated emotions and schemas need to be brought into conscious awareness for lasting change to happen, as we can only change what we are aware of.

In understanding what is causing the pain, we are also entertaining some extremely important implications. These messages will themselves positively affect the layers of additional emotional distress which people have on top of their physical pain. When you have been medically cleared of other serious conditions, these implications include:

- Your back/neck/shoulders are more than likely normal, even *with* a structural pathology.

- The chronic pain is most likely not being caused by the structural pathologies anyway.

- Even though in pain, your back is likely to be strong, powerful and resilient.

- Pain does not mean serious damage (apart from damage associated with muscle strains, which tend to be minor.)

- You are most likely not in danger of becoming crippled or highly disabled unless you cause catastrophic injury to your spine. This will not happen through normal degenerative changes, or through a normal level of use and exertion, and rarely happens with even abnormal use of the spine.

- Psychogenic pain is reversible—it is a painful but essentially *harmless* condition.

- Many people have overcome pain similar to yours.

- Like many others, you can overcome this pain and find enjoyment in life again.

Even many years after coming across these ideas, when I experience a new pain, my immediate inclination is to think physically about it. This is a reasonable response, as it may very well be that something I have done has produced an acute pain. However, after eliminating this possibility, the next step to recovery is to leave the physical explanations behind and cultivate the ability to *think psychologically* about the pain.

The strategies presented in this book will help you achieve this re-training of your natural explanations away from what merely *feels* true. As my experience with a painful foot demonstrated, if no realistic physical cause of the pain can be established, this assessment itself will likely help you in overcoming the pain.

Although some will be supportive and in agreement, it is more common for physical therapists such as chiropractors, physiotherapists and medical doctors to reject many of the notions described in this book. There are often poor working relationships between the different professions involved, with little communication about such important concepts. Some physicians believe that they would be doing their patient a disservice, or could offend them if they were to suggest a psychological cause. However, there are some physicians who have an excellent grasp of these concepts and have incorporated them very well into their clinical practice, but these are a rarity. Even some "body-therapists" and other mind/body practitioners can be either hostile towards, or often simply ignorant of the Hidden Psychology of Pain, despite having a general sense that psychology somehow matters. Although these ideas evolved over several centuries, the message has somehow not yet filtered through to many health professionals.

The problem is not all with the physical therapists. Psychology is also part of the problem, in that most contemporary psychologists are still operating within a purely cognitive-behavioral paradigm, and as such are also generally ignorant of the real connections between depth-psychology and chronic pain. And if they were to expose themselves to these ideas, many psychologists would find them so outside of their preferred model that only a minority may actually seriously consider taking them on board. As such, this is a broad cultural problem that afflicts most of the relevant professions, and it keeps reinforcing the phenomenon of chronic pain.

The Hidden Psychology of Pain can mistakenly be viewed as advocating an "alternative medicine." Sarno's view is that his approach, in assessing psychological causes to chronic pain, is simply *good* diagnostics rather than alternative or complimentary medicine. There is nothing alternative about assessing the actual causes of people's suffering, and thereby avoiding incorrect diagnoses. Where competing explanations have been eliminated through medical assessment, then the diagnosis is largely a psychological enterprise. Even though the mind/body syndrome is a physical condition, it is one that has a psychological cause. Appropriately aware psychologists and psychologically minded physical practitioners are quite able to undertake this assessment. Physical therapists who are aware of trigger point diagnoses are in an excellent position to make a sound assessment.

When I first came across the possibilities presented in this book, I spent months extensively reading a variety of sources and digesting, essentially soaking myself in them. In addition, I talked to many people about the ideas at any given opportunity. All of these actions helped me to absorb the messages, slowly teaching my mind/brain that it did not need to produce pain in order to keep distress from my conscious awareness.

In order to achieve this, I had to recognize that my spine was essentially normal, despite my body having been injured. In fact, I had to recognize that despite the advice of the chiropractor I saw soon after the accident, my spine had not been injured at all. The vertebrae not being in their ideal location may have had more to do with the muscular tension in my body resulting from emotional trauma than it had to do with the physical impact of my car accident. Muscular tension is able to pull bones out of their normal area or field of rotation. In addition to multiple cuts and wounds, only my leg, ankles and foot had been damaged. These had all healed beautifully over the coming months, as is normal for the human body. But as important as the damage to my body was the damage to my psyche. This was, however, largely ignored in the medical treatment I received. Unfortunately, I didn't have the courage or knowledge to venture there myself as a young person.

In order to recover from the chronic groin pain, I had to *repudiate* the notion that the pain I had experienced for eighteen years was due to a structural abnormality in my body, specifically in my spine or hips. I had to acknowledge the role which untreated emotional trauma had played. The last experience of extreme groin pain, when I was taking my family to the crash site many years later, enabled me to finally and fully accept that psychology was more relevant to my pain than was physiology.

The acceptance of the role of psychology is an essential component of getting better. This should be simple for a psychologist, but I can testify that it was not easy for me.

To get better, you need to retrain yourself in terms of how you think about the pain. The following are strategies to help you in this retraining process:

- Spend time reading this and other recommended books each day—and when you read, don't just skim over the words absent-mindedly, but concentrate on what is being presented. Analyze the meanings of the words, digest them deeply, and question what is being said.

- Set time aside, at least thirty minutes each day for two to three months, to think hard about how these ideas may apply to you. You must give yourself adequate time to digest them.

- Keep on reading this book, and other related books, every day for at least a month, but preferably up to three months if need be. You need to retrain your thinking about pain, and this will take a persistent effort.

- When experiencing pain, question yourself about what is going on in your life that may be emotionally challenging or threatening. How does this relate to other experiences in your life, or to the feelings that were generated when terrible things happened to you in the past?

- Think about how even positive events may bring up emotional conflicts and challenges.

- Your mind/brain could be creating chronic pain as an attempted 'solution' to what it perceives to be an even greater (psychological) problem- what could this be?

- You can subvert the brain's strategy of using pain as a distraction by instead choosing to focus on areas of distress in your life, and consciously thinking about them in relation to the pain.

- Think about your work, family and social life as well as your finances, and how you feel about aging.

- Try to go beyond the obvious problems, and be willing to speculate about other, more hidden sources of stress or inner conflicts. This may not help you to feel any happier in the short term, but in the long run it provides the best chance you have of eliminating or radically reducing chronic pain. How much happier and more able to cope with such difficulties will you be when you are no longer struggling with this painful affliction?

- Divide your list of problems into those that you can take action over, and those it seems you just have to accept.

- Remember that most people don't have to actually resolve any of these problems to heal their pain—rather, they need to just be aware that the issues are relevant to their pain.

- You don't have to be "positive" about the problems; just be realistic about them. Acknowledge their presence, and work at accepting yourself in spite of having such problems.

- Become aware of what hurts were inflicted on you as a child, and their emotional consequences in the form of anger/rage, great sadness, disappointments, feelings of unworthiness, etc.

- Think about which of your personality traits may be contributing to internally generated tension, e.g. perfectionism, the need for success and achievement, being over-conscientiousness, a tendency towards self-criticism, the need to please others, the need to always be positive, etc. Review the pressure you put on yourself with your desire to be perfect, or to avoid conflict, or to win the approval of others. We are often the hardest task-masters to ourselves.

- When you have an idea of the issues that may be causing the pain, write an essay or a story about each one. In doing so, you will be facing the depth of problematic emotions. This will subtly teach your mind/brain that you *are* able to cope with allowing this material to enter your conscious awareness. You may also want to paint or draw the issue as it relates to the pain.

- Think of the current situations which are adding to your tension, and whether it is possible for you to express your feelings about these problems, perhaps to your spouse, or to your boss. If you are not able to express your feelings, then the tension related will be suppressed and internalized, and will add to your reservoir of distress.

- Do what you need to do about the problems you can take action over, and work hard at accepting those that you can't. Acceptance of problems doesn't mean liking them (see the last chapter).

- Resort to medically prescribed pain killers during an intense bout of pain if you need to, but keep thinking about the emotions behind the pain whilst doing so. Pain relief is sometimes necessary, but don't give up the program just because you may need it.

- You may like to forcefully instruct your unconscious to increase the blood flow back into pained back, glutes, neck or shoulder muscles.

- Some relaxing guided imagery may help with this in which you envisage the muscles surrounding blood vessels to be relaxing and thereby allowing the blood to flow back into the oxygen deprived muscles or nerves. See the blood coming back into those pained parts of your body, and with it the oxygen that is needed (you may like to use my relaxation CD designed for this purpose. It is available as an MP3 download from my website, www.drjamesalexander-psychololgist.com).

- Tell your unconscious that you are aware of what is happening— *the jig is up!* You are no longer willing to be intimidated or pushed around by the pain, as you now know what is behind it. In declaring this, you have taken the purpose of the pain away and rendered it pointless.

Your goal is to think your way out of pain, using a greater awareness of what it is about. The next chapter contains a range of self-help questions and activities to assist you in addressing the above issues in a more structured way.

Rather than make people more miserable, the usual observation is that when people are undertaking this retraining process, they paradoxically reduce the negative impact of the unconscious material. When you are consciously "dealing" with such upsets, you are instructing your unconscious mind that not only can you do something different with them, but that you can cope with bringing them into your conscious awareness. Your world won't fall apart, and there is very little chance that you will either. You may not like facing difficult emotions, but there is an excellent chance that you can actually cope with this. The unconscious is terrified of these deep emotional pains and conflicts, and believes that they must be avoided at all costs. Most people, however, can cope, and the fears of the unconscious are usually found to be unwarranted.

Various forms of psychotherapy can also be of great assistance—the proviso is that the psychotherapy is informed by an awareness of psychogenic pain. Although I had wonderfully cathartic experiences whilst doing re-birthing, none of it actually eliminated my groin pain. What was lacking was simply the information that the emotional pain which I was connecting with and giving expression to in re-birthing was highly relevant to my persistent groin pain. This connection did not come to me until several years later. As such, my conclusion is that even highly effective psychotherapies can fail to eliminate chronic pain where the relevant information is lacking. Chapter 15 discusses tips for finding a psychotherapist who can help you with chronic pain, as not are all equally equipped to assist with this problem.

Exceptions as clues

Another factor to pay attention to is whether there are exceptions to your pattern of pain. People's pain tends to fall into certain patterns, e.g. "I always get pain whenever I mow the lawn," or "Whenever I fall asleep on the soft chair it hurts." These notions constitute our "pain rules," when the pain occurs in a predictable manner according to your experience of it.

Like with most rules, it is extremely unusual for pain rules to not also have exceptions, i.e. times when the pain simply doesn't occur, or is significantly less or somehow different despite having committed the same offending action. Such exceptions violate the rules of our pain experience, and are extremely important as they contain vital information which are keys to recovery.

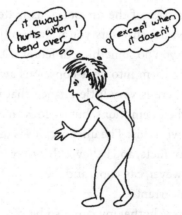

Look for exceptions to pain pattern

If your pain was entirely dependent upon structural pathology of your spine, then there could be no variation in your experience of pain—it would always be the same, as there is no "undoing" of the damage to your spine (unless caused by fractured bones that will heal with time). Bulged discs don't un-bulge themselves, nor do they un-extrude, or un-desiccate, etc. Bones usually heal, but discs do not—there is no variation to this reality. The discs that I damaged when I fractured three vertebrae in my neck remain to this day just as bulged as they were on the day of my injury.

However, when your experience of pain varies, as in pain pattern exceptions, then this suggests that your pain is dependent upon another factor that also varies, and is not dependent upon a factor that does not vary. Pain varies from day to day but disc damage does not vary, nor do most other structural pathologies of the body beyond initial healing of damage in the acute phase (inflammation from an injury will usually settle down with time). This suggests that the pain is not dependent upon the structural pathology, but rather is dependent upon something that can actually vary. Blood supply to muscles and nerves, and subsequent oxygen supply are factors which vary, and do have an impact on pain.

Some case examples help to demonstrate the point. Ronald's experience of intense chest pain demonstrated a very lengthy exception pattern to his pain—he had never experienced it until 2003, despite having lived with the structural abnormality in his chest for his whole life. The experience of having no pain contains extremely important information about its nature. Ronald's exception was longer than many others in that it lasted for most of his life. However, important exceptions can be much shorter. The most convincing example I have seen of exceptions to pain patterns was a female client that I had several years ago.

Joanne was born with an extreme curvature of her spine, giving her the classic "hunch-back" appearance, with her posture resembling the shape of a question mark. Being in her early 30s, her spine had suffered from a lifetime of unnatural pressure due to the congenital condition, resulting in the loss of virtually all of her disc matter. An orthopedic surgeon commented in a medical report that Joanne had the spine of a ninety year old, and not a very healthy ninety year old at that. She reported to me that she had several operations as a young child to try and correct the deformity, and none of them had proved effective.

Her memories of extreme back pain began when she commenced primary school. Until that time, she had been in the care and protection of her family. On beginning school, all of a sudden Joanne was exposed to the prejudices of the broader community. "Kids can be very cruel to anybody who looks different, and often their parents are no better. I was tormented at school for being a hunch-back and treated as some kind of freak." Consequently, Joanne made few friends, and had to deal with daily rejection and ridicule from her peers. This continued into high school. At a time when other students were developing interests in the opposite sex, she became even more estranged from her peers and more isolated. Needless to say, life was extremely difficult for Joanne, both emotionally and socially. This is the psychological context in which her chronic back pain began as a child.

On viewing her back and reviewing the specialist reports, it would seem a risky venture to question whether her back pain was due to her extreme physical condition. Surely, if anyone was suffering from pain generated by structural pathology, this woman was. It is likely that she did experience physically induced pain as a child, as her spine was in an early and rapid process of physical deterioration due to the extreme deformity. However, this process was well and truly over by the time I met her as an adult.

On further probing, Joanne revealed to me that there had been one notable exception to her experience of pain: five years earlier, when she had spent a year living overseas. During this time, she had lived in a small rural village, where she was engaged in doing physical work for the first time in her life (in fact, it was the first and only job she had ever held). In addition, being a novel stranger from a different part of the world, she was accepted into the community with her master identity being "the Australian," rather than just being "the hunch-back." "They just seemed to like the fact that I was an Australian, and were happy that I had chosen to spend time in their village. I was treated a bit like a celebrity, rather than as a freak. It was the first time in my life that I was special for a positive reason."

As a personal breakthrough, she had her first and only romantic relationship while living overseas. Another important exception to her normal pain pattern was when she fell and landed on her back one day, an experience that would ordinarily produce extreme pain; however, she was fine—no pain or heightened disability followed. The sad part of the story is that when she returned back home after a year away, her pain resumed, and she returned to her normal level of disability. Obviously, coming back to her home and community meant that she was again "just" a person who looked different. Overseas, she had been viewed as special in her own right by virtue of who she was—people saw past the obvious disability.

This case highlights the importance of exceptions to pain patterns. Joanne's structural pathology did not vary, however her experience of pain did, at least for one year while she was overseas. As such, her pain must be dependent upon a factor which also varied, and *not* dependent upon a factor which did not vary (i.e. her structural pathology).

What varied in her experience during the exception period overseas? Clearly, for the first time since she entered the broader world as a primary school student, she had been accepted and valued for who she was, rather than rejected because of her disability. Her experience of the world outside of her family was so hurtful that an enormous amount of psychological distress had been generated for her over most of her life.

The case studies of Ronald and Joanne are both dramatic in terms of the extent of their structural abnormalities, as well as the thoroughness of exceptions to their pain patterns. Most people whom I have helped with chronic pain over the years have not been so dramatic, but Ronald and Joanne's experiences are included here because they clearly demonstrate the importance of exceptions.

Another female client I saw had only the exception of five minutes of no-back pain over a ten-year period, but even this short exception told her that it was *possible* to experience no pain. Exceptions are valuable sources of information, and an essential component of learning to think psychologically about chronic pain.

Information as the best treatment

Professor Paul Hodges, a spokesperson for the Australian Physiotherapy Association and Professor of Physiotherapy at the University of Queensland, states that the only interventions which are demonstrated through research to make a difference with chronic pain are ones in which information provision is the main intervention.[4] In the same interview, Hodges details the poor evidence base for all of the standard physical therapies for chronic pain (for more discussion on this, see "The value of physical therapies?" in Appendix 5).

Central to the intervention programs which have proven to be of some usefulness for chronic pain sufferers are a combination of information about pain, ways to manage it, and helpful tips on becoming more active again.

The Back Book is a small publication printed by the Victorian WorkCover Authority in the 1990s, containing much of the useful information which people in chronic pain need to be aware of. It is based on the UK Royal College of General Practitioners' "Clinical Guidelines for the Management of Acute Low Back Pain," and is endorsed by most of the relevant Australian medical, orthopaedic, physiotherapy, rheumatology, surgical, psychiatric and occupational rehabilitation organizations in Australia and in the UK. As such, it reflects evidence based views of the vast majority of professional bodies that deal with chronic pain.

Notably, *The Back Book* contains none of the standard pain myths regarding structural pathology that most of the physical treatments of chronic pain are based on. There seems to be a large disconnect between what the peak professional bodies view as being essential information in the effective treatment of chronic pain, and what most of the practitioners in those professions think and do on a clinical level. The information which these specialists organizations are wanting people with back pain to understand is summarized below:

- Back pain is common, but is usually not due to any serious disease. Extreme pain does not mean there is any serious damage to the back—hurt does not mean harm.

- The back is designed for movement. The sooner the person gets back to normal activity, the sooner they will feel better.

- The spine is one of the strongest parts of the body. It is very difficult to seriously damage it.

---

4   Hodges (2004). "Exercise and Bone Strength/Physiotherapy." ABC Radio National Health Report.

- Most people with back pain do not have any serious damage or disease of their spine.

- Most X-rays of people in back pain find normal changes with age—these changes are a normal part of aging, like gray hair.

- The notion of a "slipped disc" is a physiological impossibility and a misnomer.

- The exact physical source of pain in most people cannot be pinpointed.

- Stress can increase the amount of pain felt.

- Tension can cause muscle spasms, when the muscles themselves become painful.

- Movement and exercise is the recommended response. Pain killers and other treatments can help to control pain initially, to assist the person to get active again.

- Heat or cold can alleviate pain.

- Physicians can and should assure people with back pain that they do not have a serious disease (once this has been eliminated).

- How a person's back ache affects them depends on how they react to the pain and what they do about it.

- Further back pain does not mean further damage.

As you will have gathered from reading this list of essential messages, there is a fair degree of overlap between *The Hidden Psychology of Pain*, and what the peak professional bodies have to say. The main difference, of course, is that *The Back Book* makes no statement as to *why* chronic pain arises in the first place. It simply offers evidence-based advice to people for whom pain has arisen so as to minimize the syndrome. Eliminating chronic back pain is not on their agenda; however, the more modest goal of learning to manage it is.

The reason for the oversight of *why* people experience chronic pain is that the authorities who wrote *The Back Book* are medical and para-medical specialists, not psychologists or psychiatrists with an appreciation of depth-psychology. For the most part, psychosomatic medicine is a field of which they are ignorant.

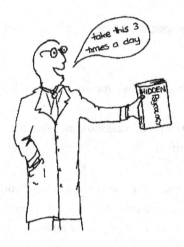

Information is the best treatment

Sarah Stewart-Brown, Professor of Public Health at the University of Warwick Medical School in the UK, conducted a large study in physiotherapy departments within the British National Health System.[5] She compared the outcomes of 1) standard physiotherapy treatment of back pain, e.g. manipulation, heat and cold treatment, and individually tailored exercises, along with *The Back Book*, and 2) giving *The Back Book* to patients in a single session of advice only. The only difference between the two treatment groups was the physical treatment which one group received and the other did not.

The results showed that a year down the track, there was absolutely no difference in the outcomes between the two groups of patients. The patients

---

[5] Stewart-Brown (2004). "Low Back Pain and Physiotherapy." ABC Radio National Life Matters.

who received the physical treatment *felt better* about the treatment earlier on, believing that they had derived more benefit when compared to people who had just been examined and given *The Back Book*. In other words, people *like* physiotherapy treatment because it feels nice to be carefully touched and treated—it feels like something is being done, and this satisfies an emotional need. However beyond this initial positive report, one year later, patients were just as likely to still be in pain regardless of the treatment they received.

Unfortunately, this means that *The Back Book* messages on their own are about as effective (and as ineffective) in eliminating pain as is standard physiotherapy treatment—the success rates for both are rather low. The messages in *The Back Book* are clearly essential ones for people in pain to understand; however, without the added element of delving into what is *causing* the pain from a psychological perspective, it remains of limited use.

In addition to this limitation, *The Back Book* contains an emphasis on the value of *coping* with pain. Part of the problem is that chronic pain sufferers are mostly copers already. This seems to set them up for chronic pain, in that they are less inclined to delve into their emotional distress in preference to just pushing on. Recovery from chronic pain needs less coping, and more preparedness to delve into the negative, as Gabor Maté suggests.

Of limited use or not, *The Back Book* is the most effective evidence based treatment for chronic back pain which the conventional pain industry has yet come up with—and it is purely information, not physical therapy. The processing of this information is a psycho-educational or cognitive approach, and in many ways it overlaps nicely with informational aspects of *The Hidden Psychology of Pain*. The ways in which it does not overlap possibly explains its only limited use in terms of reducing pain.

"Cognitive restructuring" in conventional pain management programs refers to changing people's beliefs and thinking styles, so as to become more adaptive to the situation. Most cognitive pain interventions focus on helping people to change their thoughts so that they cope better with being in pain, rather than a psychological endeavor to eliminate the pain. If a person is catastophizing about their pain, viewing it as being the end of their life, then it is helpful for them to adjust their attitude, and realize that their life really isn't over just because of seemingly intractable pain.

If coping was the only option possible, then this would be entirely laudable. However, as is apparent to clinicians who use *The Hidden Psychology of Pain*, it is actually possible to help many people radically reduce or eradicate their pain. Approaches such as CBT can help to alleviate the emotional distress associated with chronic pain, and have made a difference in many people's lives. Depth-psychology can offer more than just alleviation, however.

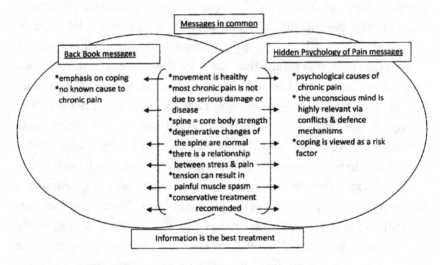

The areas of overlap between the messages from The Back Book and The Hidden Psychology of Pain

In a recent edition of *Medicine Today,* Barnsley states that, "A synopsis of systematic reviews concludes that behavioral treatment (as in CBT) versus no treatment, placebo or waiting list controls reduces pain in the short term."[6] CBT on its own would be a reasonable option if the problem it is treating were in fact a short term one. The problem is that chronic pain is not short term. By definition, it is a *long-term* problem, so any intervention that has only short-term benefits is missing the mark in the same way as an injection of analgesics misses the mark.

A purely cognitive treatment of chronic pain can certainly be helpful when it is informed by accurate information about the condition, and not by the pain myths that are promulgated by the treatment industry. Unfortunately, most of the cognitive-behavioral treatment approaches used

---

[6] Barnsley (2010 p.26). "The Significance of Chronic Back Pain." *Medicine Today.*

in conventional pain management are still operating from within these pain myths. As a result, they remain somewhat limited in their usefulness.[7]

The Hidden Psychology of Pain suggests that most people can actually get rid of their pain, not just learn to live with it. As this also has an emphasis on how people need to think about chronic pain, it is clearly a cognitive-educational approach, but paradoxically, it is a cognitive program from a depth-psychology perspective.

Chronic pain sufferers who undergo cognitive therapy are found to end up with decreased neural activity in the brain areas associated with emotional regulation and hyper-vigilance.[8] This is particularly important as chronic pain involves a hyper-vigilance to bodily pain cues, and cognitive therapy (essentially, the provision of ideas) has been shown to decrease brain activity associated with this hyper-vigilance. In learning how to change their thinking, people can so reduce their level of emotional tension that their muscles learn to relax, thereby allowing more blood and oxygen back into the pain areas, and the pain can be reduced. But we generally need instruction and guidance in regards to the most important thinking issues involved, and the most important issue is, "*Why* am I in chronic pain?"

Keith Petrie and colleagues' research on the outcomes of a conventional cognitive pain management program has demonstrated that addressing

---

[7] A former client of mine opted for a CBT pain-management approach, and rather than simply learning to feel better about being in constant pain, he greatly reduced it to the point where he was no longer disabled. As such, I am reluctant to condemn traditional CBT as being useless just because it doesn't aim for deeper distress. This particular man had experienced a great deal of grief in his life, so the prospect of changing his surface level thoughts was perhaps less threatening to him than the prospect of delving into his history of loss. The standard pain management program with a large CBT element worked for him; however, the more common experience is a more modest reduction of pain and a greater emotional acceptance of it. Many people will welcome a greater acceptance of pain, but the vast majority of them would prefer to not be in pain at all. This is what many people can actually aim for. Most of the case examples that I have presented so far in this book were people who were told that the best they could hope for was to learn to live with the pain. Had they settled for this, they would all still be in extreme pain today, although they may have learnt to accept it better. Fortunately, they chose to go beyond just coping, and instead used important information to help them find a cure for their pain.

[8] Grant (2009). *Change Your Brain, Change Your Pain.*

the cause of the chronic pain is linked to improved mental functioning for sufferers.[9] Their study shows the importance of what they refer to as "sense of coherence," or the meaning which people can make of their pain.

Low coherence, or being unable to make sense of chronic pain, is related to poor mental functioning, with the flow-on effect being increases in pain and level of disability. On the other hand, high coherence, or being able to make some kind of sense of the pain experience, reduces people's levels of distress about the pain, and ultimately, the intensity of the pain as well. When we make sense of why the pain is happening, we go a long way to curing it. From their wide ranging research studies, Petrie and colleagues have concluded that what we think about an illness actually has more of a role to play in the outcome of the condition than does its actual severity.[10]

This finding provides some explanation for the limited effectiveness of standard cognitive pain management programs, and of *The Back Book*. Both of these forms of conventional treatment address a range of very important factors, which do assist in creating some relief from chronic pain. However, they both fail to create a sense of coherence, or meaning in terms of explaining *why* the chronic pain is happening.

Lacking this essential element means that chronic pain remains a highly disturbing mystery. This sense of mystery is perhaps preferable to the physical therapists who erroneously but confidently state that the causes of chronic pain are structural pathologies. However, in the absence of *any* explanation offered (typical in most pain management programs—the message is usually "we don't know why you are in pain"), a meaning-vacuum is created.

As humans are explanation and meaning seeking beings, we will instinctively fill this vacuum with whatever explanation seems plausible. Without being equipped with the information in this book, most people settle on a structural pathology explanation, as this is still the most common explanation offered by the physical therapists who we seek help from, despite the information in *The Back Book*. As such, the structural pathology explanation becomes the default explanation, simply because the real

9   Moss-Morris et al (2007). *Patients' Perceptions of Their Pain Condition across a Multidisciplinary Pain Management Program.*

10 Petrie & Weinman (2012). "Patients' Perceptions of Their Illness: The Dynamo of Volition in Health Care." *Current Directions in Psychological Science.*

causes of chronic pain (i.e. unconscious emotional distress) is not known, accepted or presented in conventional pain management programs. Were such programs to include psycho-physiological explanations of why chronic pain happens, they would cease to be pain "management" programs, and instead could become the pain eradication programs that they should be.

Some people have raised the objection of harm that may occur to people if The Hidden Psychology of Pain does not work for them. This is a legitimate concern, but not just for this approach. Each and every psychological, surgical and medical intervention is commenced on the faith that it will be helpful.

What happens to the depressed person who does not get better in response to counseling, or antidepressant drugs? Or the surgery patient whose pain does not resolve after an operation? Should the possibility of failure prevent us from commencing interventions when our experience tells us that it is likely to be helpful? All medical and psychological interventions are commenced on good faith that the person will benefit. If we, as health professionals, don't believe in the possible benefits, then we have no business offering them. Hopefully, only interventions that have a track record of success are attempted. Problems associated with treatment failure are relevant for all health approaches, and not just this approach.

Based on outcome research and much anecdotal experience, professionals who treat people with a psychosomatic approach are also very confident about our ability to produce helpful outcomes. Around 88% of Sarno's back-pain patients in a follow-up sample reported that their pain had either decreased to a point which they felt to be a big improvement, or it was cured altogether. A further 12% were referred to short-term psychotherapy which proved effective for most of them. With the remaining 2% who did not improve, Sarno's conclusion was that they have more complicated psychological issues, often related to extreme abuse and trauma.[11]

In effect, like the pain-management program explanation for non-success, treatment resistant patients are either unwilling or unable to take on board these ideas sufficiently for them to be effective. There is always the chance that this may change and at some time in the future. People will sometimes be in a better position to process these ideas at another time in their lives.

---

[11] Sarno (1998). *The Mindbody Prescription*.

Getting active again

Another element of standard pain management programs which has proven effective is the encouragement of physical activity. Physical movement should not be confused with physical treatment or therapy, although movement per se is obviously therapeutic. Using your body in a manner for which it was designed, for either vocational or recreational purposes, is not a therapy—it is life, and a necessary part of it.

For many people suffering chronic pain, once the pain myths have been internalized, a fear of re-injuring creeps in and often prevents further movement. This in itself can create pain, as our bodies have not evolved for inactivity. Rather, we are designed for activity and movement, and to neglect this need will also increase bodily pain.

Exercise has been demonstrated to increase natural feel-good brain chemicals such as dopamine, serotonin as well as the body's own opiates, the endorphins. In addition, exercise adjusts the chemistry of the entire brain, so that it returns to a more normal state of chemical and electrical activity. Gradually building up an exercise regime can also increase a person's sense of well-being, in addition to a belief in their ability to create positive change in their lives. This is very important for people who have lost their sense of agency due to chronic pain. Regular exercise will also relieve the physical tension in your muscles, and assist in the dispersion of stress hormones. These can be very important psychological and physiological factors in countering the anxiety and depression that accompanies chronic pain for most people.

As per the statements made in *The Back Book,* pain does not equate with damage, so movement is desirable even though it may be difficult at first. It is known that excessive rest is simply bad for our bodies; however, this is what most people in chronic pain are wanting to do because of both fear and the pain itself. By being less active, we become de-conditioned, and physical movement often becomes more painful and difficult. Even if you were not in chronic pain, but just chose to be completely inactive, you could expect to be in pain upon moving again.

Disuse atrophy occurs when muscle mass begins to diminish through lack of use. In this atrophy process, skeletal muscle tissue will break down and be reabsorbed by the body. In addition, such muscles tend to get shorter and lose their tone with inactivity, making them even more vulnerable to muscle injury such as tearing. A flow-on effect of extreme inactivity is that over longer periods of time, joints, bones, blood vessels feeding the relevant areas and nerves can all be adversely affected. The saying "use it or lose it" is of critical importance here.

As such, one standard piece of advice that has been demonstrated as effective is to simply *move* again. But this can be difficult, both because of the associated pain, as well as the de-conditioning which has taken its toll. In addition, if the muscles and nerves are suffering from ischemia, then increasing the physical workload is likely to increase the gap between what the muscle/nerve/tendon needs (in terms of oxygen) and what it is actually getting. As the deficit of oxygen increases, more pain can ensue.

The answer is to neither push through the pain barrier, nor is it to concede defeat and give up. The most effective strategy is to slowly increase the amount of time spent in gentle movement and exercise, and aim to ultimately return to your pre-pain activities via a gradual process of increasing the level of activity.

Most people tend to use the "boom-or-bust" exercise cycle. On days when they feel in the most pain, they will avoid activity. On days when they feel relatively good, they will do an excessive amount of activity. The result is that they tend to suffer for protracted periods of time after the high exercise day due to over-exertion of muscles, as well as muscle tears due to disuse atrophy. More rest ensues for a week or more while they are recovering, during which no exercise is happening at all, and the de-conditioning process simply continues.

You can also feel emotional distress and worry about having pushed yourself on the good day, and upset by being back in pain again in the days that follow. This will usually produce more worry that in overdoing it you have inflicted more "serious damage" to your body. As such, "boom-or-busters" tend to not get progressively better. In fact, they may become so discouraged that they give up trying, and just sink further into more pain, more inactivity, and deepening despair.

Fear of further damage will often make it difficult for people to become more active, and we are being constantly bombarded by messages designed to induce fear of injury. The list of advice about how to move and what to avoid doing is ever growing. For people whose muscles are already compromised through lack of use or ischemia, such advice on bending and lifting may be of some use. Why stress weaker and smaller muscles that may already be suffering, when you can do the same job with larger muscles that are more able to handle the job? As such, advice from Occupational Therapists, chiropractors, or physiotherapists on lifting and bending when you are in your recovery phase can be helpful and worth obtaining. However, for people who are not in pain, such bio-mechanical advice about correct lifting can just produce a climate of fear in which the pain thrives. Keep in mind, there is no evidence that chronic back pain results from lifting or any other type of exertion, whether we be moving "properly" or not—it is all just conjecture, with very little evidence to support it.

In order to overcome the natural fear of re-injuring, you must actively retrain your mind/brain with accurate information, and thereby critically re-evaluate the fear messages. As I was already well informed by the time I heard a chiropractor tell a large radio audience that wallets in the back pocket can cause serious spinal problems, I was able to laugh-off the suggestion. But I do wonder how many people in pain were vulnerable to taking this bit of "helpful" advice seriously, and thereby became even more frightened—this time, of their wallets.

Increasing activity levels will help to reduce fear as long as you are sensible in your approach. The services of an exercise physiologist can be very helpful in training you to use your body again. To build your confidence, wait until you are substantially better (i.e. pain gone or nearly gone) before tackling your more vigorous pre-pain activities. Had my client, Max, decided to play soccer again as soon as his back pain abruptly left, he would have simply wound up in extreme pain due to his body having become de-conditioned from years of inactivity.

While you are waiting for the pain to diminish, you can slowly begin increasing your level of activity again with gentle exercises such as walking or swimming. You need to avoid the risk of muscle tears as much as possible in your gradual increase of activity. This is best done by being sensible in what to expect from your compromised body. Pain medication may still be necessary during this time, but when the pain is resolved, you are unlikely to feel the need to take them and can gradually scale down. Discuss both the use and scaling down of medications with your physician. In the meantime, slowly building your activity level in small incremental steps will help to gradually rebuild your physical condition, as well as your confidence. Confidence develops in the wake of success, so ensure that you give yourself plenty of experiences of physical movement at which you can succeed, and none at which you will fail.

"Pacing" is the approach to increasing your activity level which is more likely to succeed, as it encourages daily exercise at a minimal level. Kate, a woman in her late fifties, had been in extreme back pain for the ten years before I met her. As a result, she had become something of a reclusive invalid, relying on her dedicated husband to do most things in their household.

Her pain began when she and her husband lost their business in which she worked and had thoroughly enjoyed. Her treatment goals with me were to be able to go shopping again, and to begin meeting with friends. While she was working with me on The Hidden Psychology of Pain, Kate began a pacing exercise program. During the treatment, I asked her to work out how much walking she could do on the worst pain days without making her pain worse. She replied that she could only manage around three minutes of walking on those days. As such, I instructed her to walk three minutes each day for a week, regardless of how she felt. This is more difficult as it sounds, as there were days when three minutes of walking was quite hard for her. Just as difficult were days when she felt that she could walk twenty minutes, but had to force herself to walk only three minutes.

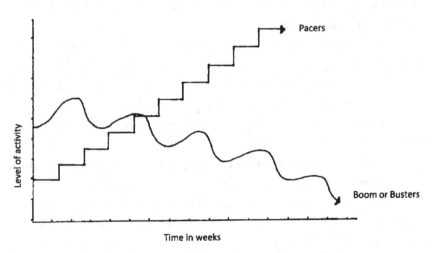

The difference in activity success between Pacers and Boom or Busters

In week two of her program, Kate decided that she was now able to walk for six minutes a day without aggravating the pain, even on the worse days. She commenced doing this regardless of how she felt. Several weeks later, continuing to gradually increase the lengths of her walks, she was able to walk for around twenty minutes at a time each day. This now meant that she was able to walk to her general store where she saw and socialized with some friends with whom she had lost contact in the years of being a recluse. Consequently, she began to take an interest in her appearance again, and enjoyed buying new nail polish for the first time in years (not a big deal to most people perhaps, but it was a significant improvement for Kate). These were important changes in her pain pattern, which until this time had included a radically shrinking social world. Rather than being confined to watching TV in her living room, she was now able to arrange to meet people at the shops and enjoy their company again.

It is worth noting that Kate engaged in this pacing exercise program even though she was still in pain. Unlike some of the more dramatic cases presented, it took a longer period of time for her to find relief from suffering. While she was busy with relevant reading, discussing with me what her pain may be about, and generally immersing herself in the ideas presented in this book, she was also gradually reconditioning her body with regular exercise. Like Kate, in order to get better, you need to gradually increase your exercise levels in small incremental steps so as to avoid straining muscles that have become unused to exertion.

Each week, re-evaluate how much you can exercise even on the worst days without re-aggravating, then stick to that amount each day of that week, regardless of how you feel. The following week, and each subsequent week, do the same thing until you find yourself exercising for longer periods of time in a consistent manner. In so doing, you will be gradually reconditioning your body and re-training your mind/brain away from expecting pain to follow exertion. This will also begin to challenge the classical conditioning which you may have undergone over the years of associating activity with pain.

However, remember that it is possible to increase your general body condition and *still* be in pain whilst working on The Hidden Psychology of Pain. It is unlikely that you will eliminate the pain just as a result of using pacing to gradually increase your body condition. The goal of this program is to get rid of the pain, not just to learn to live with it. Reconditioning your body is an important step in this process from both a psychological as well as physical perspective, but needs to be done in conjunction with learning to think psychologically about the pain.

Readiness for pain relief

For many people who use the ideas contained in this book, the processing of information will be sufficient to reduce pain. How significant this reduction proves to be is dependent on a range of factors.

- Are you able to stick to these ideas, even during times when no immediate improvement is apparent?

- Are you able to continue with the program even if those around you, family members and health professionals are arguing against the ideas presented?

- Can you ward off the invitations to be highly anxious about your pain condition, or about the chances of further injury?

- Will you dismiss these ideas as being perhaps useful for others, but not applying to you?

- Will your mind/brain intensify the pain in order to convince you that it really is physical, and has nothing to do with psychology?

- Will you be frightened by the commonly reported experience of pain moving between different locations within the body, as the unconscious mind/brain's desperate attempt to monopolize your attention with pain?

- Will you be able to think psychologically about your pain rather than physically?

- Will you mostly, but not entirely, accept that the mind/brain can produce pain and other chronic health problems?

These are all very important issues which will assist in determining the outcome.

I have introduced The Hidden Psychology of Pain to people who were so ready to get better that their pain left them within a matter of days. Other people have been less ready to embrace these ideas, often thinking, "Yes, that may be true for *them*—but *my* pain is real." They have failed to understand or process the information provided in a deep enough manner, and have only made surface-level sense of what is being proposed. Such people want to have a bet each way, continuing to believe that the pain is caused by what are essentially normal structural pathologies, but at the same time entertaining these new ideas on a superficial level only. This may be evidenced by their unwillingness to let go of physical therapies that have not yet eliminated their pain, but always promise to do so.

These are some of the individual differences which will contribute to the outcome, and they are not determined by the content of any book, including this one. However, my repeated observation is that people can radically reduce or eliminate their pain purely by processing helpful information. The deeper the level of understanding of what is being proposed, and the more thorough the understanding, the greater chance the person has of becoming pain free.

As long as people continue to seek the latest physical therapy, their ability to benefit from *The Hidden Psychology of Pain* will be limited. But, some people will just need to exhaust the entire list of physical therapies until they are ready to accept that the problem is not essentially a physical one. At such a time, they are likely to be more open to the ideas presented in this book.

My experience of working in a chronic pain unit of a hospital was that people were more likely to get better by using the ideas in this book than people whom I saw while working either in rehabilitation services or private practice. The only reason I can imagine for this is that the hospital unit was viewed as being the last option for sufferers. They had generally tried absolutely everything else on offer, all to no avail. As such, these people had for the most part stopped looking for a new physical cure.

Your current distressing life experiences may be entirely relevant to the pain as they may hit upon a vein of similarity with previous hurts: e.g. your spouse or boss speaks to you in an unkind manner. You may note that your emotional response seems to be somewhat out of proportion to the "crime," and your pain increases. This may be similar enough to how your abusive parent spoke to you as a child. The current experience has tapped into a vein of similarity such that the gas is now turned up on the reservoir of distress in your unconscious, and these feelings begin to heat up.

On a surface level, you will probably be aware that you feel stressed because of how you have been spoken to, and that this is similar to how you were spoken to as a child. However, deeper than this level of awareness could be the unacceptable feelings of shame and self-rejection. As a child, you may have been so often spoken to with disdain that you learnt to believe in your unworthiness as a human being. As an adult, you have done all you can to demonstrate your worth, and have developed a very positive outlook in life. However, deep down there may be a sense of unworthiness which is still haunting you.

These may be the types of feelings which threaten to erupt into your conscious awareness as a result of your spouse or boss being unkind. You may even consciously deny the possibility that deep down you still feel unworthy. Some additional help may be needed to assist you in cutting through the defenses that we all routinely use to deflect our attention away from distressing psychological material. The next chapter discusses a range of strategies which have been found helpful in the quest to diminish emotional and physical pain. You will note that they are all psychological strategies, and that they are all addressing psychological issues. By now, this should come as no surprise.

CHAPTER 9

Self-Help Strategies

THIS CHAPTER PROVIDES YOU WITH a range of self-help approaches that have proven effective in alleviating chronic pain by addressing the emotional causes behind it. Firstly, the goal of this chapter is to help you address these issues with a range of specific questions which you are asked to answer in the spaces provided. The healing process is an active one. You need to do more than just passively read the concepts presented to you.

Self-analysis questions

Try to maximize the potential benefit of this by honestly answering the questions. Add extra sheets of paper, or better still, use an exercise book where there is not enough room provided here for your answers. Go over the questions and re-answer them as many times as you need, as often your answers will deepen to a new layer each time you ponder the questions. The goal is to raise your level of awareness about your feelings, and then to see the possible connection between these and your pain.

There is considerable evidence that writing about distressing experiences is an effective therapy for many people. Create a habit of writing your thoughts and feelings about the issues raised, as well as your answers to the questions posed in this chapter on a daily basis. Doing this writing exercise for at least thirty days is likely to be of great help to you.[1] This may seem self-indulgent or unnecessarily negative; however, such reflection is an essential component of getting better, and is a strategy which you are able to engage in without professional guidance.

Each question is aimed at helping you bring to awareness issues which may be lurking in your unconscious. By bringing them into your consciousness, your mind/brain can begin to learn that it is a safe activity, and that pain is not necessary to prevent this from occurring.

As there are many questions presented here, give yourself permission to not answer them all at once You may decide to keep reading the book and return to answering a couple of the questions each day. It may make sense for you to re-answer the questions at different times over the next few months as well.

Mind/Body Health Issues

1) On the 1-10 scale below, how well does the possibility of a psychological cause to your condition sit with you? Do you totally reject the possibility, or are you very open to it?

very uncomfortable   somewhat open   very comfortable
1_____2_____3_____4_____5_____6_____7_____8_____9_____10

Detail and explain your answer in the space below.

_____
_____
_____
_____
_____
_____
_____

---

[1]   Mind/Body medical practitioner, Dr. David Schechter, provides a series of questions for chronic pain sufferers in the form of a thirty-day workbook, in which people are required to answer questions on a daily basis for a month. This can be ordered through his website, http://www.mindbodymedicine.com

2) What type of responses have you received so far from family members, friends and treating professionals when you have raised the notion of psychology having a role to play in chronic pain? What do you think is the intention of their response? What impact have these responses had on you?

_____

_____

_____

_____

_____

_____

3) A standard observation is that mind/body health problems appear to occur in clusters within individuals. It is quite common for people to be afflicted by a range of such conditions, and this observation is an important clue as to what is going on. Of the conditions mentioned in Chapter 1, which other conditions have you suffered from?

_____

_____

_____

_____

_____

4) Were you given any clues by your examining physician that these conditions could have been examples of mind/body complaints? Was anything said to you that suggested a role for psychological factors in these conditions?

_____

_____

_____

_____

_____

_____

5) If you have undergone imaging studies (e.g. X-ray, scans) or pathology tests regarding your condition, were the results inconclusive, inconsistent, or showing a benign condition? Did the results *exclude* a serious pathology (e.g. cancer or infection), and/or support the possibility of a mind/body condition?

_____

_____

_____

_____

_____

_____

_____

Attachment styles

Reviewing the description of attachment styles (in Chapter 7) which parents/care givers show towards their children, do you have a sense of which style was applied to you as a child? Searching your memory as far back as it will go, can you remember any behaviours from your care-givers that would indicate their attachment style? If you have no early recollections of your own, did you observe your care-givers with younger siblings or grandchildren? Could this be an indicator of their attachment style? If you can get a sense of it, which attachment style do you think was applied to you as a young child?

- Secure
- Avoidant
- Ambivalent
- disorganised

_____

_____

_____

Can you recognise your own attachment style of care-giving towards your children? This could be a clue as to how you were raised.

_____

_____

_____

What sort of impact do you think this attachment style has had on your emotional development, as well as your emotional approach to life now as an adult? Have you received feedback from friends or partners that would indicate a consequence of your care-givers attachment style?

_____

_____

_____

_____

_____

_____

_____

Problem schemas

Reviewing the description of problematic schemas in Chapter 7, which of the following do you relate most to?

- Disconnection & rejection
- Impaired autonomy & performance
- Other directedness
- Over-vigilance & inhibition.

_____

_____

_____

_____

_____

What examples of these schemas can you see in your life and how you have experienced events?

_____

_____

_____

_____

_____

_____

_____

How do you know when one of these schemas is active? As an indicator, what is the emotional state that is associated with the schema?

_____

_____

_____

_____

_____

_____

What impact do you think these schemas have had on your life?

_____

_____

_____

_____

_____

_____

Exceptions

It is common for people to begin experiencing more variations in their pain pattern (exceptions—see Chapter 8) when they begin entertaining the ideas presented in this book. These initial changes are extremely important, and you need to make a proper sense of them to obtain their full potential benefit.

If your pain really was due to structural abnormalities which do not vary, then you would experience no variation in your pattern of pain either. The fact that your pain varies means that it must be related to something else which also varies, such as your beliefs about pain, your emotions and inner conflicts.

1) Take a few minutes now to write down any variations or exceptions to your pain pattern that you have noticed since you started reading this book. These may include times when the pain was absent, or times when the pain was less than what you thought it should be. If you can't think of recent exceptions, think about other times when the pain was in some way different

than what you expected. Also, think about other times in your life when you experienced unexpected differences in your pain.

_____

_____

_____

_____

_____

_____

Make a daily habit of thinking about and writing down such exceptions and variations in your experience of pain, as these are essential clues as to what is going on for you.

Fear

This difficult emotion is often a significant part of the chronic pain problem, and may actually prevent people from seriously looking at the issues presented in this book.

1) What negative possibilities in your life are you the most fearful of? How much time do you spend thinking about these fears?

_____

_____

_____

_____

_____

_____

2) How do these fears dictate what you do, and how you do them? Do they prevent you from taking risks or striving for important things in your life?

_____

_____

_____

_____

3) How do you avoid facing these fears in your attempts to keep things "safe"?

_____

_____

_____

_____

_____

_____

_____

4) Is it possible that you may be in denial of some of your fears? You may maintain a brave face, but lurking deep down, are there fears which are kept repressed? Imagine for a moment that there were such fears— what might they be?

_____

_____

_____

_____

_____

_____

_____

5) What is the biggest fear that you have in regards to pain? Do you worry about where it may be heading; a high level of disability; the inability to earn an income; the effects on your family; medical interventions; having to rely on others for basic self-maintenance? What are you most frightened about in regards to the pain?

_____

_____

_____

_____

_____

_____

_____

Personality Factors

Personality factors appear to be important in the causation of chronic pain, as these reflect habitual patterns of dealing with the world. Looking at the below list, tick the personality traits which you think apply to you.

___ perfectionist
___ highly conscientious
___ control oriented
___ self-critical
___ very thorough
___ overly responsible

1) As these aspects of your personality may predispose you to psychosomatic problems, think and write about how these characteristics generate stress and tension for you.

_____
_____
_____
_____
_____
_____
_____
_____

Responsibility

Being highly responsible appears to be a personality trait related to chronic pain. Sufferers are often people who will repeatedly put other's needs first and their own needs second out of a sense of responsibility. This goes along with a desire to be viewed as "good" by authority figures.

1) What were the messages about responsibility which you received as a child? Were your parents highly responsible people, always putting others first in order to fulfill their perceived obligations?

_____
_____
_____

_____

_____

_____

_____

_____

2) How were you treated if you acted in a less-than-responsible manner?

_____

_____

_____

_____

_____

_____

_____

3) What does responsibility mean to you as an adult, and what pressures do you feel as a result of taking responsibility?

_____

_____

_____

_____

_____

_____

_____

4) How does this create additional stress and frustration for you?

_____

_____

_____

_____

_____

_____

_____

5) What issues do you take responsibility for, which others may not see as being yours to take?

_____

_____

_____

_____

_____

_____

_____

_____

6) Would you hold others as responsible in the same situations? What would you say to them?

_____

_____

_____

_____

_____

_____

_____

_____

7) How do you feel when you take responsibility for such issues?

_____

_____

_____

_____

_____

_____

_____

_____

8) Is there any way you can challenge taking such a level of responsibility for issues which are arguably not yours?

_____

_____

_____
_____
_____
_____
_____
_____

Self-Criticism

Another common personality trait amongst sufferers of chronic pain is a tendency towards being highly self-critical. When combined with a heightened sense of responsibility, and perfectionist expectations, self-critical people will usually generate a great deal of internal stress.

1) Have there been times in your life when you have been extremely self-critical? What were the related events, and how did you run yourself down about them?

_____
_____
_____
_____
_____
_____
_____
_____
_____

2) Is there a particular theme to your self-criticisms (e.g. "I am stupid/ugly/incompetent/worthless.")?

_____
_____
_____
_____
_____
_____
_____
_____

3) Where did you learn this theme, and from whom? How do you keep reinforcing this theme?

_____

_____

_____

_____

_____

_____

_____

_____

4) If you had a friend criticizing themselves in the same way (in the same situation) would you agree with them? If not, what would you say to challenge their self-criticism?

_____

_____

_____

_____

_____

_____

_____

_____

Anger & Rage

We typically learn how to conduct ourselves, and how to respond to the world in the context of our families of origin. Part of this influence is no doubt genetic, and part of it is picked up through a process of social learning—we observe how our parents or caregivers behave, and usually replicate what we have seen over many formative years. Repressed anger and rage often play a significant role in chronic pain.

1) Thinking of your family of origin, what was the way in which anger was expressed? How did you know if your parents or siblings were angry? Did they express it calmly, explosively, repress it, or bury it with substances?

_____

_____

_____

_____

_____

_____

_____

_____

2) How did your parents or caregivers respond to you when you were angry as a child or teenager? Did they allow and accept it, or punish your expression of anger?

_____

_____

_____

_____

_____

_____

3) How do you find yourself expressing anger now as an adult? Is it the same style as your parents, or have you been influenced by your partner or other life experiences?

_____

_____

_____

_____

_____

_____

4) What about your work/homemaking/parenting/relationships do you get most angry or frustrated about?

_____

_____

Anger can be dealt with in such a way as to prevent it going deeper as a form of suppressed rage. If we deny, ignore or deflect our anger, there is a very good chance that we have not adequately dealt with the situation which caused the feeling to begin with. The situation is likely to remain the same, or to get worse to the extent that it remains unaddressed.

An important step in changing this pattern is to become aware of it. Use the following chart as a method to help you raise your awareness about anger, and thereby prevent it from being driven deeper into your unconscious where it can just add to your burden of distress.

Summarize the anger	When did it happen?	Source of the anger?	How did you let it go?
e.g. Phone company invoiced me for services I didn't use	Received the invoice yesterday	Phone company	Complained vigorously; demanded the supervisor; worked out how to prove my case. Meditated to calm down; listened to soothing music.
Summarize the anger	When did it happen?	Source of the anger?	How did you let it go?

It is essential that you allow the anger to be there, that you acknowledge the feeling within yourself, and that you take appropriate action about it if possible. Note that expressing anger may at times be entirely appropriate, but at others times getting vigorously angry with a boss or a police officer may simply make things worse for you. You need to exercise some discretion about what level of expression of anger is appropriate to the situation.

If you feel unable to let go of the anger, despite self-soothing activities like meditating, calming music, warm baths, emotionally ventilating or exercising, then you may need to use another approach. Also, if giving more and repeated expression to your anger is simply making things worse for you with your boss, spouse or a Magistrate, then another option is called for.

NLP process for anger reduction

Neuro-Linguistic Programming (NLP), an innovative approach to psychotherapy developed by Richard Bandler and John Grinder in the 1970s,[2] introduced an approach to voluntarily changing the nature of memories in order to reduce their emotional impact. Anger associated with memories can be reduced with this method.

To use this process, sit quietly in a place where you are not likely to be disturbed. Allow yourself to bring up the memory of the experience which produced the excessive anger.

Begin by seeing the situation as you saw it at the time, and take note of how distressing it feels while you are doing this on a scale from 0-10 (0= not at all upsetting, 10= fully upsetting). Once you have recreated the scene in your imagination, begin to change some of the aspects of the memory as per the following suggestions.

- Where you have been seeing the image from a first person perspective (from your own eyes), allow yourself to now see it from the view of a person watching this situation happening to someone else. Once you have achieved this view, again rate how disturbing it feels from 0-10. Then return back to the original first person perspective.

---

[2] Bandler & Grinder (1975). *Patterns of the Hypnotic Techniques of Milton H. Erikson.*

- Next, experiment with altering the brightness of the scene, as though you have a TV remote control. Make the scene brighter as though you have altered it with the remote. Again, gauge how distressing this feels from 0-10. Then, use the remote to make the scene more dull, turning the brightness right down. Rate how upsetting it now feels from 0-10. Then, return the brightness now to how it was initially.

- Alter the color of the scene as though you are turning the color control all the way up. See the other person and the scene in all extreme colors, and rate how upsetting this feels from 0-10. Now, turn the colors all the way down so that the person and the scene becomes black and white. Rate how disturbing this feels from 0-10, and then return it to normal.

- Experiment with bringing the other person in the scene up very close, saying the things they were saying, but this time right in your face. Notice how this feels, and rate the distress from 0-10. Now, have this person move far away, right out of your personal space and way over there in the distance. Rate how this feels from 0-10, and then allow the scene to return to normal.

- Allow the other person in the scene to grow in size, until they become extremely tall. Rate how upsetting this now feels from 0-10. Then, shrink the person down to a very small size, like that of a ten-year-old, and rate how upsetting this feels. Then return them to their normal size again.

- Think of a person, either one you have known, or someone you know of, who represents strength to you. It may be a good friend, or someone who you view as being very powerful in some way. Imagine this person in the scene, there to support you. It could even be a superhero. They may be standing between you and the other person, or perhaps behind you with their hands on your shoulders. When you can see this strong person, rate how disturbing the scene now feels from 0-10. Then allow this person to fade out of the scene.

- Now, think of a comical circus monkey standing on a wooden box behind the other person in the scene. This monkey is imitating perfectly the mannerisms and gestures of the other person who you are angry with. See this monkey imitating all that the other person is doing, and then rate how distressed you feel from 0-10. Then let the monkey fade away from the scene.

- Next, alter some of the auditory aspects of the memory. Turn the other person's volume right up so that their statements are all very loud. Rate how distressing this feels from 0-10. Then, using the remote, turn their volume down very low so that you can barely hear them at all, as though they are whispering. Again, rate how upsetting this now feels from 0-10, then return the volume back to normal.

- Think of a comical cartoon character, and have the other person in this scene now speaking with the character's voice, e.g. Donald Duck or Porky Pig. Have the person saying all the same things, but now with the cartoon character's voice. Tune in to how disturbing this now feels to you from 0-10. Now, allow their voice to return to normal, and again rate the level of distress.

- Finally, see the impacts of different types of self-talk. Imagine the scene while telling yourself negative statements, such as "I can't cope with this," "This is shocking and I can't handle it," etc. As you are doing this, rate how disturbing it feels from 0-10. Then, swap these negative statements for coping statements, e.g. "I don't like it, but I can handle this," "I am strong and resilient," etc. While repeating these statements, rate how upsetting the scene feels from 0-10.

You will find that some of these variations make more of an impact on you than others—everyone is different. Take note of which ones allow you to decrease the level of distress the most, and practice this exercise until you feel that the anger has dissipated. As stated earlier, rather than just using psychological strategies to make you feel better about bad situations (a form of denial and suppression), this type of exercise is best done when you have already tried to address the injustice done to you and you are left with residual and persistent anger, and/or when your vigorous expression of anger is only going to get you into further trouble and make the situation worse for you. Where possible, change the situation you are reacting to as the first option.

Conflicts

Conflicts with others are usually stressful in their own right, and they can be doubly so when they trigger feelings which relate to other episodes from earlier in life. As such, a current conflict can be a clue as to what feelings have been kept in the unconscious for a long time.

1) Have you had any serious conflicts with family members, friends, or work colleagues lately? What are your feelings about the conflict?

_____
_____
_____
_____
_____
_____

2) Has this conflict reminded you of problems that you experienced in previous relationships, e.g. with parents, teachers, siblings, friends?

_____
_____
_____
_____
_____
_____

3) Can you see any relationship between the current conflicts, the old feelings of distress from previous relationship problems, and your pain?

_____

_____

_____

_____

_____

_____

_____

Summary

1) In answering the questions so far, look for examples, both in your recent and distant past, which typify the most important emotions that are highlighted in your answers. Describe how you felt and your reactions to the experiences. Write down the lasting effects which you feel these experiences have had on you.

_____

_____

_____

_____

_____

_____

_____

2) What are the possible connections between these feelings/experiences and your pain? Have you noticed flare-ups or decreases in your pain as you recall, think and write about these experiences and feelings? What do you notice going on in your body as you engage in this process?

_____

_____

_____

_____

_____

_____

_____

3) Now is a good time to reflect on your answers and try to obtain an overview. Review all the questions and answers so far and gauge your sense of how important each issue is to you. Write down the issues that seem to resonate the most with you.

_____

_____

_____

_____

_____

_____

_____

_____

_____

CHAPTER 10

Psychological Trauma & Depression

T‍HE ROLE WHICH PSYCHOLOGICAL TRAUMA plays in the causation of chronic pain has been underappreciated by the mental health and medical professions alike. In order to overcome many chronic pain syndromes, we need to develop a greater understanding of trauma and the role it plays in many people's lives.

As a psychologist in clinical practice, it has become increasingly apparent to me that beneath the many presentations of people complaining of depression and anxiety (often referred to as the "common colds" of mental health problems), not to mention chronic pain, are underlying traumas which remain unaddressed, and consequently unresolved. In fact, I have come to the conclusion that in varying degrees, trauma is so prevalent that it is the best kept secret of our culture.

The medical notion of depression

The cultural discussion of mental health issues in the last twenty-five years has been overly determined by the marketing branches of pharmaceutical companies, which has filtered down to the language and concepts that the medical profession uses in making sense of human distress. As such, the notion of depression (as a "medical" condition, rather than a problem in living) has taken hold. As a result, around 5% of the Australian population are currently on antidepressant drugs, and around 11% of the American population are on them.

Like the flu, depression has become conceptualized as a medical condition which you either have or don't have, rather than an experience that you may pass in and out of at various times in your life (which is a reality for many people).

Add to this, the "illness" of depression is hypothesized as resulting from aberrant brain chemicals, primarily serotonin. The problem is not with the *theory* itself, but that the theory has been promoted to the status of established fact. This has been done not by science, but by the marketing branches of drug companies.[1] When neurologists who study the brain are asked about the evidence for the serotonin theory of depression, they reveal that there is as much evidence to suggest that the problem is too much serotonin as there is evidence suggesting that the problem is not enough serotonin.[2] This is further complicated by the fact that, unlike cholesterol, it is not possible to take a measure of serotonin in a living person. Levels of serotonin can be indirectly inferred from other biological markers; however, they can only be directly measured through analysis of a dead brain. How then can anyone know what is a normal level of serotonin, much less what is an abnormally low or high level?

However, the theory has been very useful in the marketing of antidepressants. If we are convinced to believe that we are depressed because of a too-low level of serotonin, then we may also be convinced to buy SSRI antidepressant drugs. This marketing exercise has been stunningly successful, especially in America where the rates of people on these drugs has increased by around 400% since 1988.[3]

A study recently published in the *Archives of General Psychiatry* reveals that around half of Americans receiving antidepressants aren't even being treated for depression.[4] These people are being prescribed the drugs for issues such as back pain, nerve pain, fatigue, sleep difficulties, or other problems. As stated throughout this book, pharmaceutical solutions to chronic pain problems are of unproven benefit, and most come with a range of potentially serious adverse side effects.

[1] Healy (2004). *Let Them Eat Prozac.*
[2] Kirsch (2010). *The Emperor's New Drugs: Exploding the Antidepressant Myth.*
[3] Lloyd (2011). "Antidepressant Use Skyrockets 400% in Past 20 Years." *USA Today.*
[4] Szabo (2009). "Number of Americans Taking Antidepressants Doubles."

No drug has ever been proven to heal people of either trauma, or of the wounds from bad childhood events, although "forgetting pills" are currently being researched.[5] Rather than have painful memories simply lose their emotional charge, these forgetting-chemicals (PKMzeta inhibitors called zeta-interacting protein, or ZIP for short) could eliminate the memory altogether. There are some very significant moral, ethical, social and political implications for such a venture. Most people would agree that we actually need to have our memories, even of events that were highly distressing. Certainly, for highly traumatized people, especially while they are in a distressed state, some may prefer having the memory wiped-out. However, most people feel a need to know what they have experienced in their lives. Our experiences, both positive and negative, constitute an important part of who we are and lead to the learning of important information about life.

I view my vigilance in road safety as being a useful outcome of nearly being killed in a car accident as an eighteen-year-old, and I have passed this vigilance on to my children. If this traumatic memory had been erased with a drug like ZIP, then it is quite likely that I would have also lost an awareness of the need to remain careful of others on the road. I might also have lost an awareness of the seriousness of trauma, and the need to help people who are suffering from it. It seems hard to imagine an outcome other than *Groundhog Day* with such a forgetting-pill. The use of ZIP in humans could also make it possible for governments to "treat" combat veterans after a battle with the drug, thereby increasing the chances of them signing on for yet another tour of duty. The memory of awful battle experiences probably helps some

---

[5] The protein PKMzeta is highly involved in the memory process. Lehrer (2012) reports on experiments in which rats have been traumatized and then exposed to the alarming stimuli. They naturally show a reluctance to approach the noxious stimuli, however this is overcome when they are injected with a PKMzeta inhibitor, ZIP—then the rats forget that they were ever frightened. Lehrer seems to think this is potentially a great break-through for humanity; however, no consideration is given to the ethical issues or for the considerable differences between rats and humans. Cannaboids and purer strains of the recreational drug Ecstasy are also being trialed with PTSD and are said to be showing promising results. However, the experimental methodology is often poor and the outcomes are contributed to by psychological support which is administered in addition to the drug. This means that it is not the drug alone which is being tested, and the results could be just as attributable to the emotional support.

soldiers to stay alive. The use of such a drug may simply mean that soldiers keep on fighting new battles, until they are killed.

Due to the lack of a viable pharmaceutical agent to ease the emotional pain associated with awful life events, trauma has been largely ignored in the cultural discussion of mental health issues. In fact, it could be argued that our entire culture has been in a state of radical denial in regards to trauma. Instead of focusing on the bad experiences which create depression and anxiety, we discuss these conditions as though they occur in some kind of experiential vacuum. This makes the widespread use of pharmaceuticals appear a sensible option.

There are several extremely viable psychological theories of depression, none of which need view the experience as an illness, nor resort to mythical or correlative chemical imbalances. From a psychological perspective, depression is essentially a persistent low mood (which also entails bodily experiences) that results from "learned helplessness."[6] Learned helplessness is a psychological state of despair which occurs when a person views themselves as being unable to escape a punishing situation or experience, regardless of what they do. Where in the past they may have tried a range of strategies to change their circumstance, these strategies are given up one by one as they are found to be ineffective.

The result is a profound sense of being unable to escape bad circumstances, resulting in helplessness with a negative view of the self, the world in general, and of one's future. These are the psychological precursors to depression, and many chronic pain sufferers can relate to them. Is this an illness in any medical sense, or simply a human tendency in the face of unrelenting bad situations and resultant despair? Those who define depression as an illness generally have a large financial incentive to do so, rather than a scientific incentive—they make huge amounts of money by doing so.

Not everyone who has been traumatized will experience depressed mood to the same degree. Many people who have experienced highly disturbing events are more vulnerable to both an increased frequency, as well as intensity of depressive experiences. Effective therapies for depression usually involve a psychological process of helping a person to restore their sense of being able to create positive change in their lives. Psychologists refer

---

[6]   Seligman (1991). *Learned Optimism.*

to this as self-efficacy. There are many ways of going about doing this, and most psychological approaches appear to be equally effective.

Where trauma is the underlying factor, and depression is one of the "symptoms," trauma focused psychotherapy such as Eye Movement Desensitization and Reprocessing (to be discussed in a chapter 16), Cognitive Control Techniques (see Chapter 11), or exposure therapy are the treatments of choice. Merely talking with a sympathetic counselor about the trauma *may* be helpful, especially if you have had no opportunity in your life to talk to someone about what you have been through. However, there is little research evidence to suggest supportive counseling alone will significantly reduce or eliminate trauma symptoms. People will often appreciate feeling better in the short term, but in the long run, pure "talk therapy" does little for the alleviation of trauma. Instead, trauma focused therapies are required, and these often involve very little talk.

With a greater awareness of trauma and how to heal it, I now rarely see people in my practice who I would primarily conceive of as being depressed or anxious. I see the same type of people, but I no longer make sense of their experience in terms of anxiety or depression, other than as aspects of what is often untreated trauma. These symptoms may very well be part of their experience and presentation, but I don't see much point in thinking of clients in such terms. A focus on depression and anxiety can preclude a focus on the trauma, which is usually underlying their distress. Why focus on a symptom when we really need to address the root cause?

The study of trauma

Prior to the social and cultural changes of the 1960s and '70s, people rarely spoke about their traumas. It was clear that many World War I and World War II veterans were highly traumatized by their combat experiences; however, this was rarely ever discussed openly. Vietnam veterans returned to a society that was equivocal about their war service, and at times actively hostile. But because of the social changes that were happening at the time, they also returned to what was becoming a more open culture.

Despite the misdirected anger metered out to them by parts of the protest movement, our culture in general become more interested in discussing people's experiences and distress. The stoicism associated with the Victorian stiff upper lip as a cultural ideal was in decline, challenged by social changes such as the "counter-culture," the women's movement, and the civil rights movement.

It took many years before the Vietnam veterans were actually encouraged to talk of their experiences and to share their pain. Society first had to recognize the damage which blaming the young soldiers for the political wrongs of the Vietnam War had caused. But their trauma, perhaps added to by the societal rejection they experienced, was so extreme and widespread that it was undeniable. More American Vietnam veterans have committed suicide (100,000 or more) than were killed in the war (approximately 58,000 in Vietnam). [7] It was in this context that the formal study of trauma became a more serious academic endeavor.

Samples of Vietnam veterans suffering from Post Traumatic Stress Disorder (PTSD) have been studied in great detail. One of the prevailing conclusions is that the experience of terrible combat was generally not enough for a person to wind up with PTSD. In fact, around 80-85% of men who experienced combat did not suffer PTSD in an ongoing sense. The vast majority of them remained in a highly emotional state after the battle, experiencing a mix of emotions including anger, shock, fear, hyper-vigilance, anxiety, etc. For the majority of them, this response settled down over the course of weeks and months, even though they may never have returned to base-line levels. Many veterans would still agree that life has never been the same since, and they struggle to view themselves or the world in the ways they did before combat. However, most of them managed to somewhat settle down emotionally over time.

The remaining 15-20%, however, did not succeed in this settling down process. These men remained as emotionally affected for months and years after the event as they had in the days immediately following combat experience. They report to having regular flashbacks of the distressing scenes, nightmares and obtrusive thoughts about the incidences, heightened physiological arousal for much of the time, and an overactive startle response. Their distress is easily triggered by stimuli such as sounds

---

[7]   Over 100,000 US Vietnam Vet Suicides To Date! http://rense.com/general77/
       hdtage.htm

or sights associated with their military service. They generally try to avoid such triggers, as they are unable to manage their responses to them. They will often seek to self-medicate the emotional pain and heightened responses with alcohol and other drugs. Many of them become reliant upon substances in order to just "cope."

Research also indicated that the factors which distinguished between those who did wind up with PTSD from those who did not were not just the nature of their combat experiences. Two soldiers, shoulder to shoulder in the same fire-fight, could experience radically different responses in the months and years that followed.

It appears that the distinguishing feature was the amount of trauma which the soldier had *already* experienced as a child and adolescent. If he was highly upset from negative events in his life (e.g. parents separating, domestic violence, abuse, sibling or parent dying), then his "distress-cup" was already relatively full by the time he experienced combat. If a soldier had experienced a relatively trouble-free childhood and teenage years, then his distress-cup was relatively empty when he arrived in Vietnam.

When experiencing combat, all soldiers' cups received a fill-up of distress. For those who were already traumatized young men, the level of distress reached such a point that they were simply overwhelmed. Those who were up to that time relatively un-traumatized soldiers were also highly distressed from combat, but it did not reach this overwhelm point—they managed to recover better over time. As such, they were more able to settle down in the weeks and months following the combat experiences. From this, the importance of early childhood and adolescent upsets can be seen.

The effects of early trauma can also be seen in the brain. Researchers at the Anna Freud Center in London have recently examined the brain effects of trauma on children who have experienced physical abuse and domestic violence.[8] The functional MRI (fMRI) scans of a sample of children (average age of twelve) who had been referred to protective services were compared with children who had not experienced abuse or family violence. The results showed that two brain areas of the traumatized children were highly active when they were exposed to pictures of angry faces. This pattern of activation,

---

[8] McCory, et al (2011). "Heightened Neural Reactivity to Threat in Child Victims of Family Violence." *Current Biology*.

in the anterior insular and the amygdala, was not seen in the children with no history of violence. The researchers noted that the pattern of brain activation seen in the traumatized children was actually similar to that seen in soldiers who had been exposed to violent combat situations. Both groups show brain activity which is typical of people who are hyper-aware of danger in their environment, and this factor is highly related to the subsequent development of significant problems with anxiety.

It is common for people with chronic pain to have experienced some form of trauma in their childhood or adolescence. The relationship between trauma and psychosomatic pain is even evident during childhood.[9] Swedish researchers have found that physically abused children are more than twice as likely to exhibit symptoms which are viewed as psychosomatic, such as stomach ache, headache, sleeplessness, dizziness, and back pain. These traumatized children grow up to become adults who are carrying a large burden of distress within them, and thus a higher likelihood of chronic pain.

The amygdala memories (covert recollections) referred to in Chapter 7, can produce a physical reminiscence or "body memory," resulting in the physiological body state that arose with the original experience, complete with racing heart and sweaty palms. At its extreme, these memories can, if burnt into the amygdala with enough force, trigger such dramatic bodily reactions that a person re-experiences the terrible event with full sensory replay. As far as their mind and body are concerned, they are back in combat again.

Understandably, most survivors of abuse and trauma have a very strong goal to overcome their adversity and to be more than just a perpetual victim. This resilience is an entirely admirable quality and demonstrates their personal strength. However, in this desire to overcome are often the seeds to deny self-doubts, terrifying fears, and debilitating beliefs about the self and the world in general. The observation of over a hundred years of depth-psychology is that just because we deny the existence of such fears, feelings and beliefs, it does not mean they don't exist. Such feelings do not

---

[9] Jernbro et al (2012). "Multiple Psychosomatic Symptoms Can Indicate Child Physical Abuse—Results from a Study of Swedish Schoolchildren. *Acta Paediatrica. Current Biology.*

easily go away with denial. Survivors of trauma and abuse are perhaps more vulnerable to denying the existence of these thoughts and feelings, as for them the stakes are very high. The fear is that giving in to them could mean psychological collapse, with potentially catastrophic consequences. No wonder their mind/brain wants to keep it from their conscious awareness.

The traumatic experience itself may not be the material that needs to be worked with in psychotherapy. It may be the *implications* of the experience— the meaning which the experience has for them, such as "I am a bad person because ____ happened." In such cases, I would highly recommend contact with a competent psychotherapist to assist with delving into the meaning of traumatic experiences in your life, and then stimulating your innate ability to adaptively process the experiences. As this can be very difficult and emotionally demanding work, it is unlikely that you will be able to undertake it on your own without the assistance of a capable psychotherapist who is trained in effective means of helping you to resolve these issues. Where you are less overwhelmed by the ongoing implications of the trauma, but suffer more from the bad memories, then self-help strategies (described later in this chapter) can be quite useful. Seek advice if you are not sure on the need for professional help.

Traumatic life events can often reverberate within us for many years afterwards, and can be associated with deep levels of distress. I am often astonished in counseling when clients casually tell me of terrible life events, and then genuinely wonder whether these may have had some impact on them. They will usually state that other people have been through so many worse experiences, so they think it is unlikely that the violent death of a family member, or sustained sexual or physical abuse is likely to have made much of an impact on them.

Think of your own experiences as though someone who you care about is telling you that these happened to them. In such a case, would you be more likely to recognize the damaging effects if you were hearing it from someone else, say a child? If so, then also consider the potential damage which these experiences could have had on you.

Thinking of significant events in your life (like major crises or losses) that keep "repeating" within you, to such an extent that they still feel current in some way, is a step towards healing. Some additional self-analysis questions are important in helping you to address traumas.

Dr Nancy Selfridge, in *Freedom from Fibromyalgia*, offers the following way of plotting these events.[10] These charts can help you develop more awareness about the impact of significant events in your life, and their possible relationship to chronic pain.

Historical Record of My Key Milestones

Event	Month	Year	Emotional Impact 0 = most pain 10 = most pleasure
Earliest event I can recall			
Leaving high school			
Completing university or other training			
Marriage(s)			
Birth(s)			
Separation/divorce(s)			
Death of father/grandfather			
Death of mother/grandmother			
Death of sibling/friend (name)			
Death of significant other person(s)			
Highly negative event in my life (not stated elsewhere)			
Highly negative event in my family (not stated elsewhere)			
Chronic pain probably started			
Diagnosis of _____ was made			
Major accident(s) or trauma(s) involving me (name the event)			

---

[10] Selfridge & Peterson (2001). *Freedom from Fibromyalgia.*

Major accident(s) or trauma(s) involving family members (name and event)			
Major illnesses			
Major illnesses of family members			
Start of major jobs			
End of major jobs			
Being fired from jobs			

If you are still struggling to get a sense of traumas which you have experienced in your life, try the "Floatback" exercise, as described by psychologist Dr Francine Shapiro.[11]

1. Think of a recent event which you found emotionally distressing.

2. As you "tune into" the experience, become aware of the negative thought or belief about yourself which this experience brings up. Typically, such negative self-beliefs will involve at least one of the following:

   - issues of responsibility ("I did something wrong"; "There is something wrong with me") or
   - lack of safety ("I am in danger"; "I cannot trust anyone") or
   - lack of control/power ("I am helpless"; "I have no control").

3. As you think of the recent incident and the negative self-belief, notice the feelings in your body. Where do you feel the distress? e.g. in the shoulders, or neck, or stomach, or chest, or throat, etc.

---

[11] Shapiro (2012). *Getting Past Your Past: Take Control of Your Life with Self-Help Techniques from EMDR Therapy.*

4. As you hold this awareness, allow your mind to float back to earlier years, such as your childhood, adolescence or early adulthood. What memories come to mind of when you felt that way before?

5. If earlier experiences come to mind, write them down in the chart above, and include the negative self-belief as well as the emotional impact.

The next step is to take the emotionally significant events from your Milestones chart and enter them onto the following Chronic Pain Timeline chart in chronological order. Remember, even positive or pleasurable events can stimulate chronic pain as a result of the "flip side of the coin" phenomenon discussed earlier.

Chronic Pain Timeline

Event & emotional reaction:	Month	Year	Emotional Impact 0= most pain 10= most pleasure

Once you become more aware of traumatic experiences, the question is what can be done with them? Are we simply "stuck" with the reverberations of past traumatic events? It is important to note that humans appear to have an innate capacity to process and digest upsetting experiences. Although we are rarely aware of it, this capacity represents much of our natural self-healing ability, as will be revealed in the next chapter.

CHAPTER 11

The Healing Power of Dreams

RESEARCH RECENTLY REPORTED IN THE journal *Current Biology* indicates that the dream stage of sleep provides us with a form of "overnight psychotherapy" in that it allows our mind/brain to process or sort out experiences.[1] While we are dreaming, the normal stress reaction that goes with upsetting memories and associated stress chemicals are suppressed. This allows our brains to reactivate, put in perspective and integrate pleasant as well as disturbing experiences, largely without the interference of normal stress hormones that often make upsetting memories overwhelming. As such, the distressing aspects of the experience can be processed while we sleep so that it can lose some of its negative emotional impact on us.

When we sleep, our brainwaves move through regular cycles of measurable electrical activity. During a normal night of undisturbed sleep, we cycle through four stages of sleep in which distinctly different brain wave patterns can be measured by electroencephalographs (EEGs).

From being fully awake, our brain enters a state of transition in stage one, during which we are somewhere between wakefulness and sleep. During this stage, our brain waves are of low voltage as measured by EEGs. On an EEG graph, the brain waves look like small ocean waves with little space in between them. Stage two of sleep, in which we spend around half of each night, is characterized by theta brain waves. Both stages one and two are referred to as shallow sleep, with relatively fast brain waves being observed.

---

[1] Van der Helm et al (2011). "REM Sleep Depoentiates Amygdala Activity to Previous Emotional Experiences." *Current Biology*.

Your brain slows to delta waves as you sink deeper into stages three and four of sleep, with stage four being characterized by very slow and high voltage brain waves. If these were ocean waves, they would look like large waves with big spaces in between them.

When in these deeper stages of sleep, it appears that restoration of both the immune and the energy systems is occurring.[2] With this decrease in activity, the brain is simply "idling" rather than working at full speed, and very little limbic area or emotional activity is happening. As such, resting the brain during stages three and four is a necessary function to allow energy to rebuild. During the slower stages of sleep, there is a corresponding decrease in heart rate, blood pressure and respiration.

After some time in stage four, our brain enters a stage of sleep in which most dreaming occurs. Dreaming is associated with a set of brain activities which are quite different to non-dream sleep. Firstly, the visual association cortex becomes highly active as we see things happening in our dreams. The anterior cingulate also shows heightened activity. If a dream is frightening, as in a nightmare, activity in the amygdala becomes observable. The hippocampus, highly involved in memory, becomes active as our mind/brain replays recent events. The pathways which carry alerting signals from the brainstem and auditory processing areas of the brain become active. All this occurs while activity is radically *decreased* in the reality testing and thinking pre-frontal cortex.

The consistent observation of people who are dreaming is that their eyes move rapidly back and forth. As such, the dream stage of sleep is referred to as rapid-eye-movement, or REM sleep. While dreams do occur in the other stages of sleep, it is during REM sleep that our dream-life is most active. The few dreams that occur in the other stages of sleep tend to have no real story line, are less emotional and have less of a visual content. Whereas the dreams that occur during REM sleep generally have a story line, are often emotionally charged and are more easily recalled.

The brain is highly active during REM sleep, as evidenced by the low voltage and fast brain waves—looking like small ocean waves with little space in between them. At times, our dreaming brain is even more active than when we are awake. As an indicator of the amount of activity associated

---

[2] Arden (2010). *Rewire Your Brain.*

with dreaming, our brain uses more oxygen during REM sleep than it does when we are either physically or mentally exercising.[3] Even though it constitutes only around 3% of body weight, the brain consumes around 25% of the body's energy, so what the brain is doing while we dream is highly relevant for the entire body. Heart rate, blood pressure, respiration and oxygen consumption are all elevated during REM sleep—this is the pattern of arousal seen when we are in a state of "fight or flight" (see Chapter 14). As is the case with the hyper-aroused fight-or-flight state, rather than having a great deal of involvement from the thinking cortex, our emotional limbic system is highly active while we are dreaming.

Despite this high level of activity, similar to that seen when we are awake, we are actually in the *deepest* stage of sleep when we dream. As such, REM sleep is often referred to as "paradoxical" sleep—both highly active *and* deeply asleep.

Over the course of a night, the initial stages of REM sleep are generally quite short, but as the night progresses, seeing us go through five to seven of these cycles, the stages of REM get progressively longer. Our brain tends to repeat this cycle around every ninety minutes. Overall, REM sleep amounts to around 25% of time spent asleep in healthy adults—about two hours of each night spent asleep.

The emotional limbic system, as well as areas involved in memory and sensory processing, can be busier while we are dreaming than when we are awake. Whilst awake, the limbic areas are active, as are parts of the midbrain-brainstem junction, which take messages directly to the cortex (this allows our rational thinking brain to be involved as well). Both of these brain areas wind down during the earlier slower stages of sleep. But while we are dreaming, the pathway between the pons and medulla (in the brainstem) to the cortex becomes *deactivated*, and only the limbic area remains highly active. As such, the neo-cortex can exercise less control over the dream than does the emotional limbic system.

With the inhibiting functions of the frontal cortex becoming inactive, the "brakes" that are usually applied to control our emotions are taken off, allowing our emotional and imaginative brain to have a free reign

---

[3] Norden (2007). *Understanding the Brain: Course Guidebook.*

in the context of the dream.[4] This is why dreams can be so bizarre and outlandish—no reality check from the frontal cortex is operating. As such we can often fly in dreams or breath under water, with no voice saying, "Hang on—you are going to die if you jump off that cliff!" However, the neo-cortex must still be playing some important role, as REM sleep occurs only in mammals that have a neo-cortex. The limbic areas that remain highly active during REM sleep also connect to the cortex via a structure called the thalamus, even though the more direct route to the cortex is turned off.

There are many different theories about what is happening when we dream, most of which have some kind of evidence in their support. Despite the various theories, it is apparent that dreams result from a combination of sensory input occurring while we are asleep; some images generated from random fluctuations in electrical activity in the brain; as yet undigested aspects of that days experiences; and the reprocessing of memories that are still needing some kind of consolidation.[5]

This consolidation involves the processing of lessons learnt during the day, wishes, and vital survival information, all culminating in the formation of long-term memories. Some evidence suggests that the consolidation process can take up to three years to complete.[6] Experiences are reviewed by the brain and linked in with other useful information that is relevant to the issue being processed. As a result, our brain is able to take a negative experience with our boss that day, link it up with other experiences with the boss in which we saw him rip into other employees, and allow us to conclude that this is a reflection of his management style. The emotional distress which we felt from being spoken to harshly by her can be released, as we are now able to depersonalize the altercation, realizing that the altercation says more about her than about us. This is the psychological digestive process, so essential for our emotional well-being that dreams appear to facilitate for us.

---

[4] Sapolsky (2004). *Why Zebras Don't Get Ulcers.*
[5] Siegel (2011). *Mindsight: The New Science of Personal Transformation.*
[6] Takashima et al (2006) "Declarative memory consolidation in humans". *Proceedings of the National Academy of Sciences.*

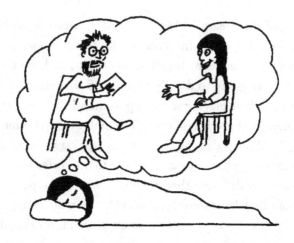

Dreaming- our nightly psychotherapy session

Through many years of creative studies, sleep researchers have concluded that while we are dreaming, our mind/brain is highly active in reviewing and sorting out such experiences. Part of this process entails deciding where things need to go—integrated in a storage process, or tossed out as less useful information? Dreams are our mind/brain's vehicle for such transferring and integration of information into existing memory networks, and letting go of less useful information. During dreams, there are often discoveries of new and valuable associations between older memories—this would explain the creative outcomes of dreams which geniuses often describe.

William Dement, now at Stanford University School of Medicine, conducted groundbreaking research in 1960 in which subjects were awakened every time they entered REM sleep. Over the course of the study, they were permitted to get all the stages—two, three and four—sleep that they wanted, but every time they began to dream, they were woken up. During the course of the study, subjects were also put through a range of learning experiments. They were given, for example a list of words to remember and then recall the next day and puzzles to solve.

When people are deprived of REM sleep, they are unable to learn and integrate new information as well as they can when getting adequate REM sleep. When another group of subjects are allowed to get all the REM sleep they need, but are woken up whenever they are in stages two, three or four of sleep, they tend not to lose their cognitive functions to the same extent.

While no doubt getting sick of being regularly woken up, they don't lose their emotional stability, as the REM deprived subjects tend to. Not surprisingly, studies also demonstrate that REM sleep alleviates depressed mood, such that a decreased amount of REM sleep makes us more vulnerable to mood problems.

More recent researchers report similar findings to Dement's.[7] Subjects who undertake a puzzle on two occasions, each time a week apart, are able to perform better on the puzzle the second time as a result of having "digested" some of the implicit strategies of the task. One group of subjects are given alcohol the night of doing the puzzle for the first time. As alcohol inhibits REM sleep, these people show no improvement in their puzzle performance a week later. This indicates that the lack of REM sleep interferes with natural digesting of the winning strategies—these subjects failed to learn the gist of the puzzle from their previous experience.

In addition, subjects who are deprived of REM sleep over the course of several days generally show a deteriorating emotional state with increasing anxiety, irritability and difficulty concentrating. Research has also demonstrated that the ability of stem cells to grow and become new brain cells is also compromised as a result of sleep deprivation.[8] There is not a lot to be said for a lack of sleep or dreaming.

Both long-past experiences and those of the most recent day are reactivated during REM sleep so that they can then be consolidated into existing meaning structures. Less than useful elements can be discarded, while important pieces of information can be processed to form long-term memories. Fear about situations that are no longer occurring, or childhood guilt from a lack of mature understanding could be viewed as less than useful elements of past experiences which dreams are able to help us discard. Computer oriented people will see the analogy between what our brain does whilst we dream and the "defragging" of computers—eliminating all that is unnecessary for efficient processing of information.

When considering the findings of sleep research, it could be said that dreams represent our specie's innate capacity for the psychological digestion

---

[7] Stickgold (2008). "Sleep-Dependent Memory Processing and EMDR Action." *Journal of EMDR Practice and Research.*

[8] Arden (2010). *Rewire Your Brain.*

of experience, thus their "psychotherapeutic" nature. If we fail to partake of this digestive process, emotional and psychological problems result. It appears that this is as essential for our emotional well-being as is the digestive process of food for our physical well-being. To the extent that either form of digestion breaks down, we suffer, either physically or psychologically, and usually both.

Unfortunately, our culture is chronically deprived of adequate dreaming due to the ingestion of substances which interfere with this process. The average Australian consumes around 15 standard alcoholic drinks per week. Americans are amongst the lowest consumers of alcohol in the developed world, while British people and Europeans consume around the most. Only around two standard alcoholic drinks per night are required to interfere with REM sleep. In addition, commonly prescribed antidepressants, more used in America than elsewhere, also interfere with our ability to dream. The MAO inhibitors (such as Isocarboxazid (Marplan), Phenelzine (Nardil), Tranylcypromine (Parnate), Selegeline (Emsam or Selgine) block almost all REM sleep; Tricyclic antidepressants (such as amitriptyline (Anafranil, Endep), desipramine (Norpramin), doxepin, imipramine,(Tofranil, Tofranil-PM), maprotiline, nortriptyline (Pamelor), protriptyline (Vivactil), trimipramine (Surmontil) block around half of REM sleep; while SSRI antidepressants (such as fluoxetine (Prozac, Lovan), venlafaxine (Effexor), paroxetine (Paxil, Seroxat, Aropax),sertraline (Zoloft, Lustral), citalopram (Celexa, Cipramil, Celopram), escitalopram (Lexapro, Cipralex, Lexapro), fluvoxamine (Luvox, Faverin) block around a third of REM sleep.

As the term REM suggests, while we dream our eyes move rapidly back and forth. It is also noted that when we access either memories or feelings, our eyes tend to move to the side. There appears to be something highly pertinent about the movement of our eyes to the processing of experience, memories and feelings. Several highly sophisticated neurological theories have been developed to account for this relationship, however, the fine details of these need not concern us here.[9]

David Mamet, a playwright with a depth-psychology bent, compares our capacity to dream with the psychological aspects of theatre. He states

9   Stickgold (2002). "EMDR: A Putative Mechanism for Action." *Journal of Clinical Psychology.*

that, "In dreams we do not seek answers which our conscious (rational) mind is capable of supplying, we seek answers to those questions which the conscious mind is incompetent to deal with."[10] In other words, we (as our conscious mind) are quite capable of dealing with many of the difficulties which come our way. These generally do not constitute the deep, conflicted difficulties which give rise to the Hidden Psychology of Pain. Comparing our own inner dramas while asleep with theatrical drama on stage, Mamet goes on to say that, "Only if the question posed is one whose complexity and depth renders it unsusceptible to rational examination does the dramatic treatment seem to us appropriate, and the dramatic solution become enlightening."

It is ironic that psycho-philosophy in theatre is more aware of the healing power of dreams to arrive at solutions to seemingly un-resolvable psychological problems than is much of contemporary psychology. Mamet can obviously recognize that dreams are our own internal theatre in which we are the main actors and our unconscious is the playwright, director and producer, utilized for the solving of deep and perplexing problems.

Although our mind/brain is attempting to process experience while we are dreaming, this is rarely apparent to us. Firstly, most of us don't remember too many of our dreams. But, it is a mistake to think that just because we don't remember our dreams we do not dream at all. If we sleep well, we typically just don't remember much of what was going on while we dreamt, other than the dreams we had immediately prior to waking. Most other dreams are lost to our conscious recall, unless we happen to wake up and take note of them either mentally or with pen and paper.

Substances that affect the brain, both illicit and prescription drugs, also affect our ability to obtain REM sleep. It is possible that some people will have less REM sleep than others if they are regularly taking drugs, including alcohol, cannabis, and prescription psychiatric drugs.

The other obscuring feature of our dream life is that they are usually in a highly symbolic form, so much so that we may not be able to make immediate sense of them even when they can be recalled. A child who is being bullied at school may dream about being chased by a pack of wild wolves through a forest rather than have a literal dream about the school

---

[10] Mamet (1986 p8). *Writing in Restaurants.*

bullies. It is likely that he will wake up in a nightmare, and not associate it with his actual experience.

I remember, as a small child, having a recurring nightmare of being chased around suburban streets by large farm trucks with no drivers. Having never had this experience in real life, it must have been symbolic of other things that were happening at the time—possibly a fear of being punished, with the associated feelings of helplessness and powerlessness. I recently had a dream of being in the central business district of a city when a huge dinosaur was terrorizing and killing everyone in sight. As I have never had an experience remotely like this, it must also have been highly symbolic of something else.

When I was first studying psychology in the early 1980s, it was suggested in text books at the time that dreams were just the result of random electrical activity in the brain as an attempt to explain their often bizarre nature. I found this explanation highly unlikely. So many of my dreams seemed emotionally relevant to my life, even if I could not immediately pinpoint their exact meaning. The emotions which they generate are entirely real, and the dreams often relate to important issues in my life.

The fact that my dinosaur dream happened the night after I had spent an entire day (8:30 a.m.-11:00 p.m.) grappling with the huge task of organizing several thousand family photos into new albums was not unrelated to the dream. It was a painful and laborious task. Every time I thought I had the chronological order of the photos worked out and in their albums, I would discover another batch of photos and have to start the whole process again. What do old family photos and dinosaurs have in common? They are both history, and I was grappling with both—perhaps the dinosaur was symbolic of history, which for me was proving to be very difficult.

The view that dreams represent no more than random electrical activity could only be proposed by people who have never remembered any of their emotionally significant ones. Most normal people are generally able to see the relevance of at least some of their nocturnal dramas. As stated above, while dreaming, the limbic region will usually be highly active. If we are dreaming about something unpleasant or threatening, this can be associated with feelings of anger which go with fight, the anxiety associated with flight, or the despair associated with freezing.

In order to prevent an extreme level of disturbance while we are dreaming about bad events in our life, which would probably result in waking, the secretion of stress-hormone noreadrenaline (norepinehphrine) is suppressed while we dream.[11] This chemical alteration associated with REM sleep creates a chemically safe environment in which our mind/brain is more able to reactivate distressing memories in order to re-process and integrate them without being overwhelmed by stress hormones. If the dream is so upsetting or frightening, it seems that this chemical suppression of the stress response is not enough to prevent a high level of disturbance, and you may still wake up in the middle of a nightmare.

I had a client whose dream demonstrated these points perfectly. He told me that he had been beaten up a couple of times in the previous few years by an obviously sociopathic neighbor. The neighbor was involved in criminal activities, and had guns and savage dogs to assist him. He told my client that if he went to the police, he would kill both him and his children and would burn down his house to destroy the evidence. My client was so terrified by this man that the intimidation worked and he lived in fear for several years, unable to take appropriate action.

He reported that prior to us meeting, he had a dream one night in which he saw the neighbor coming towards him in an aggressive and abusive manner. My client, a man who was not at all violent, told his neighbor to go away and leave him alone. The neighbor kept advancing towards him, unperturbed. My client grabbed the man's arm, threw him over his shoulder in a judo move, pinned him down on the ground and shouted at him to go away and to never bother him again. The neighbor got up and ran back to his own house, after which the dream ended. My client woke up feeling very different about the entire situation.

Being nonviolent, he was not going to attempt this stunt in reality. However, he reported to no longer feeling intimidated. He simply knew that if there was another threatening incident he would just call the police and report this man's activities. This solution had always been available, however due to his distressed emotions, he could not access it. Any time he thought of the situation he had been overwhelmed with fear and his mental processing

---

[11] Van der Helm et al (2011). "REM Sleep Depoentiates Amygdala Activity to Previous Emotional Experiences." *Current Biology.*

got no further. As a result of the dream taking him through stages of fear and anxiety, and then anger resulting in winning a physical altercation, my client was no longer intimidated. The solution, which had been there all along, presented itself as a realistic option—just call the police.

It is likely that during the course of the dream, his secretion of stress hormones was suppressed, allowing his mind/brain to continue with the dream without being overwhelmed by fear and anxiety. Also, because his neo-cortex was deactivated in the course of the dream, the thinking part of his brain that would otherwise say, "Hang on—if you try to throw him over your shoulder, he'll kill you!" was not active. Instead, no reality check was operating. As a result, he was able to go through the entire dream and have it arrive at a point where he no longer felt frightened or intimidated by his neighbor.

The above is an excellent example of the power that dreams have in solving our emotional problems. It is a built-in function which aids in our emotional well-being and makes sense of the reports of people deteriorating in their cognitive and emotional faculties when they are deprived of REM sleep.

One of the astonishing things about the healing power of dreams is the fact that most of us, most of the time, are completely unaware that this is happening at all. Nevertheless, it is occurring for most of us each night, and is one of the keys to our psychological functioning and well-being. Even for people who are still carrying trauma from a distressing incident, if they are managing to function in any manner at all, it is probably because their mind/brain is still able to make sense of some of their experiences and sort through them each night while they are sleeping—filing away what they do need to keep, and expelling what they no longer need in this psychological digestive process.

Clearly, this remarkable function does not work equally well for all people all the time. The fact that there are people who remain carrying significant traumas, as evidenced both by their emotional and physical symptoms, is an indicator that this process is capable of failing or at least under-functioning. If the mind/brain feels the need to create a physical pain to take attention away from unresolved emotional pain then clearly this sorting process has not worked thoroughly enough. The pain is there because this emotional digestion has not worked and you are experiencing the "repeating" of upset in a similar way to indigestion of food—thus the need for your mind/brain to generate pain as a distraction. Where you are not aware of the distressed emotions, as these are operating at a less than conscious level, chronic pain is a fairly good indicator that such distressed emotions do in fact exist.

What could be going wrong with this built-in emotional digestive process? As stated, while the electrical activity associated with distress in a dream is located in the limbic system areas, the person in the dream will experiences the very real associated emotions. If the dream is an attempt to digest a traumatic event which actually occurred, then the distressed emotions which are activated can be so intense that the dream simply becomes a nightmare from which the person awakes in a frightened state. When this happens, the digestive process, which the dream is, has stopped and any chance of processing that distress has stopped with it. The distress remains in an undigested state within the person's neurological system. It therefore keeps on reverberating or repeating on them in the form of emotional upset and/or chronic physical pain.

The presence of PTSD is associated with increases of stress hormones, such as adrenaline and noreadrenaline (epinephrine and norepinephrine). This is seen in sufferers of PTSD both while they are awake as well as when they are asleep.[12] The normal dream-state suppression of noreadrenaline, seen in most people while they are dreaming, does not seem to operate as well in people suffering from PTSD. As such, these people are more likely to show a greater stress-response while they are dreaming and therefore are more likely to be woken up in the middle of extreme nightmares. For them, the softening of the upset associated with the memory has not been sufficient.

This failure of the noreadrenaline (norepinephrine) suppression function during the sleep of PTSD sufferers interferes with the integrative processes which the mind/brain usually engages in during REM sleep. Brain imaging research shows that the parts of the brain activated during REM sleep are also the same parts of the brain that are highly active PTSD

---

[12] Carter (2010). *Mapping the Mind.*

sufferers.[13] As various brain structures are not able to perform their usual roles required for integration and processing of traumatic memories, the innate psychological digestive system stops working. This is one of the reasons why PTSD sufferers struggle to "get over" their trauma.

Where people have repeated nightmares, it would seem that the mind/brain is repeatedly attempting to deal with or process the distress. However, this function keeps on failing due to the person being woken up by extreme distress in the dream. Of course, repeated nightmares are one of the hallmarks of PTSD. They are usually reported by people that have been traumatized in harrowing experiences such as combat, severe car accidents or crimes of violence.

Children are especially susceptible to blockages in reprocessing while dreaming. As small people with little social power, few life experiences or coping resources to draw upon, they are easily overwhelmed by the negativity of a bad situation or experience. What you could cope with as a fifteen-year-old is generally a whole lot more than what you could cope with as a five-year-old; and what you could cope with as a twenty-five-year-old is again more than what you could cope with as a fifteen-year-old. Some children are simply born more sensitive compared to others, and as such are more likely to be frightened and highly anxious from negative experiences.

Most children, having very limited coping resources are more easily swamped by distress, resulting in higher secretions of associated stress hormones when awake *and* asleep. This means that when their mind/brain is trying to deal with difficult emotions from a bad experience in the course of a dream, it is more likely that they will not be able to cope with the upsets that are experienced in the dream and will subsequently wake up with a nightmare. As a result, it is not uncommon for people to be carrying undigested emotional distress with them well into their adulthoods from experiences that they had as children. Where these experiences and related feelings would be extremely difficult to cope with on a conscious level, our mind/brain is likely to employ defense mechanisms to ensure that they remain below the surface.

---

[13] Stickgold (2002). "Sleep-Dependent Memory Processing and EMDR Action." *Journal of Clinical Psychology.*

Notwithstanding failed attempts in nightmares, our capacity to dream generally has such power to resolve emotional problems that the solution seems relatively simple—just program ourselves to dream about particular experiences and let our unconscious do the rest while we sleep. While possible, it is rarely that simple. Although we may never be able to have total control over dreams, it is possible with concerted effort to harness their healing potentials.

In using any self-help strategy to assist with trauma, it is important to recognize both the possible benefits and limitations. The processes described below may prove helpful if you do not feel overwhelmed by the difficult memories which you may address. If you do feel overwhelmed by distress when thinking about the bad experiences, it is likely that you will need additional help and should seek it from a psychologist or psychotherapist who is experienced in dealing with trauma.

Also, keep in mind that simply using techniques from a book takes them out of the helping context which you would experience were you to see a psychologist. There are many useful aspects of seeing a psychologist such as "normalizing" your experience, especially important when people think that they are the only one experiencing the reaction. Psycho-education about human responses to traumatic events is very useful for most people. If we can understand what is happening, it tends to be less bewildering and frightening. Other humans are able to provide much needed reassurance and support which no book or computer program is able to. As such, what is being presented throughout this book is not intended as an alternative to seeking professional help. It is likely to be useful for many people whose psychological suffering is not at the extreme end of the continuum, and as a potential adjunct to therapy which you may seek if your distress is at the extreme end.

Healing emotions with dream awareness

Dr Nancy Selfridge describes a set of dream-work procedures which often help to reduce the pain associated with fibromyalgia.[14] With effort, these

---

[14] Selfridge & Peterson (2001). *Freedom from Fibromyalgia.*

strategies allow us to firstly gain some insight into dreams, and secondly, to harness their healing capacities. This approach offers the possibility of actively engaging in the mind/brain's natural healing capacity as described above. As emotional distress can be a causal factor in the experience of chronic pain, it follows that healing work with dreams can also have implications for the healing of chronic pain.

The initial discipline with this method is training yourself to remember your dreams. This will require your willingness to record the main aspects of each night's nocturnal adventures. If you embark on this process, you will need to write down key episodes of dreams each time you wake up, regardless of the time of night. The discipline involved in this can put a lot of people off immediately, however, it may prove a very helpful part in your recovery if you persevere with it.

Place a pen and paper on your bedside table and decide to record each of the dreams you remember whenever you wake up. Make a commitment to yourself, prior to falling asleep each night, that you will try to remember each of your dreams. Each time you wake up, spend a little time reviewing the dream while you lie still, and then write down any element which you can remember. Include details about people, places, situations and the emotions felt.

If this is not done until the next morning, we tend to forget the contents of dreams as new ones occur during the night, and wake-state experiences begin to compete with memories of dreams. If you can't remember the exact contents of the dream, try just imagining what it was about, and there is a reasonable chance that you won't be far from the mark as long as you do this upon waking. If all you can remember are only fragments of the dream, try thinking of those fragments as you go to sleep the next night. People often report that they are then able to remember the dream in more detail within a few minutes of falling asleep.

With practice, you will become better at remembering your dreams within a relatively short time. Many people will experience a sense of emotional relief simply from training themselves to be more aware of their dreams and remembering them. It may be that as we become more conscious of what is going on in our dream state, the emotional pressure that can drive chronic pain is finding another outlet for expression. By remembering dreams, we are becoming more conscious of material that had until that time been primarily unconscious. Allowing this to happen gives the mind/brain the message that we can actually cope with allowing unconscious material into our conscious awareness. No emotional "meltdown" occurs, and the protective pain is not actually necessary.

Learning to remember and write down dreams can lessen the distressed emotions which are responsible for both upsetting dreams and pain. It is also possible that you will see the healing work of dreams in action, and this can dissipate upset emotions as well. Anything which reduces deep emotional distress is likely to have a positive impact on your experience of pain, as well as on your ability to cope.

You may need to think creatively about the symbolism inherent in your dreams. Some of your dreams will be quite literal, but many will be symbolic representations of other experiences which may or may not be readily apparent. Try to look for what the dream is representing, and use the emotions which are generated in the dreams as a clue. Threatening dinosaurs and driverless trucks, for example, are likely to be symbolic representations of something else. Try having a 'conversation' with an object from the dream which calls your attention to it. Why is it there, and what is its purpose?

People will often report that with this additional focus on dreams, their dream life becomes more active, emotionally alive, and vivid. Of course, it may have been like this all along, but we are for the most part unaware of many of our dreams unless we actively choose to remember them.

When embarking on this process, it may also be that your dreams become more threatening or disturbing. With the help of the questions posed in the last chapter, there is a good chance that you are becoming more aware of past hurts and repressed emotions. You may find many of these emotions presenting themselves in the context of your dreams, as well as in your waking state. Themes of extreme anger, trauma, or sadness may become more evident and pronounced in your dreams as you are choosing to become more conscious of them—this book is also likely to stir things up at an unconscious level, and your dreams can be an expression of this process. This is likely to be therapeutic in that it encourages unconscious material to come to the surface in a gradual manner.

Challenging experiences in your current life may also provoke the re-emergence of older bad dreams that went underground for many years. The old dreams most likely relate to negative experiences which have been stored away in the memory banks of your unconscious. They may reflect the emotional challenges you felt at the time. The associated distress, and feelings like fear or helplessness, have been stored away for many years. New experiences can trigger these old feelings, which may again find expression in distressing dreams with themes from your past.

The distressing nature of your dreams is likely to settle down as your mind/brain goes through the process of using them as a vehicle for self-healing. You are also likely to become more comfortable with these feelings over time. Your mind/brain may be effectively working through a backlog of distress, reducing the overall burden, until it reaches a point where much of it has been cleared.

After developing the habit of recording your dreams, the next step is to deliberately influence the nature of our dreams so as to encourage and harness the natural healing capacities which they entail. You may want to take it to this next level of "dream-seeding" if you feel that you have unfinished emotional business with an incident or person in your life.

Dream-seeding

This process is not so much telling your unconscious how to end a dream (resulting in a preferred outcome, or resolution), but is more about setting up the conditions for the dream to allow your natural healing capacities to come to the fore. Our mind/brain has an incredibly creative capacity for working out answers to emotional problems without our deliberate instruction.

When preparing for bed, you can start the dream-seeding process by choosing to think about the situation or person, the place or incident which you feel is still unfinished or disturbing within you. There is no need to script or dictate what will happen in the dream, but you can think about key elements which you feel are highly relevant. Get a sense of what elements are the most important—people, places, situations, the time in your life, etc.

As you are going off to sleep, visualize the aspects that you want to have present in the dream. In a sense, this is a bit like adding ingredients to a cake mixture, and then trusting the process to sort itself out and result in a cake. It is likely that your mind/brain will use the ingredients that you have added to create a dream, which then acts as a vehicle for the resolution of the outstanding issue. Remember to write down your dreams so as to capture what happened while you were asleep. With a greater ability to remember dreams, you will be astonished with their creative and healing capacities. I am regularly amazed at the creative intelligence of my unconscious in 'reworking' situations from my life during dreams, usually in a manner that my conscious mind would have no hope of doing.

If the dream-seeding works, you are likely to wake up feeling somewhat relieved of the issue which had felt unfinished—it will feel like you have been through a journey in which resolution has occurred. This is what is happening quite naturally for us most nights anyway, we just usually aren't aware of it.

The suggestion is that you can become more aware of this natural healing capacity, and that you can then deliberately program yourself to dream about certain topics. The actual resolution of the issues in the context of the dream is highly creative and is best not manipulated—just trust that your unconscious is able to work out what needs to be done with the distress once you have indicated a need for resolving it.

If you have a repeated nightmare, this may indicate a need which your mind/brain has to resolve a particular distress deep within you. Rather than the process reaching fruition, the emotions which are generated in the dream are so intense that you wake up in fright, and the processing consequently stops. If it is a repeated nightmare, you don't need to be dream seeding it—your mind/brain, recognizing the need to heal it, will keep coming back to the same dream. In this situation, it can make sense to undertake some deliberate "rescripting" of the dream, so as to assist your unconscious in the resolution of the distress.

Dream rescripting

Rescripting involves consciously choosing a different scenario or ending for a dream. A couple of years ago I had a very frightening dream in which my teenage son and I were about to cross a road busy with traffic. My son was a few steps in front of me, and began to cross the road with his school bag slung over his shoulder. I saw a car coming towards him at great speed as he stepped onto the road. Being unable to watch the moment of impact, I turned away and heard the sickening thump instead. With this sound, I woke up in fright, feeling extremely distressed with my heart nearly bursting out of my chest. When I eventually settled down, with the aid of deep breathing, I began to rescript the dream. Even though it was only a one-off nightmare, I had found it so disturbing that I simply couldn't tolerate it happening even just the once, or being left with its terror for the rest of the night.

In the rescripted version, I kept looking at the moment of impact, rather than turning my head away in fright. What I saw happening was my son stepping back from the path of the car, however the school bag on his shoulder was hit by the car as it sped past him. This created the impact sound. Having his bag pulled away from his shoulder threw him on the ground next to the road, dazed but essentially unharmed. With this rescripted version of the dream, I was able to emotionally settle down and then fall back asleep. Had I not done this, I think the amount of distress from the dream was too strong to have allowed me to resume sleeping at all. As far as I am aware, I have never had the dream again.

Some important questions to ask yourself are, "Why did I have this dream?" and "Why now?" In answering these questions, you will need to reflect on the nexus of themes between your waking life and your dream. If we discount the idea that high emotional impact dreams are just random electrical activity in your brain, there must be issues which led your unconscious mind to reveal these emotions in the dream which are bubbling away at a deep level. What events occurring in your waking life now remind you of events from your past? Your unconscious mind is using the dream as a vehicle to bring attention to these issues, as it recognizes the need for healing.

As stated, this approach to rescripting can be particularly useful for reoccurring nightmares. With a greater awareness of dreams, it is possible to develop the ability to stop the dream while it is happening, and rewrite the script. In so doing, we are assisting our unconscious mind in its efforts at updating our inner story and sense of who we are. This is done by the dream bringing to our awareness the negative and demoralizing aspects of the circumstance, and then searching our memory for images of strength and competence. These more positive images can then be activated and incorporated into the dream, to allow a change in our conscious experience.

The changes in our self-image, e.g. from being a victim to being a strong person, allows the mind/brain to imagine different and better ways of being.

The mind/brain does not care that these new self-images are not real. Judged from the perspective of physical reality, no dreams are "real" anyway. Their reality is never the issue, even though the emotions and physiological reactions which they create within us are entirely real. Where dreams can spontaneously create different scenarios which feel healing, we can learn to actively create these changes in the dreams with the same results.

"Dream therapy," which research has demonstrated does work in changing distressing dreams, can be done using the following four steps.[15]

- Recognize when you are having a bad dream *while* you are in the dream. Such a capacity is called lucid dreaming. This will be easier when you have been dream journaling for some time.

- Identify the distressing aspects of the dream. What about it makes you feel bad, helpless, ashamed, guilty, weak, incompetent or frightened?

- Stop the bad dream. You need to develop the capacity to exercise a degree of control while in the dream state. Again, through regular dream journaling and becoming more attuned to dreams, you can develop the ability to be more in charge of them. You are not compelled to let a disturbing dream continue. You can develop the ability to recognize when an upsetting dream is happening, and call a halt to it while in the dream.

- Change the most disturbing aspects of the dream. As I did with the dream of my son being hit by a car, you can be creative in deciding on different things that need to happen in the dream. I had to wake up to be able to do this; however, with practice, you can develop the ability to do this while you are still asleep and in the dream. Even if you are not able to do this while dreaming,

---

[15] Cartwright & Lamberg (2003). "Directing Your Dreams." *Psychology Today.*

as I found, there will be benefits for you in doing it while awake. You may also get a sense of the emotional flavor of the dream, and deliberately choose to script the opposite dimension. For example, if the dream has you being weak and easily bullied, re-script it so that you become powerful and assertive—see yourself taking these actions in the dream.

If dreams are our mind/brain's efforts to heal emotional hurts, and if repeated nightmares are repeated efforts to heal, then it stands to reason that aiding the unconscious via dream scripting can help in the processing of negative experiences and emotions. This is yet another way in which we can retrain our mind/brain away from the strategy of creating chronic pain as a means to distract us away from deep emotional pain.

Cognitive Control Training

Cognitive Control Training are two additional self-help options.[16] These techniques, and related variations, have been seen over many years in different approaches to psychology under a range of different terms. Psychologist Wayne Somerville refers to them collectively as Cognitive Control Training (CCT), which he has researched as treatments for PTSD. His studies indicate that these cognitive-imaginal strategies may be as effective in treating trauma as many of the more established trauma therapies.

The strategies involve two variations of using one's imagination to alter the experience of the memory. This can result in different feelings and physical sensations which then accompany the memory, replacing the normal distress. This may be particularly helpful when the natural psychological digestive abilities have not worked effectively, such that the memories remain stored in a "raw" or unprocessed state, continuing to produce disturbed emotion. The person will usually seek to avoid triggering

---

[16] Somerville (2004). "Cognitive Control Training for PTSD." *Psychotherapy: Theory, Research, Practice, Training.*

the memories, thereby further reducing the chance of digesting the upset through more exposure to it.

Rescripting the movie

Rescripting is a strategy which has been discussed in relation to changing distressing dreams. It can also be used very effectively to assist in decreasing the level of trauma associated with distressing events. As with rescripting dreams, the negative experience is deliberately given a new ending, however, we need not wait until sleeping in order to do this.

Firstly, create the space and time in which you are not likely to be disturbed by anyone. Close your eyes and get in touch with the memory that is still causing you distress. Allow yourself to see all of the images and hear the sounds that went along with this event. If, while getting in touch with the distressing memory, you feel overwhelmed or upset, it is worth considering seeking professional assistance.

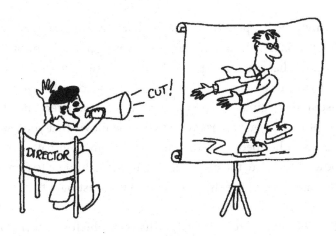

Direct your own movie with rescripting

Being overwhelmed indicates against the advisability of self-help strategies. If you are able to tolerate the distress, rate it on a scale from 0-10, with 0 being not at all upsetting, and 10 being completely upsetting.

- Visualize the image of you sitting in front of a large blank movie screen, on which you will be able to see the images of the event, just like in a film.

- Next, imagine that you are a movie director, able to literally call the shots of what is to be filmed and presented on the screen. As the director, you will be able to make any changes to the film that you like. Allow yourself to see on the screen a new version of the movie which includes the changes which you prefer. You can have yourself, and the other people involved, taking completely different actions, and saying different things to what happened in reality. As the director, you are able to add any new elements you desire, create any changes, and bring the story to a completely different ending if you wish—you are in charge.

- If anything happens in the movie that you don't want, call out "Cut." Then rewind, and start the action again, this time in the manner that you would prefer. The new action or outcomes do not have to be at all realistic. As a creative director, you can use your imagination, and incorporate any computer generated graphics that you so desire to make the movie that you want. You or other people in the new movie can even have super-powers to create the preferred outcomes. Continue to remake this movie until it feels, looks, and sounds just right to you.

- Finally, again rate the level of distress which you feel from the memory now on the scale from 0-10. Usually, the level of distress will have gone down. If it has not, you may try repeating the exercise until it does—perhaps you have more rescripting to do before it creates the desired result.

Resourcing the younger you

The next trauma-focused procedure involves more rescripting, this time allowing your adult perspective to remain present while you are in touch with an upsetting memory from your past. This is especially important when the distressing event happened to you at an earlier time in your life when you had fewer coping skills, less social or physical power, and a limited opportunity to make positive choices for yourself. As a result, the distress which gets stored away in us for years is usually the distress, perceptions and feelings of a younger person. Now, as an older person with more experiences and coping skills, the benefit of hindsight, an overall life perspective, as well as greater physical and social power, we no longer need to feel like the frightened or overwhelmed child we once were. Our experience of ourselves, as well as our self-concept, can be updated to make it more appropriate to who we now are. Rescripting, in which we maintain an adult perspective, can help with this updating.

- Begin the process by getting in touch with the distressing event that you want to work on. Rather than see the experience from the perspective of the younger you, this time watch it happening to the younger you from the distance of an adult looking on.

- Rate how upsetting this feels now on the scale from 0-10.

- While you are watching the event, retain the knowledge that in reality, it is now years later, and that you are watching this experience as the adult who you are now with greater coping skills, social and physical power, knowledge and wisdom. Retain an awareness of where and who you are now.

- When you feel that you have seen the entire episode, gauge if you have an understanding of what happened to the younger you. If you need to continue looking at the incident in order to gain as full understanding as possible, then do so until you feel that you have got a solid adult comprehension.

- The next step involves transferring your adult resources to the younger you in the memory. As an older person, you now have more wisdom and understanding from life experiences; you know how things will unfold for that younger person; and you now have more social and physical power. Very importantly,

231

you know that the younger you did actually survive that and other bad experiences. See if you can work out a way to transfer this knowledge and these qualities to the younger you.

You may see yourself as the adult you are now being with the younger you and providing the comfort and reassurance which s/he needs. You understand how the younger you is feeling in that situation, and how s/he is making sense of the experience. This may involve some self-blame, or denigrating his/herself in some way, or thinking that the torment will never end. As an adult with experience, strength and wisdom, you actually know better. Allow a picture of you tuning into the young person's needs, and providing the reassurance and support they need. Do you hold their hand, hug or hold them? What do you say to help them with how they are feeling about the situation, and about themselves?

If you find this difficult to do, imagine this young person is someone other than you—a younger person who you care a great deal about, like one of your children. What would you say to help them? Is their perspective, often involving self-blame, right? Would you allow a young person to hold on to this belief, seeing the pain that it causes them? Or would you challenge the belief in a loving and reassuring manner? If you are now a parent, you may have had to help your own child in similar ways. Trust that you know how to do this, and use the same skills you would use with your own child. Stay with the younger you, providing the adult perspective with reassurance and support, until you can sense the difference this makes to him/her.

Get a sense of how the younger you is now feeling, possibly receiving the messages and support which s/he needed at the time but didn't get. Is there a sense of relief? Does s/he feel less fearful? Have you been able to tell them that as unpleasant as the experience is, they did in fact survive it? Does s/he now know, from the benefit of your experience, that they will reach a time when they no longer have to put up with the bad situation, and are able to make a difference to it, or get themselves away from it? What difference does it make to them to know that they will get through this? That they are not to blame for bad things that happened to them?

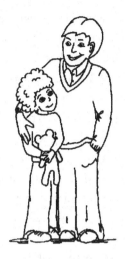

Resourcing and comforting the younger you

Work out for yourself if you still need to hang on to the upset and tension associated with the memory. If you feel that you don't need to hang on to these outdated feelings anymore, then let them go. It may feel appropriate for you to again see the younger you, and allow who you are now to blend with that younger person, merging together. You may also devise a letting go ritual of writing or drawing these feelings, and then releasing them in a fire.

If it does not feel right for you to let go of the tensions associated with the memory, this may indicate that you still feel the need for some protection which the tensions may provide. Try to tune inwards and work out the reasons that you may need to retain some of the old feelings. If not all of them, would it be appropriate for you to let go of some of the old feelings? If the same feelings are needed, but not to the same degree, see if you can let go of the element which is no longer needed. If the tensions are still there, get a sense of whether the younger you is able to explain why you need to keep hold of them. Again, this may indicate that you need some professional help to address the need for protection.

After this process, again take a measure of how distressing all this feels on the scale from 0-10. When they have been able to let go of the old upsets, most people will find that their distress rating goes down as a result. You can also use this procedure with unpleasant situations which may have happened in your more recent past. Now, only days, weeks or months later, you are likely to have more perspective over the situation, and a greater understanding of it. Often, when in the middle of a bad event, it is difficult for us to gain a proper comprehension of what is happening due to the confusion and inhibited mental functions which usually accompany heightened stress. You now know how the situation unfolded, and perhaps ended. As such, you are at least equipped with this more up to date knowledge now, and can impart the benefit of this to the only slightly younger you.

Some people may object that as these procedures are all happening in the imagination, none of it is real, and the improvements are therefore illusory. We need to be aware that no memory is real at all, if by "real" we mean something that is happening now. Memory is viewed by psychologists as a *creative* process, and not as the laying down of exact recordings of what happened. Our mind/brain is able to creatively fill in the missing pieces of memory episodes, and also alter them according to a particular need.

I have a vivid memory of visiting a gold-rush ghost town with my family as a young child. I can still easily recall a scene out of something like a Western movie, complete with an empty saloon-style hotel with dust covered tables and empty glasses. Many years later, my mother told me that it was nothing like that at all. Obviously, my mind/brain filled in the gaps and created something which was a lot more interesting than the actual place at the time, even though I "remember" walking in the abandoned hotel. My imagination was captured at the time as a young child, and it is this imagination which has been rehearsed as a memory over the years, rather than the reality of the actual experience. However, neither my memory, nor my mother's memories of this place are "real," as we are not currently there walking around the town. For both of us, these are just traces of the actual experience. I do, however, trust her memory of it more than mine, even though mine feels very real.

All memories are internal, psychological representations of events, and not the events themselves. Some of these internal representations can be stored within us in a manner which incorporates a range of distressing elements. My ghost town memory is a pleasant and exciting one, but most people who have experienced abuse will still feel tension and distress around their abuse memories. Their internal representations of those events will continue to generate emotional distress when they are in touch with the memory, and oftentimes, even when they are not in touch with it. The unconscious is the repository for all of these experiences and associated feelings. As stated throughout this book, the unconscious distress is often there, whether we are focusing on or aware of it at the time or not.

If the internal representations of bad experiences are not real in any present-moment sense, then there is no reason to *not* alter them for therapeutic outcomes. Each time a memory is revisited, it becomes changeable to a certain extent, as the mental and emotional state you are in when you bring up the memory gets combined with it. The memory is then stored again, this time under the influence of the newer thoughts and feelings. It takes on an apparent "solid" quality again until the next time it is brought out and re-experienced, this time with additional new thoughts and feelings. As such, memory is more like writing over a re-writable DVD than it is like making a solid recording of an event. Each time we remember an experience, it isn't the actual event we remember, but is in fact our memory of the last time we remembered it—this is the ongoing re-writing quality of memory.[17]

Distressed emotions in relation to memories can be changed by bringing them into consciousness and then overlaying them with a new vision, such as the rescripting suggested above. As such, a new internal representation can be created in place of the old one. The new version is no more real or unreal than the old one. It is merely more adaptive in being far less distressing, and allows the perceptions of the self (and associated emotions) to become more updated according to your current life.

You are able to practice both of these procedures with a range of troubling memories, and continue to gauge the emotional impact of these changes. As stated earlier, if you find that these approaches are not working for you, or if you feel emotionally overwhelmed when thinking about the upsetting experiences, then you may need to consider obtaining professional help.

---

[17] Bridge & Paller (2012) Neural Correlates of Reactivation and Retrieval-Induced Distortion. *Journal of Neuroscience.*

CHAPTER 12

The Promise of Energy Psychology

"ENERGY PSYCHOLOGY" IS DESCRIBED AS comprising of a set of physical and cognitive procedures designed to bring about therapeutic shifts in targeted emotions, thoughts and behaviors.[1] It represents a blending of traditional healing and spiritual systems of the East, along with elements of Western psychology. In terms of its legacy from the East, many forms of energy psychology have borrowed practices and concepts from acupuncture and acupressure, whereas others have borrowed from yoga, meditation, qigong, and other traditional practices for well-being. In regards to their legacy from Western psychology, energy psychology therapies can be conceived as being within the tradition of "exposure" therapies, a form of behavioral psychology.

There are more than two dozen different variations of energy psychology. Typically, they entail undertaking a physical procedure while you are psychologically focusing on target emotions, thoughts or behaviors. As will be presented in this chapter, energy psychology can be well used in conjunction with The Hidden Psychology of Pain.

---

[1] Feinstein (2008). "Energy Psychology: A Review of the Preliminary Evidence." *Psychotherapy: Theory, Research, Practice, Training.*

Acupuncture & acupressure

A form of energy psychology, Emotional Freedom Techniques (EFT), can be thought of as type of "psychological acupuncture" in that it involves tapping on acupuncture points while engaging in a psychological process. There are various ways of making sense of how EFT works. The most accessible explanations do not rely on notions of "energy," other than the fact that electro-chemical processes within the brain *are* ultimately a form of energy. As no piercing of the skin with needles is involved, EFT is referred to as a form of *acupressure*, with repeated light taps applied to specific acupuncture points while the person repeats a verbal phrase about the problem he or she would like to address.

While it is commonly thought to have originated with the work of psychologist Dr. Roger Callahan, as is usual for important "discoveries," there is a rich and long history to the development of this technique. Traditional Chinese Medicine (TCM) has been developing the practice of acupuncture for thousands of years. In short, the TCM suggestion is that "life energy," traditionally referred to as *chi* or *ki* energy, runs through our body along flow-lines, referred to as meridians. As these meridians do not entirely correspond with any known structure in the body, Western medical science has found it hard, if not impossible, to endorse and incorporate such concepts.

Much harder to dismiss, however, has been the amount of positive reports of acupuncture outcomes, even when research is conducted under Western scientific standards. The results have not been supportive of the application of acupuncture with *all* health conditions that its enthusiasts claim; however, the amount of supportive findings have surprised many scientists. The World Health Organization has identified twenty-eight medical or psychological conditions where evidence strongly supports the efficacy of acupuncture, and sixty-three more conditions where the evidence is promising but still inconclusive.[2]

Is acupuncture merely wishful thinking—a placebo effect—or is there a property specific to particular points on the skin? Research has revealed

---

[2] Feinstein (2008). "Energy Psychology: A Review of the Preliminary Evidence." *Psychotherapy: Theory, Research, Practice, Training.*

that stimulation of specific acupuncture points produce observed changes in specific parts of the brain. For example, needling a toe acupuncture point used to treat eye disorders activates the occipital lobes of the brain which are responsible for vision, as seen in fMRI images of the brain. When non-acupuncture points that are two to five centimeters away are needled, no activation of the occipital lobes is observed. This suggests a relationship between the stimulation of acupuncture points and the activation of particular areas of the brain. This makes sense, as every part of the skin is intimately connected with specific parts of the brain which are responsible for detecting nerve stimulation from those areas.

Other researchers have found correlations between the pathways on which acupuncture points are situated and interstitial connective tissue. A very high level of correspondence (80%) has been found between acupuncture points and the "channels" in intramuscular connective tissue planes that connect the internal organs to the outer surface of the body.[3] It is thought that the semi-conductive properties of the body's connective tissue allow acupuncture stimulation to rapidly send electromagnetic signals to specific areas of the body and brain.

Brain researchers at the University of Michigan have demonstrated that the neurological and chemical processes involved with pain relief from acupuncture are very similar to the processes involved in pain relief from opioid drugs.[4] In a study with twenty women who had been diagnosed with fibromyalgia, position emission tomography (PET) scans during their first acupuncture treatment, and then again after their eighth treatment, revealed that the treatment increased the binding availability of mu-opioid receptors in parts of the brain which can dampen pain signals. The brain structures involved in this observation were the cingulate, insula, caudate, thalamus and amygdala. Similar imaging research conducted in Germany used fMRI scans to establish brain activity during the application of a painful stimuli, both while acupuncture was being used, and when it was not. The researchers

---

[3] Feinstein (2010). "Rapid Treatment of PTSD: Why Psychological Exposure with Acupoint Tapping May be Effective." *Psychotherapy: Theory, Research, Practice, Training.*

[4] Harris et al (2009). "Traditional Chinese Acupuncture and Placebo (sham) Acupuncture Are Differentiated by their Effects on U-opioid Receptors." *Journal of NeuroImage.*

reported that the brain areas that are associated with pain perception, such as parts of the motor area, somatosensory cortex, somatomotor cortex and the insular, showed reduced activation under acupuncture. With no acupuncture, these brain structures were observed to have a higher level of activation with painful stimuli.[5]

To complicate the picture a little, researchers note that "sham" acupuncture points are found to work as well, but they do not create the same observed changes in neuro-chemistry or brain activity. British and Korean researchers, through an extensive systematic review of the studies conducted on acupuncture, concluded that high-quality randomized controlled trials show that both legitimate *and* sham acupuncture are *more* effective in reducing chronic low back pain than standard care.[6] This finding is echoed in regards to prevention of headaches and migraines in a systematic review by Cochrane Researchers—both legitimate and sham acupuncture points performed better than standard medications.[7]

The fact that both genuine and sham acupuncture treatments appear to produce the same impressive results suggests a process that is responsible for the beneficial outcomes, other than that offered by TCM involving meridians. Notwithstanding the high correspondence found between meridians and intramuscular connective tissue planes, an alternative explanation may have more to do with neurology and psychology. This possibility will be explored further, particularly in relation to acupressure.

Is the use of acupressure, in the form of pressing or tapping, as effective as puncturing the skin with needles? The *British Medical Journal* (BMJ) reported a study in which 129 sufferers of low-back pain were randomly assigned to either acupressure treatment or standard physical therapy from a specialist orthopaedic clinic. The patients were recruited from the clinic, and were assessed on a standard disability questionnaire immediately after the completion of treatment, and again six months later. Pre—and post-treatment measures of both groups showed that those who received the

[5] Kyung-Eun Choi et al (2010). "Acupuncture Changes Brain's Perception and Processing of Pain, Researchers Find." *Science Daily.*

[6] Ernst, Myeong, Tae-Young (2011). "Acupuncture: Does it Alleviate Pain and Are There Serious Risks? A Review of Reviews." *Pain.*

[7] Linde et al (2009). "Acupuncture for Migraine Prophylaxis." *Cochrane Database of Systematic Reviews.*

acupressure treatment ended the study with a lower average disability score when compared to the physical therapy group. These results were found to be statistically significant, meaning that it was the different treatments themselves which were responsible for the lower pain and disability scores and better functional status in the acupressure group, rather than just random chance. The better outcomes for the acupressure group was also found six months later when they were again assessed.[8]

Acupressure is also seen to be effective in treating emotional or psychological complaints. A survey of evidence conducted by the Harvard Medical School in 2008, which included a literature review of forty-five peer-reviewed studies published since 2000, found at least preliminary support for the efficacy of acupressure with a majority of the conditions for which the World Health Organization found acupuncture to be effective, including anxiety, depression, addictions, insomnia, and hypertension.[9]

Emotional Freedom Techniques (EFT)

The application of acupuncture to emotional issues was aided by chiropractor George Goodheart who, in the early in 1960s developed what he referred to as "Applied Kinesiology." Goodheart discovered that he could get equally impressive results by stimulating the acupuncture points with either pressure or tapping. The next step in the development of what ultimately became EFT was the work of psychiatrist John Diamond, who in the 1970s created what he referred to as "Behavioral Kinesiology." Diamond applied Goodheart's approach to emotional difficulties, having his patients repeat affirmations while stimulating specific acupuncture points. This became a forerunner to what has since been called energy psychology.

In the early 1980s, as a psychologist specializing in the treatment of anxiety states, Roger Callahan had undergone training in behavioral kinesiology as well as acupuncture. He treated a woman who experienced an extreme phobia to water, so much so that even seeing water on TV would

8   *British Medical Journal* (2006).
9   Feinstein (2010). "Rapid Treatment of PTSD: Why Psychological Exposure with Acupoint Tapping May be Effective." *Psychotherapy: Theory, Research, Practice, Training.*

lead to a large anxiety response. As part of his treatment, Callahan was attempting to desensitize her to water by having her sit on the edge of a swimming pool. When the woman complained of stomach pains whilst attempting this, he suggested that she tap a point on her cheekbone which corresponds with the "stomach meridian." The woman reported that not only did her stomach pain quickly go away, but so did her phobia of water. In fact, she began joyously splashing it on her face. None of the other standard psychological approaches to reducing her anxiety over the previous two years of treatment had helped this woman at all.

Callahan investigated and researched the potentials of this discovery further, arriving at a process which he called Thought Field Therapy (TFT). As stated, this involved tapping on a range of acupuncture points whilst mentally focusing on specific thoughts. Gary Craig, a minister of religion who studied TFT under Callahan, concluded that the process was unnecessarily complicated and convoluted. While learning these procedures, he observed many occasions when the person administering the taps accidentally did it out of the supposedly correct sequence, however the person's symptoms still improved. From these observations, he decided to modify TFT into a more simple sequence of taps which could be applied to a very wide range of presenting problems, including pain.

Craig titled this reworking of Callahan's approach "Emotional Freedom Techniques," and created an extremely thorough website dedicated to it in which he gave EFT away for free. More than a million people have downloaded the beginners' manual for EFT, and have benefited from the enormous archive of reports which have accumulated over the years in which both health professionals and sufferers of various conditions have reported their findings. I have had clients report an almost immediate departure of persistent pain when they have undertaken the simple and brief EFT procedure (to be described below), and there are scores of such accounts on the EFT website, http://www.eftuniverse.com/

As I have no training in either Traditional Chinese Medicine or behavioral kinesiology, such energy psychology theories are simply not the language that I use to make sense of how EFT works. However, as a treating psychologist, I do have a need to understand these remarkable outcomes, especially as I often introduce the process to clients. Whilst not a neurologist or a neuropsychologist, I am more able to develop some understanding of what may be happening with EFT from a very basic neuro-psychological point of view. As such, my way of making sense of EFT has less to do with Chinese medicine, meridians or life-energy, and more to do with conventional psychology and neurology.

While neuroscience has developed rapidly in the last couple of decades, and produced some remarkable insights in the process, one is still left with the impression that we know relatively little of what goes on inside our black box of a brain. However, there are neurological observations from studies which pinpoint specific brain changes that occur as a result of actions and experiences. Where the knowledge is incomplete, we are able to hypothesize about the possible neuro-psychological components of the changes that have been observed from processes like EFT. It is still somewhat speculative in that, despite recent advances, there are few absolute certainties when dealing with the human brain. The interested reader can find more extensive examples of this psycho-neurological understanding of EFT on the Net.[10]

Other people who use EFT may not have the same need to understand its ability to produce results, and therefore may settle on the acupuncture and/or energy psychology theories. Or these explanatory systems may be inherently meaningful to them. In the end, I suspect that acupuncture/energy psychology explanations on the one hand, and neuro-psychological explanations on the other, are simply different languages used to describe the same phenomenon. As such, I am not too concerned about the different explanations. The results are the same, regardless of how one makes sense of them.

Involving both emotional causes and physical symptoms, chronic pain is perhaps *the* mind/body health condition. As such, it makes good sense that an approach which works with both physical and emotional issues would be useful to sufferers. *The Hidden Psychology of Pain* suggests that the mind/brain is highly implicated in the production of chronic pain, as well as a raft of other chronic health issues. This is evident from the repeated observation that people who internalize relevant information are able to become pain-free. This would simply not be possible were the mind/brain *not* generating the pain. The information itself has no direct impact on blood vessels, nerves

---

[10] Ruden (2005). "Why Tapping Works: A Sense of Healing." www.healingthe mind.net

or the muscles surrounding them, nor on tendons and ligaments; and the information certainly has no impact on existing structural pathologies. However, the information does need to be mediated by the mind/brain in order to produce a beneficial flow-on effect to bodily functions and tissue changes.

Acupuncture has been demonstrated in scientific research to change the electromagnetic field of the skin surface. Other forms of sufficient stimulation, such as the application of heat, mild electrical current, pressing or tapping, also impact on the surface of the skin. Through an elaborate system of sensory nerves, our mind/brain is highly aware of changes in the skin caused by different forms of stimuli. Put your hand in either cold or hot water, and the part of your brain which processes sensory input from your hand will become electro-chemically activated in order to make sense of the nerve experience. The same is true for other forms of stimulation to your skin as skin tissue is being manipulated, including the insertion of acupuncture needles, or the sensations derived from tapping, pressing or massage.[11] Change the stimuli experienced by your hand, and you will also change the corresponding parts of your brain (sensory cortex) in their attempt to make sense of the physical experience.

Acupuncture theory suggests that in order to produce the greatest response, and corresponding change in the meridian, the stimuli needs to be applied to specific points on the skin. Neurological theory would suggest that the type of stimuli applied during either acupuncture or acupressure will produce corresponding alterations in the brain.

It is possible that the benefits seen with EFT may derive from its ability to create such alterations in the brain. A range of sensory stimuli, via tapping, are being presented while the person is engaging in essentially a psychological process of repeating phrases about the problem they are wanting to change. It is also possible that the observed high level of correspondence between "meridians" and the "channels" in intramuscular connective tissue planes may make specific points on the skin even more able to produce changes in the brain than non-acupuncture points. No definitive answer to this question is yet available.

---

[11] Butler & Moseley (2003) *Explain Pain.*

We have multiple neurological pathways which correspond to all of our experiences and actions, taking in the actions of millions of neurons. For example, we have "driving a manual car pathways," "brushing my teeth pathways," as well as a "feeling anxious" or "feeling back pain pathways." In fact, it is likely that each of these simple experiences and actions actually require hundreds of neural pathways in getting us to anticipate and prepare for the action (such as brushing your teeth) then in executing and controlling the action.

Multiple pathways in the brain will be activated and associated with each of these activities, in which the brain cells connect with other brain cells via their "tentacles" (axons and dendrites) to form specific patterns of connection (see Appendix 2).

Any experience that we repeat on a regular basis, either internally or externally generated, will have a pathway which is "well-travelled," involving multitudes of neurons. If we regularly drive a manual car, the neural pathway for changing gears is very well established after many years of use, such that it is rare to make a mistake. If we are regularly anxious, upset or in physical pain, then likewise, the neural pathways for these experiences are also very well-travelled. It is not unusual for people to follow a typical emotional course of sinking into despair or anxiety once they commence the very familiar route to becoming anxious or despairing, e.g. when a regular argument with a spouse begins.

The brain works on a "use it or lose it" principle, meaning that neural pathways which get a lot of traffic typically become very well established, and like driving a manual car after many years, a regularly rehearsed action or emotion requires very little effort to engage in. For this reason, it can feel like the emotion or behavior takes on a life of its own. After years of doing it, you don't have to think about changing gears in a car, or how to make yourself miserable.

Having an overactive mind, as while ruminating about distressing events, is a key component of low mood. Many people feel that once they start ruminating over their misfortunes, they are simply unable to stop, despite their desire to do so. When experiences are similar enough to another distressing event, or are related in theme to a well-rehearsed distress, then the electro-chemical activity in the brain is likely to follow the well-travelled pathways that are most relevant for that experience.

For example, if you were often belittled by a parent when you were a child, it is likely that the neural pathways relating to this experience (and all the self-doubts that it may entail) will be activated again when your boss speaks to you in the same way. People will often report to feeling like a hurt child again under such circumstances, as the feelings and thoughts which the experience triggers are all too familiar. This is also very common in intimate relationships.

If, as this book suggests, your mind/brain is generating chronic pain in order to distract attention away from emotional distress, then it is worthwhile trying to gain a sense of what the emotional issue is in order to combat the pain. After much pondering, you may conclude that your pain is related to abuse you experienced as a child, for example.

I recently had a conversation with a woman who was repeatedly sexually abused by several people in her childhood. Although she had successfully engaged in psychotherapy to assist in processing the trauma related to these experiences, she remained in extreme physical pain in most of her body. In discussion with me, it became apparent that she believed that she had somehow been the cause of the unwanted sexual attention of these men. She revealed a belief that she was a "sexually provocative child," otherwise the abuse would not have happened, and she would not have 'invited' their sexual attention. To convince me, she cited examples of the types of behavior which she *"must have"* engaged in, e.g. rubbing herself against the men's legs, which somehow gave these sexual predators a green light to abuse her. When I asked her for specific memories in which she engaged in this sort of behavior, she revealed that she didn't actually have any memories of doing such things. It is highly unlikely that she could remember the acts of abuse against her, but have forgotten her own sexually provocative behavior. But nevertheless, she was convinced that she must have behaved in this manner, and felt to blame for the assaults, even though she could not remember ever behaving in a "provocative" manner.

This was clearly a deeply ingrained belief system with attached feelings of shame, and no doubt had corresponding neural pathways which were created within her as a child while she was trying to make sense of her experiences. As stated earlier, children will often blame themselves for the terrible actions of adults. Ironically, it can help them to minimize anxiety if they distort reality and believe that they are responsible for the bad behavior of adults. At least they feel at the mercy of their own bad behavior, which theoretically at least they can do something about, rather than at the mercy of a psychopathic adult (which they can often do nothing about).

Neural pathways, in which are contained beliefs like "I am responsible for the sexual abuse," are good targets for interventions like EFT. Being very well-travelled, it is often not so easy to change these pathways purely by conscious choice. People can intellectually recognize that, as a child, they weren't responsible for the behavior of dysfunctional adults around them. However, at a much deeper level, this belief and associated feelings can be highly resistant to change, as they are emanating from a much deeper part of the brain than the thinking neo-cortex, i.e. the limbic system.

Often the person may recognize the folly of such an idea while all is well, but when a current life experience is similar in some way to the childhood trauma, the old well-travelled pathways are very easily activated again. And then the person can *feel* shame, even if intellectually recognizing that they aren't to blame for the situation. The electro-chemical activity can simply whiz around the old pathways, intensifying as it goes and increasing the level of distressed feelings with each circuit it completes. Again, you may simply feel unable to stop this vicious cycle of distressed thought and feeling, and find yourself ruminating endlessly about it. EFT can be thought of as a useful circuit-breaker in this type of scenario.

There are several metaphors to help you make sense of how EFT works. If you have ever lived on a dirt road, you will be familiar with what happens to it with torrential rain. Water will generally run across the road at the lowest point, and cut something of a channel across it. The way of rectifying the problem is not to simply fill the channel with a wheelbarrow load of gravel, as with the next heavy downpour of rain, the same channel will again be cut across the road and the gravel will be washed away. The answer to the problem is to firstly cut what are referred to as "feather-drains" near the low point. These are a series of smaller drains, taking water away from the main channel and dispersing it from the direction of the road. When the next rain comes, rather than simply follow the old pathway towards the deeper channel, water will now be dispersed in different directions along the feather-drains. You can now fill the main channel in with gravel and be confident that it won't just be immediately washed out, as long as you maintain the feather-drains.

The deeper channel across the road is analogous to the well-travelled neural pathway of "I am responsible for the abuse." Any time there is an "emotional storm" with torrential rain (electro-chemical activity), the energy associated with the storm will travel down the usual channel and result in distress.

EFT can be thought of as giving the brain a range of alternative pathways (like feather-drains) through which the electro-chemical activity can travel, dispersing the energy and diluting the negative power of the experience. With each component of the process, a new 'feather-drain' is being dug, so that when the next storm occurs, the brain has a range of pre-established pathways which the electro-chemical activity can travel down, rather than simply remain stuck cycling in the old pathway.

This proposed neuro-psychological change is supported by the now established reality of neuro-plasticity, wherein it has become apparent that the brain is highly able to develop new neural pathways in place of older ones. With more use of these alternative neural pathways, the use-it-or-lose-it notion begins to work for you, and with regular practice of EFT, electro-chemical activity is now routinely dispersed away from the problematic pathways, and with it the distress dissipates.

The EFT webpage (http://www.eftuniverse.com) reveals that this procedure has been researched in more than seven countries, by more than fifty investigators. The results of these studies have been published in more than fifteen different peer-reviewed journals, including prominent journals such as *Journal of Clinical Psychology*, and *Psychotherapy: Theory, Research, Practice, Training*, as well as the *Review of General Psychology*. In America, the Harvard Medical School, the University of California, the City University of New York, the Walter Reed Army Medical Center, and the Texas A&M University have conducted such research on EFT. Research institutions in universities from other countries have contributed to the growing evidence base, including Sweden, Turkey, The Philippines, England, Peru, and Griffith University in Australia.

Such research has found EFT to be effective for a range of conditions including anxiety, athletic performance, depression, pain and physical symptoms, phobias, PTSD and weight loss. Despite the research, as well as the abundance of anecdotal reports of positive outcomes, it has not been around for long enough or attracted enough research interest to yet reach a critical mass of positive findings that allow it to qualify as a "Well-Established Treatment."

On the basis of research that has been conducted to date, the American Psychological Association has given EFT the status of a "Probably Efficacious Treatment." In America, EFT is increasingly being used in traditional health care settings such as Health Maintenance Organizations, disaster relief efforts, and Veteran's Administration hospitals.[12]

Practitioners of energy psychology have provided services to traumatized people in Kosovo, New Orleans, Rwanda, South Africa, and The Congo with impressive results. Training in energy psychology qualifies as continuing education for psychologists, physicians, and related professions in several European countries such as Germany, Austria, and Switzerland.

Despite the slowly accumulating evidence, there are critics of EFT and other energy therapies within psychology. One can only presume that as more people learn of EFT, and more researchers decide to investigate it for themselves, the amount of positive findings will continue to mount until it does reach the critical mass required of a well-established treatment. I suspect this is simply a matter of time, as the level of interest appears to be growing rapidly, with subscribers to an email newsletter, *EFT Insights*, increasing by around seven thousand per month.

EFT & pain

The EFT process begins with establishing an appropriate target for change (see Appendix 8 for a brief guide to the process). If you are doing EFT to decrease chronic pain, it is helpful if you have an idea of what the pain could be about. As with the woman described above, her pain was about the issue of blame.

When you can develop a reasonable sense of what the pain is about, then you will need to use EFT with this in mind. If you are not sure what the pain or other chronic health issue could be about, it can be useful to consult with a book such as Louise Hay's *Heal Your Body*. Rather than a

---

[12] Feinstein (2008). "Energy Psychology: A Review of the Preliminary Evidence." *Psychotherapy: Theory, Research, Practice, Training.*

set of explanations, this book simply lists a large range of health and pain issues with corresponding suggestions regarding what emotional issue the symptom could relate to. Another option, if you cannot arrive at a sense of what the pain is about, is to simply focus on the pain itself in the EFT procedure, rather than its presumed meaning. Any of these approaches can prove helpful.

The first step in EFT is to tap on the "karate-chop" point, or to rub on the "sore-spots" in the upper chest while repeating a phrase about the issue you are wishing to address. This statement, referred to as the Set-Up Phrase, may follow the standard formula:

> "*Even though I have this* _____, *I deeply and completely accept myself.*"

The blank is to be filled with a statement about the issue you are wishing to change. For example, if you suspect that your pain is about feeling responsible for sexual abuse as a child, you could state,

> "*Even though I feel responsible for my childhood sexual abuse, I deeply and completely accept myself.*"

There are variations of this standard phrase; however, when beginning it is best to stick to this, or a modified variation of it that makes sense in regards to the issue you are wanting to address. If you don't have any idea of why you are in pain, you can just focus on the pain itself with your Set-Up Phrase:

> "*Even though I have back pain, I deeply and completely accept myself.*"

The logic of just focusing on the symptom is that while you may not consciously know why the pain is happening, if it is being generating by your mind/brain as per the suggestion of this book, it is safe to assume that the part of your mind/brain responsible for creating the pain *does* know. The pain has been created without "you" (your conscious mind) knowing why, so your mind/brain can *un*-create the pain, also without you knowing why. In fact, when people are unaware of pain's hidden psychology, this is what is already happening on a regular basis with repeated flare-ups and exceptions to the normal pain pattern. You can also combine your *suspicion* of what is causing the pain with a reference to the pain:

> *"Even though I have back pain which I think is related to my sexual abuse as a child, I deeply and completely accept myself."*

In summary, there are at least three suitable Set-Up Phrases for pain:

i) Focus on the actual quality of the pain:

> *Even though I have this dull pain in my back . . .*
> *Even though I have this shooting pain in my neck . . .*

ii) Focus on how you feel about the pain:

> *Even though I am upset about this back pain . . .*
> *Even though I am frightened by this neck pain . . .*
> *Even though I am frustrated by this shoulder pain . . .*

iii) Focus on an emotion which you think relates to the pain:

> *Even though I have this fear in my sinuses . . .*
> *Even though I feel this burden in my back . . . .*
> *Even though I have this shame in my neck . . . .*

If you are unable to work out what the pain could be about, you may state:

> *Even though* I can't understand why my back hurts, *I deeply and completely accept myself.*

Why the emphasis on accepting oneself at the end of the Set-Up Phrase? It is normal for us to be highly critical of ourselves, and even more so when things aren't going well because of an episode of distress or pain. Our tendency to beat ourselves up with self-condemnation, particularly when things aren't good for us, will only exacerbate the associated emotional distress, which can further entrench physical pain. More emotional tension from self-punishment, because we are having problems, may lead to more muscular tension, and thereby to more oxygen deprivation and consequent pain. Making an overt and deliberate statement about accepting ourselves, *in spite of* having the problem, is a powerful message about our worth as human beings. It is possible to be a worthy person at the same time as feeling overwhelmed by a problem. The Set-Up Phrase reinforces this reality, and also represents a different neural pathway to the usual self-condemnation pathway.

The Set-Up Phrase is repeated three times while continuously tapping on the karate-chop point, or rubbing on the sore spots. On a neurological level, repeating a phrase about the thing you are wanting to change will create a small electrical storm in the pathway of neurons which relates to that experience.

If you have nearly choked on a ham sandwich, the casual mention of ham sandwiches in a conversation is likely to be more distressing to you than it is to a person who has never had this experience. The neural pathways relating to the near death experience, most likely with associated limbic system activity, will be electro-chemically activated with further experiences which trigger this response. A person who has only ever enjoyed ham sandwiches will have fairly different neural pathways relating to them than the person who nearly choked to death on one.

A Set-Up Phrase that is meaningful to you, by virtue of it referring to a genuine problem in your life, will stimulate neurological activity in the pathway of neurons which relate to that experience. As the issue or memory being worked on is typically a distressing one, the pathway of neurons relating to that experience will most likely be related to limbic system activity, as the fight/flight/freeze response has probably been instigated by the memory.

Plasma Ball model

Another metaphor for understanding how EFT works is the Plasma Ball. These are the home novelty lamps which became popular in the 1980s, and which resemble a round glass orb with an electrical core from which multi-colored streaks of light shoot out in all directions. A much smaller orb in its center serves as an electrode. Contained within the larger orb are various electrically charged gases with particular properties, referred to as plasma because of their brilliant colors when electrically charged. These dancing beams of light extend from the inner electrode to the outer glass insulator, giving the appearance of multiple constant beams of colored and waving streaks of light. Placing a hand on the glass alters the high-frequency electrical field, causing light beams to migrate from the inner orb to the point of contact on the glass ball. The glass does not block the electromagnetic field created by the electrical current flowing through the plasma, although it does block the current itself. With a hand placed against the glass, an electrical pole is created with the beam of light heading towards the hand, which allows the electrical charge to "earth" via your body.

In using this as a metaphor for how EFT works, consider the glass orb to be a model for our brain. The electrical core at the center of the orb is analogous to the pathway of neurons which becomes electrically activated when you think of the ham sandwich that nearly killed you, or the sense of shame felt in relation to sexual abuse. (Note: this model is admittedly simplistic, as all memories will involve a *range* of neural pathways in different parts of the brain which reflect the actual experience—for the sake of explanation, the plasma ball model will relate to a presumed single neural pathway relating to the experience. This model is presented not as literal, but merely as a tool to aid understanding).

The level of activity in this pathway of neurons is evident by the emotional distress (or in the plasma ball, by the amount of colored light strands being thrown out from the central electrode). If the goal is to decrease the emotional distress, then we want to decrease this electrical activity in the part of the brain responsible for it.

Imagine that the plasma ball is powered by a battery rather than mains electricity. The goal in this analogy is to deplete the battery so that the electrical storm—or "lightning bolts"—cease. At that point, the electrical core (or neural pathway relating to the distress) has become inactive. The storm has passed, and the person is able to feel calm rather than emotionally distressed.

The initial Set-up Phrase has the effect of creating an electrical storm in the pathway of neurons relating to the distress or pain. This is referred to as "emotional activation." In effect, this is like turning the plasma ball on, and is a necessary step to achieving the goal of flattening the battery. It is common in traditional exposure therapies for the person to activate stressful imagery and feelings, so as to allow the process to then desensitize them to these images and emotions.

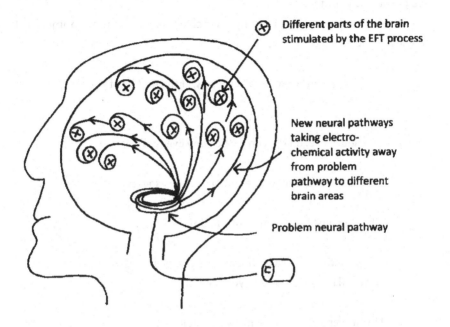

Different parts of the brain stimulated by the EFT process

New neural pathways taking electro-chemical activity away from problem pathway to different brain areas

Problem neural pathway

Plasma ball model of the effects of EFT on the brain

After activating the distress with the Set-up Phrase, the next step in the EFT process is tapping on each of the energy points around seven times, or for five seconds, while repeating the "Reminder Phrase." The Reminder Phrase is simply the part of the Set-up Phrase that you filled the blank in with, e.g. *"frightened of ham sandwiches"* or *"feel responsible for my childhood sexual abuse"* or *"feeling back pain."*

If there were several elements to your Set-up Phrase, you can break these down to one element for each tapping spot, e.g.

point 1— *"feel responsible for my childhood sexual abuse"*
point 2— *"feeling back pain"*
point 3— *"feel responsible for my childhood sexual abuse"*
point 4— *"feeling back pain,"* etc.

The taps should be generally light, but hard enough to be felt. If you question the impact of these light taps on your body, and therefore on your brain, try doing it with ear plugs in and you will get some sense of the stimulation created by the taps—they will sound like *boom, boom, boom* when tapping the points on your face.

The Sequence involves tapping on each of the following acupoints while repeating the Reminder Phrase.

EB (at the beginning of the eyebrow, at the middle of your forehead end)

SE (side of eye, on the rim of the bony eye socket)

UE (under eye, also on the rim of the bony socket)

Ch (chin, just below your bottom lip)

CB (collarbone—where bulb of bone is, at the beginning of your collarbone, closest to your center)

UA (under arm, in line with your nipples)

BN (below nipple—an inch beneath it)

Th (on your thumbnail at the place where your two thumbnails are closest if you put your hands together in a traditional prayer position)

IF (index finger, at the same place of the nail)

MF (middle finger—same place on your middle finger nail)

BF (baby finger—same place on your little finger)

KC (karate chop—back to the karate chop point again, the place where your hand would impact on something were you to give it a karate chop).

My preference is to tap on the opposite side of my body so as to engage my brain in some bilateral stimulation (see the discussion on EMDR in Chapter 16, which suggests that stimulating the different sides of the brain in an alternating manner is a powerful means of self-soothing). I also tap with two fingers together so as to double the surface area of the tap, which also doubles the chance of hitting the "right" acupoint (assuming that the research suggesting actual spots are more effective than fake spots is accurate—no harm in having a bet each way).

The next part of the EFT procedure involves a range of eye movements while you are still tapping on an acupoint on the surface of your hand (the "Gamut Point"), and repeating the Reminder Phrase. I make sense of this part of the process in reference to stimulating the occipital lobe at the back of the brain by creating unusual visual stimuli. Essentially, it is just another way of stimulating a part of the brain that is not associated with the problem. For example, our eyes and brains will actively attempt to keep our perception of our visual field relatively stable while we are running. When you roll your eyes in different directions, your occipital lobe is being bombarded by your cascading visual field. Again, this is just another way of creating a lot of brain stimulation in different brain locations.

Likewise, when the procedure requires that you hum the melody of a tune that you knew before five years of age, e.g. "Happy Birthday" (choose a song that has no negative associations), a large amount of brain structures become activated by virtue of: thinking of childhood memories; thinking of a tune with associated emotions; and turning that tune into a melodic vocal behavior. Each component of the music (pitch, melody, and rhythm) is instigated separately, and the parts are reassembled along with the emotional flavor of the song, derived from limbic area activity, along with the memories it elicits. Counting from one to five then activates left hemisphere activity for most people, so that both hemispheres are getting a decent work-out.

The Gamut Point can be found by locating the tendons of your little finger and the next finger as they travel up your hand. Follow these tendons up, just past your knuckle and close your hand. You will be able to feel a small indentation on the surface of your hand just behind the knuckle and in between the two stated tendons. This is the Gamut Point. Tap on this point around seven times while performing each of the following, and still repeating the Reminder Phrase:

1)Eyes closed 2) Eyes open 3) Eyes hard down to the right 4) Eyes hard down to the left. 5) Roll eyes in one direction 6) Roll eyes in opposite direction 7) Hum two seconds of a song 8) Count rapidly from one to five. 9) Hum again.

On completion of the Gamut Procedure, go back to The Sequence and complete this again, starting with the eyebrow and ending with the karate chop point. (See summary in Appendix 8):

EB, SE, UE, Ch, CB, UA, BN, Th, IF, MF, BF, KC.

When repeating the reminder phrase, the electrical activity associated with the problem you are wanting to change simply goes around the neural pathways relating to that experience or distress, with the electricity travelling along the axons and dendrites. As stated earlier, there are thousands of possible directions for the electricity to travel, as each axon has thousands of branches. The well-travelled pathway of repeated distress is merely one of many pathways which the electrical activity *could* travel down, however it tends to travel along the most used pathways.

While you are repeating the Reminder Phrase, you are also creating a host of other forms of brain stimulation by engaging in the tapping procedure. Tapping is a motor activity, and every motor activity is initiated by electro-chemical activity in particular areas of the brain. The back part of the frontal lobe allows us to take physical action via the motor cortex. Just in front of the motor cortex is the pre-motor cortex, where proposed actions are rehearsed before they are actually carried out. Typing on a key board or tying your shoe laces all entail corresponding areas of brain activity which enable you to perform these actions—these simple actions would take pages to describe from a neurological perspective in that the amount of brain areas involved are numerous and highly complex.

Whilst tapping on the acupoints, different parts of the brain are activated with each different location of tapping. If tapping with your right hand, the corresponding areas of brain activity will be in the left cerebral hemisphere. At the same time as executing the tap, you are also stimulating nerve endings in the area of the tapping point. As these nerve endings are being stimulated, they are sending electrical messages through the spine and into the brain where other cerebral locations are becoming electro-chemically activated by virtue of receiving the nerve stimulation. With each different point tapped, different parts of your brain are becoming activated as they register and make sense of the nerve stimulation. If you are using your right hand to tap on the left side of your body, areas in your left cerebral hemisphere will become activated by the motor activity at the same time as areas in your right hemisphere will become activated by the nerve stimulation.

As such, when you are going through the procedure, you are activating multiple locations within both hemispheres of your brain at the same time as you are activating the "problematic" neural pathways with repeating the Reminder Phrase. One of the possible results of this is that with each circuit of electro-chemical activity that sweeps around the neural pathways, some of the electrical charge is siphoned off and away from the regular pathways and out towards the parts of the brain that have been activated by the tapping procedure.

As with the plasma ball, where placing your hand on the glass surface sends lightning bolts to that location because an electrical pole has been created, the EFT procedure allows the electrical charge associated with the problem to deviate away from the normal paths, and create new pathways out to the areas of the brain that are being activated. Each new tapping point stimulated creates other alternative pathways for the electrical activity to travel down, and therefore takes some of the electrical charge away from the usual pathways.

As with trying to flatten the battery of a 12volt plasma ball, the more you create electrical poles by placing your hand on different locations of the glass orb, the more the electrical charges will be sent to that place and the more the energy will be dissipated. Repeating the EFT tapping procedure will likewise dissipate the amount of electrical charge racing around the problematic neural pathways, as it is now being dispersed into a range of other brain locations.

And as with the dirt-road-with-a-channel analogy, the electrical energy is being sent away from the well-travelled pathway (deeper channel) and dispersed in a range of different directions by the new pathways (feather drains) that have been created by the tapping procedure. Consequently, the next time it rains heavily (or there is an emotionally distressing event), the water is able to move away from the old channel and not exacerbate the problem. The electrical energy now has a range of alternative pathways that it can travel down, rather than just the well-travelled problematic pathways. In this way, an entrenched emotional or physical problem can be decreased both while it is happening (by "flattening the battery") and also in anticipation (creating different pathways in advance that the electrical energy can travel down when the problem arises again).

Overall, the entire EFT process can be thought of as a means of creating a large amount of neural activity in parts of the brain that are not associated with the problem which you are wanting to address, and thereby taking electrical energy away from the "problem" pathways which have also been activated in the process.

This is not what the originators of EFT had in mind, and it is not the language or concepts that they use to make sense of the procedure. However, from a basic neuro-psychological perspective, it makes perfectly good sense that a person undertaking the procedure would feel less distress than when they started. The procedure creates a very effective circuit-breaker, taking the excessive electrical charge away from the usual areas of neural activity, allowing the brain to refocus on other things.

Reading the EFT webpage will give you a good idea of the range of problems which it has successfully been applied to. If the brain is centrally involved in the regulation of all bodily functions, including the perception of pain, why wouldn't such a procedure alter the process and experience of other phenomena which the brain is involved in? The archive of reports on the EFT webpage make it clear that there is a substantial amount of anecdotal evidence in favor of its ability to create significant change with many different issues. Some of these reports are provided by health professionals, including physicians as well as psychologists amongst others who have used it with their patients; other reports are provided by people who are presenting the results of their own use of the procedure.

The question of whether it is a placebo effect becomes a moot point. If a chronic back pain diminishes as a result of a few rounds of EFT (as I have seen happen with clients to whom I have taught this), and even if this is merely the result of wishful thinking, then this alone demonstrates the point that the pain is being generated by the brain, and not by the structural pathology. No amount of EFT tapping or wishful thinking will alter a structural pathology such as a bulged disc. Yet people will often report a significant decrease in the pain, as is evident from the EFT webpage.

Some people suggest that EFT works to reduce pain simply by virtue of the distraction which it offers the person. No doubt there is an element of truth to this; however, does this mean that nothing therapeutic is actually happening while the distraction is occurring? German research recently reported fMRI observations of people undergoing painful procedures while they given a mental distraction. The study results show that when such a distraction is provided, the incoming pain signals from the spinal cord to the higher-order brain regions are inhibited. Variations in the experimental design allowed the researchers to conclude that this blocking of pain signals is via the secretion of endogenous opioids in the brain, resulting in relief from the pain. Mental distractions are able to trigger this blocking of pain signals, not only in the brain, but also as early in the pain process as the spinal cord itself. As such, even just distraction is not just a psychological phenomenon, but involves active chemical processes in the spine and brain which can reduce the experience of pain.[13]

Robyn was a client of mine who had been sexually abused during her childhood. As an eight-year-old, a man grabbed her as she walked on her way home after school. As far as sexual abuse of children goes, her experience was not so physically traumatic, as it involved fondling rather than penetration. Amongst the more emotionally damaging aspects of the experience was that when he had finished with her, he put her in a *rubbish bin*. She presented to me as an adult with ongoing back pain, which flared up whenever she was under extreme stress in her relationship, or with work.

Amongst the interventions I used with her, one day we went through the EFT procedure in regards to her back pain. Each time we repeated it, her

---

[13] Spengler et.al (2012). "Attention Modulates Spinal Cord Responses to Pain." *Current Biology.*

back pain lessened until she reported no pain at all. This can only happen if the pain is being caused by the brain, and the brain is being somewhat "altered" by the tapping procedure. If the pain is essentially an "opinion" arrived at by the brain, as suggested by Doidge, then it makes sense that a procedure that changes brain processes can also change the pain.

My initial personal view was that EFT was not as powerful tool as some preferred psychotherapies, however this perception was radically challenged when I viewed one of the EFT training videos. Vietnam veterans who had suffered extreme post-traumatic stress since their war experience, and had been in psychiatric hospitals ever since, were treated using a particular application of EFT. One such veteran reported that he had barely stopped shaking in the decades since the war, and had also suffered from chronic insomnia. This man's post-traumatic stress had remained resistant to all of the treatment approaches which psychiatry and psychology had been able to throw at it over several decades. He was interviewed again the day after the EFT treatment, and was able to report that he'd had his first good night sleep in years. In addition, he had stopped shaking for the first time since the war. This is a remarkable outcome for any treatment approach.

A study conducted in Rwanda with children left orphaned after the "ethnic cleansing" of 1994, which saw between 500,000 and one million people murdered, produced similarly remarkable results on a larger scale. One hundred and eighty eight orphans were treated with a one off session of Thought Field Therapy (the highly related precursor to EFT), combined with brief relaxation training. Seventy two per cent of them were assessed as suffering from PTSD prior to the treatment, with around 50 of them suffering trauma to the highest degree possible. These adolescents experienced PTSD symptoms such as intrusive flashbacks, nightmares, difficulty concentrating, aggressiveness, bedwetting, and withdrawal during the twelve year period following the ethnic cleansing. Immediately after the treatment, only 18% scored within the PTSD range, and this had reduced further to 16% one year after treatment.[14]

---

[14] Fenstein (2008). "Energy Psychology: A Review of the Preliminary Evidence." *Psychotherapy: Theory, Research, Practice, Training.*

While the EFT universe webpage contains descriptions of many varied applications of the procedure, the issues where I have personally seen EFT most helpful include chronic pain, anxiety problems and sleep problems. As sleep disturbance and anxiety often accompany chronic pain, I will describe the application of EFT to these issues over the next two chapters.

CHAPTER 13

Improving Your Sleep

Around eighty percent of people living with chronic pain experience sleep disturbances. Research also shows that poor sleep patterns make people more sensitive to pain, so a vicious cycle of poor sleep due to pain and intensified pain due to poor sleep easily established.[1]

Sleep plays a vital role in emotional well-being in terms of our ability to cope with life in general. It also plays a very important role in our ability to cope with pain. Getting less sleep, or poor-quality sleep, will result in a heightened sensitivity to pain, and a reduced ability to cope. The ability to sleep is somewhat regulated by the actions of neurotransmitters, which are highly effected by stress. As most people in chronic pain are highly stressed by their experience, it makes sense that sleep problems are experienced by most people with this problem. Improving the quality of your sleep is often vital to addressing both acute and chronic pain.

One of the ongoing effects of the car accident in which I was injured as an eighteen-year-old was that I became a relatively poor sleeper. Where I had been a sound sleeper before, after the accident I became a very light sleeper, and for years experienced being awake for hours on-end during the night. It was not unusual for me to wake in the very early hours of the morning, and stay awake until I needed to get out of bed four or five hours later. Nor was

---

[1] Buenaver et al (2012). "Evidence for Indirect Effects of Pain Catastrophizing on Clinical Pain among Myofascial Temporomandibular Disorder Patients." *Pain.*

it unusual for me to miss the opportunity to fall asleep easily at the start of the night, and to then remain awake for most of it.

As I never had any recollection of the impact moment in the head-on car accident, I used to tell people it was not unlike going to bed one night believing that everything in your world was safe and under control, and then being shaken awake during the night to be told that you had been in a bad accident and that you were still trapped in the car wreck, in lots of pain and bleeding to death. Needless to say, this was an enormous fright, and perhaps explains why from that time onwards I became a light sleeper.

As is typical for people who have experienced trauma, I lost the ability to trust that all would be well. I am still a light sleeper, but since coming across EFT, it has become extremely rare for me to wake up and stay awake for a lengthy time during the night, or to have a problem drifting off to sleep. As a result, I have really had to redefine myself as a person who *used* to have a problem with sleeping. In addition, most of the clients to whom I have introduced this procedure have much the same experience: a large improvement in their sleep, often after an entire adulthood of night-time frustration.

Sleep is a multi-factorial issue, and pain is often a significant factor which interferes with it. If you are having an extreme attack of chronic pain, you may need to resort to the temporary use of pain killing medication in order to help. Do this in consultation with your physician, and remember that while it is reasonable to try and control painful symptoms, the real cure is in addressing the ultimate cause. Keep on thinking psychologically about your pain (as long as serious physical health issues have been excluded) and following *The Hidden Psychology of Pain* program in the ways described in earlier chapters, even if you need to temporarily resort to symptom management with pain medication. In addition to these interventions, you may need to take steps in regards to all of the following issues in order to improve sleep.

Sleep environment

The quality of the sleeping environment is very important. If it is too loud, too hot, too cold, too light, too active, etc, you can struggle with sleep. There is a reasonably narrow bandwidth of environmental conditions which some people can sleep in, although there are obvious individual variations in this. Where some people are fussy, others are more easy-going with these conditions. You need to work out for yourself what your requirements for noise, light, background activity, and temperature are, and then do what you can to maximize these factors. This may mean gaining assistance and cooperation from family or friends who live with you. If people care for your well-being, they will usually take your needs somewhat seriously. You may need to be assertive in making your requirements clear to others, and you may also need to take some responsibility for your own needs. For example, you may need to explore a different amount of blankets to your bed-partner; ear plugs; eye covers, the use of white noise, etc.

Evening excitation

Secondly, our quality and ability to sleep is often a function of what we have been doing prior to going to bed. Rich and spicy foods eaten just before bed time can create sleep problems for some people, as can being too hungry or too full. If you insist on exciting yourself with action packed TV programs, movies or engaging computer games, expect your central nervous system to be highly aroused when you actually want it to settle down. This may also be true for exciting novels that you are reading prior to sleep. Again, if you are exciting yourself, expect to be excited. This is not likely to be conducive to sleep.

The exception to this is sexual excitement. If it results in satisfaction of your needs, it will be conducive to sleep; however, if it does not lead to satisfaction, then sexual activity will have the opposite effect, and can make it more difficult to sleep. Take responsibility for what you are exposing yourself to, and manage these forms of stimulation in regards to your goal of sleeping better. Be in charge of what you will or won't do, and what you will and won't expose yourself to prior to going to bed.

Substances and sleep

Another pre-bed trap people often unwittingly fall into is relying on substances such as alcohol and/or cannabis to help them sleep. Alcohol is a depressant on the central nervous system, meaning that it will suppress brain functioning. Despite being a depressant, people often act in a highly excitable manner whilst getting drunk at a party, displaying more extroverted behavior. This is because the parts of the brain that are being suppressed first are the parts that usually keep the brakes on their extroversion. As these inhibitory parts are shut down before other brain areas, the net effect is that the person becomes more excited. However, if they keep on drinking, the rest of the brain will also become progressively shut down, and their behavior shows signs of obvious suppression of a larger range of brain functions.

The active agent in cannabis, THC, is somewhat different than alcohol. Rather than just being a simple depressant, it acts as a stimulant in low doses. However, in medium to higher doses, THC acts as a depressant, and in very high doses, it acts as an hallucinogenic. It is harder to establish the effect of a dose of cannabis as the dose strength varies greatly. One small joint of very powerful cannabis may have the same effect (depression of the central nervous system) as do several joints of less powerful cannabis; whereas a joint of less powerful cannabis may act as a stimulant. People who are smoking cannabis to assist with sleep are generally aiming for a sedating effect, in which case their brain functioning is being depressed, making sleep more likely in the short term.

When people use alcohol and cannabis together, the effects tend to "cannonball" and intensify beyond the individual effect of either substance alone. This will produce a higher level of sedation via more suppression of brain functioning. This sedation is what people are looking for if they are using depressants to help get them to sleep. The problem is that the effects of these substances is relatively short lived, and people tend to wake up much more alert in the middle of the night, and are then unable to get back to sleep. This comes about as a result of a brain process called the "rebound effect."

Our brain has an equilibrium level of electrical activity. There are normal variations in this level of excitation, but they tend to fall within a range which is natural for us. When sedation has been caused by a central nervous system depressant (like alcohol or cannabis), then the brain is aware that its normal level of electrical excitation has been artificially suppressed. The level of brain arousal has been dragged downwards in a way which is recognized as externally caused. It appears that the brain's goal is to maintain its normal level of arousal, and therefore acts to overcome the effects of introduced agents. As such, a brain that is being sedated will react by *increasing* its own level of excitation in an attempt to overcome the effect of the depressant. There are many brain chemicals for it to change levels of in order to stimulate itself as part of a rebound effect, rather than experience the sedation.

When the hours required for your body to process and metabolize the substance have passed, so that the substance is no longer having the sedating effect, all that you will be left with is your brain's efforts to stimulate itself. This is the time in which people report they wake up, entirely alert and feel "wired," with their minds racing a thousand miles an hour. Often, this occurs in the very early hours of the morning, but the time will depend on a range of factors such as the person's tolerance for the substance, the amount and strength of the substance, and the time of taking it. If people are taking a very large dose of alcohol and/or cannabis, they may essentially knock themselves out and sleep through the night and avoid an early morning rebound effect, but this just means that other nasty consequences will await them later, e.g. a savage hangover.

Many people who do not have a substance abuse problem, and take just small amounts of depressants in order to help themselves fall asleep, will repeatedly experience this rebound effect and regular waking. For this problem, they often further self-medicate with more depressants, and thereby create a vicious cycle. People who do this are often unaware of how they are actually interfering with their brain's natural ability to sleep with substances like alcohol or cannabis.

The other problem with relying on substances, including prescription drugs such as minor tranquillizers or sleeping pills, is that any substance that affects the functioning of your central nervous system will also interfere with the natural brain processes associated with dreaming. Researchers in sleep laboratories have demonstrated that alcohol taken on the night of engaging in learning experiments interferes with the natural brain processes responsible for integrating new information.

If dreams are our species' natural process for digesting our experiences, anything that interferes with this ability is likely to have deleterious effects on a range of psychological functions. If emotional stress is keeping you awake at night, and you are relying on substances to help you cope and sleep, then you are likely to be interfering with your natural ability to resolve the emotional component of your problem. This is likely to reduce your overall ability to cope. Most substances like alcohol, cannabis and medically prescribed tranquillizers or antidepressants are double-edged swords, apparently giving us something to help us cope, whilst at the same time taking something away and diminishing our overall ability to cope.

The manufacturers of Prozac acknowledge that up to 33% of people taking this popular SSRI antidepressant report an increase in insomnia as a result of the drug.[2] They also acknowledge that up to 5% of people will have an increase in abnormal dreams (often nightmares) as a result of being on the drug. Independent research would suggest that most figures of adverse side effects given by the pharmaceutical companies are likely to be underestimated.[3] The real number of people who find it increasingly hard to sleep while on SSRIs could be much higher. The SSRI antidepressants create an increase in the availability of serotonin, and as a result of being on the drug, more serotonin stimulation occurs in the person's brain. This unnatural increase in serotonin stimulation of brain cells could be responsible for worsening sleep problems.

The rebound effect discussed above is also true for other substances, such as amphetamines and the host of "party drugs" such as Ecstasy, Fantasy, etc. These stimulants may produce euphoria in the period of intoxication; however, as they are artificially increasing the level of brain arousal above the normal baseline level, the brain will fight back with a rebound effect. This time, the brain will alter neurotransmitter levels in order to drag the level of arousal down, closer to its normal level, by depressing itself. Again, when the stimulant has been metabolized and processed by the person's system, they will be left just with the rebound effect of depressed brain functioning. As such, it is common for people "coming down" from amphetamine and other stimulant use to "crash" in the days that follow, whereby they simply feel an unshakable depression.

Louise was a young client of mine who struggled with various issues. For the most part, she was able cope with the challenges with great courage. However, she resorted to using Ecstasy one night to lift her mood after a relationship break-up, and two days later she was so miserable that she attempted suicide. Sadly, this is not an uncommon occurrence. Many people remain unaware of rebound effects, and how recreational drugs can result in utter despair.

If a person's ability to sleep is being hampered by drug reactions as discussed here, then this is essentially a neurological problem that needs

---

[2]   Breggin (2001). *The Antidepressant Fact Book.*
[3]   Kirsch (2010). *The Emperor's New Drugs.*

to be addressed at that level. Drug reactions need to be understood and appropriate action taken before sleep is likely to improve. Sedative pain-killing drugs are also likely to produce their own rebound effects. As such, they too can interfere with sleep, unless they are taken at such high dosages that they simply render the person unconscious. Doses at such a level are likely to produce a whole raft of other problems, including accidental overdose, thus the importance of developing other means of addressing chronic pain. You should never take yourself off prescription medications without first discussing this with your physician and being alerted to the issues involved. A well thought-out and monitored withdrawal plan is necessary to avoid further problems.

Daytime activities

What we do during the day is also likely to either enhance or hinder our ability to sleep. Excessive amounts of caffeine during the day or evening can obviously produce such a level of arousal to make sleep difficult. On the positive side, being physically and psychologically active is important in optimizing the chances of good sleep. If you are able to go to bed physically tired as a result of a high level of activity during the day, then this is likely to help. As such, getting into a good exercise routine is an important part of not only reducing chronic pain, but also of enhancing the chances of sound sleep. Research indicates that increasing your body temperature with vigorous exercise or a hot bath around three hours prior to sleep time will also help to create a physiological readiness for sleep at bed time.

If you are going to bed highly anxious about the day's events, or perhaps anticipating the worst of the next day, then you are less likely to sleep well. If this is a regular occurrence for you, then you should again develop an exercise routine which will help to dissipate the build-up of stress hormones which accumulate in your system during the day. In addition, it would make sense for you to create an evening ritual of being still and quiet in the form of meditation, yoga, prayer or relaxation exercises. Some people will find the same meditative stillness and pleasure in quietly playing an instrument, or listening to enjoyable music. People respond differently to these options, with some feeling that they can most relax in reflective prayer or contemplation, while others prefer to focus just on their breath or yoga, and others respond well to guided imagery as found on relaxation CDs (available as an MP3 download, from my website www.drjamesalexander-psychologist.com). Experiment with a range of calming options until you find one that works for you, and then incorporate it in your evening ritual, perhaps as an alternative to watching TV.

Waves of sleep

Sleepiness tends to come to us in waves. If we have taken care of all the factors discussed above and we are in a state of readiness for sleep, then it is likely that the next wave of sleepiness will simply take us with it. The understanding of sleep as coming in waves is totally opposite to the notion of trying to *make* yourself sleep. Like digestion and circulation, sleep is a function of our organism that requires no conscious effort to make happen. In fact, any effort to make sleep happen will most likely interfere with our ability to be taken by the next wave of sleepiness.

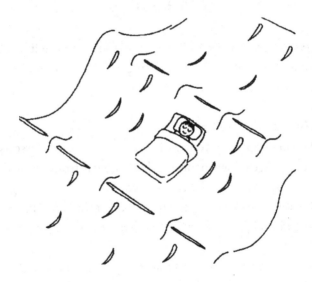

Sleepiness comes in waves

People can make themselves entirely anxious about sleep, such that they end up trying too hard to make it happen. Being taken by a wave of sleepiness does not always occur, particularly if you have become anxious about sleep, and have incorporated into your self-concept "I have a sleeping problem."

Fortunately, EFT is an excellent remedy for this, once you have created the right conditions to allow sleep to occur.

As with other problems, when your experiences have led you to the view that you have a sleep problem, you will also have pathways of neurons which reflect both this experience and the self-concept of being a poor sleeper. On trying to sleep, this pathway of neurons will be highly activated to the extent that you are anxious about not being able to sleep. As such, it becomes something of a self-fulfilling prophecy which is constantly being reinforced in a circular manner. The longer it goes on, the more deeply entrenched these pathways become, and the more difficult you find it to get to sleep. Again, EFT can act as a perfect circuit-breaker, allowing the next wave of sleepiness to take you with it.

EFT for sleep

There are two ways of using EFT for sleep. One is to use it preemptively, before you have the experience of not being able to sleep, and the other is to use it *while* you are having a problem sleeping.

Pre-emptive use

In using EFT pre-emptively, you need to repeat the procedure so as to create and reinforce a range of new neural pathways, away from the well-travelled pathway of "I can't sleep well." My experience is that in wording the Set-up Phrase, I don't want to make a certain statement that I *will* have a problem sleeping tonight, so I phrase it in terms of *may*. For example,

> "*Even though I* may *have a bad night sleep tonight, I* may *wake up with a racing mind, and I* may *find it hard to get back to sleep, I deeply and completely accept myself.*"

I would suggest doing the procedure several times during the day so that the alternate neural pathways can be established and reinforced. It is also very important to do this procedure several times prior to going to bed.

Each time I have slipped back into a poor sleep pattern, perhaps waking up too many times during the night and staying awake for long periods of time, I have had the same experience. On the first night that I do the procedure, I will generally still wake up at the usual unsatisfactory time, as my body clock has become used to this. However, my observation is that with using EFT, I tend to wake up less alert, and therefore find it easier to get back to sleep again. The next night, I will have the same experience, finding myself even less alert again and getting back to sleep easier. By the third or fourth night of using EFT, I generally don't wake up at all. If I do wake up, I am so sleepy and un-aroused that I will very easily fall back asleep again. Each time I have undertaken this process after finding myself in a bad sleep pattern, I have the same experience of progressively sleeping better each night, until I am totally satisfied by around the fourth or fifth night. At that point, I generally don't see the need for the pre-bed EFT procedure and cease doing it.

While experiencing the problem

The second application of EFT with sleep involves doing the procedure on the nights when you do happen to wake up fully alert in all the wrong hours. I soon discovered that performing the procedure at 2:00 a.m. was not only making me more alert due to the physical activity, but it would also wake my wife up. As such, I resorted to doing the procedure in my *imagination*, seeing myself in my mind's eye starting with the Set-Up Phrase and tapping on the karate-chop point and going through the steps until I reached the karate-chop point again.

In doing this, I was inspired by professional athletes who regularly imagine themselves performing the perfect action—Olympians would not use their imagination as a training tool if it were ineffective. Research has been conducted in which subjects were able to increase their finger strength by 21% simply by *imagining* each day for a month performing strength-building exercises of their finger. Note that these people did no exercises in reality to build their finger strength, but simply imagined themselves doing the exercise.

It appears that the brain is not differentiating between what it does in creating motor activity, and merely imagining the same motor activity. The same parts of the brain become activated, apparently to such an extent that cellular changes that are usually associated with muscular exertion are created. If this is possible, then it also makes sense that imagining oneself undertaking the EFT procedure at 2:00 a.m. will also be engaging much of the same brain activity as if you were actually doing it.

In terms of the plasma lamp analogy, you want to flatten the power supply of the device so that it stops throwing out electrical energy, and instead arrives at a state of inactivity. Having the plasma lamp operating with a fully charged battery will ensure that the abundant supply of electricity will result in the lightning bolts being highly active. A state of readiness for sleep, in this analogy, will be achieved when the power supply has been exhausted by placing one's hands all over the surface of the lamp (analogous to tapping on the energy points, this time in your imagination). Sleep can then result when the electrical charge in the lamp (or in the over-active neural pathways) is no longer active, and a state of inertia is reached.

There are several benefits to imagining doing the EFT procedure. Firstly, you are not waking yourself up with a physical activity. At 2:00 a.m., doing EFT in your imagination is incredibly boring. Unlike counting sheep, however, it is a procedure that you actually need to *think* about. When I can't sleep due to a racing mind, I often think that my mind/brain is like a thousand screeching piglets running in different directions. Forcing myself to undertake the EFT process is like throwing a large net over them and slowly drawing them in, constricting their erratic behavior and decreasing the general chaos until it ceases.

Because EFT is a step-by-step procedure, you actually have to think about where you are in the process, and what comes next. This is akin to blotting paper absorbing spilt ink. Your brain is racing with too much energy, and the procedure absorbs this excessive amount of energy as it is engaged in the necessity of thinking about the process and what comes next.

As the procedure itself is repetitive and boring, it will not arouse your interest or create mental stimulation—rather, it will have the opposite effect. When your mind is racing with too much energy, EFT will give you an uninteresting focal point for your mind's activity. My experience is that this tends to have a calming and sedating effect, which is of course conducive to sleep. The next wave of sleepiness to come your way is then more likely to catch you.

In wording the Set-up and Reminder Phrases whilst struggling to sleep, I like to focus on what my actual experience is. If I have woken up worrying about something I expect to happen the next day, I will state this in my Set-up Phrase as:

"Even though I am worried about tomorrow and this is interfering with my sleep, I deeply and completely accept myself."

My experimenting with the phrases has led me to the following standard set which works very well for me:

"Even though my mind is racing, and I am finding it hard to get back to sleep, and I am becoming frustrated, I deeply and completely accept myself."

I repeat this Set-up Phrase three times internally while I imagine tapping on my karate-chop point. I have found that having at least three components of the Set-up Phrase, which then become three different Reminder Phrases (each stated in turn while "tapping" on the different points) is necessary to hold my attention. One or two elements to the phrases just don't seem to be enough if I have woken up with a racing mind, but three aspects to the phrases does the trick perfectly, as it give me more that I have to think about. You will need to experiment with the number of aspects to the phrases and the actual wording for yourself, but ensure that the wording reflects your actual experience in that moment.

After the Set-up, I then proceed to imagine tapping on each of the energy points, starting with my eyebrow, and following the standard procedure all the way until I reach my karate-chop point again. At each energy point, I am internally repeating a different Reminder Phrase, such as:

point 1— *"Racing mind, racing mind, racing mind"*
point 2— *"finding it hard to sleep, finding it hard to sleep, finding it hard to sleep"*
point 3— *"becoming frustrated, becoming frustrated, becoming frustrated"*

and then cycling back through the phrases again with each new acupoint.

When doing this in my imagination, I choose to leave out the Gamut procedure which involves rotations of the eyes, humming a tune and counting. My main reason for this is that I find it impossible to imagine rolling my eyes without actually doing it, and I have found doing this is a little arousing as it is a physical action. As such, I simply leave out the Gamut procedure when undertaking the procedure in my imagination, and after each round, just go back and start again at the eye brow point.

My experience is that this is so effective in "capturing" the excessive amount of electrical activity in my brain, that I generally only need to repeat the procedure for a relatively short period of time. Usually, within around five minutes my mind/brain has been lulled into something of a sleep-enhancing stupor. I can recognize this is happening when my now unfocused mind/brain makes mistakes in the wording of the Reminder Phrases. It will begin making nonsense statements such as, "*I am tree is made of marshmallow,*" or any other such nonsensical statement, rather than "*finding it hard to sleep.*"

At that point, I know that I am extremely close to sleep, and the last vestiges of my remaining awareness tend to snap me back to the actual Reminder Phrase. Typically, I will simply drift off to sleep as my mind/brain loses its grip on the procedure. When this happens, the excessive amount of electrical energy in my neural pathway responsible for keeping me awake has been exhausted, absorbed and/or spent, and sleep will naturally result.

The only times I have not found this to be effective are the occasions when I have come down with a cold or a flu on the day following the restless night. It appears that before I am aware of any symptoms, my immune system is already working hard at battling the bacteria or virus. As such, there is a heightened level of activity going on within my system as it is at full alert to beat the pathogen. This immune response is arousing my mind/body, and so I struggle to sleep due to the heightened arousal.

On such occasions, I persevere with the procedure and incorporate additional elements, adding to its complexity. For example, I will begin imagining conducting the procedure with my right hand on the left side of my body. Once I have completed this, then I imagine doing it again but this time with my left hand down the right side of my body. I may continue alternating this for a while, and if it is still not working, I will add another element of reversing the order of the Reminder Phrases. Phrase 3 becomes Phrase 1, Phrase 1 becomes Phrase 3, and Phrase 2 remains where it is. I will then do this reverse order phrasing using my right hand down the left side, and then using my left hand down the right side. If this is still not lulling me into less mental activity, I will add an additional Reminder Phrase, bringing it to four statements. I can then reverse the order of the phrases with even more complexity.

The effect of these modifications to the basic procedure is that they all require an extra level of concentration and thought. In that sense, they are more absorbing to the extent that you need to think more about them. Although becoming more complex and requiring more thought, it does not actually become any more interesting or mentally arousing. The procedure remains repetitive and boring, despite being more complex.

On the occasions when my system is apparently battling a pathogen, I need to persevere with the procedure until my mind/brain simply gives up. This will take longer than when my immune response is not highly activated, however I have noted that if I persist, it still eventually works. It can mean the difference between being awake in the middle of the night for one hour compared to four hours, and this is a substantial improvement for me.

You may also find benefit from using the Relaxation for Sleep CD which I have prepared. Such relaxation CDs are useful for also creating a circuit breaker when the mind/brain is too busy and racing from topic to topic while you are trying to sleep. Try listening to the CD and just allow yourself to focus on the words and the relaxing sounds. This can be an excellent adjunct to EFT for sleep.

Circadian problems

If you have addressed all of the issues detailed above, and have used EFT to address the contribution which a racing mind can make to poor sleep, but the quality of your sleep has not improved, then it is likely to be a problem relating to your circadian cycle.

The circadian cycle is your body's natural body clock. Through a complex interplay of various hormones, your body gets used to falling asleep and waking up at certain times of the 24-hour cycle. If you have a regular sleep time, your brain will excrete "sleepy" hormones into your blood supply when this time is approaching, and will create the opposite effect when it is your regular wake-up time.

Jet-lag is a problem relating to your circadian cycle being in the opposite hemisphere to where you find yourself. If travelling between different time zones, either east or west, then your body clock will still be on your normal time for the first days. When everyone else in Australia is waking up for a new day, if you have come from the U.K or the U.S, you will find yourself feeling extremely tired and ready for sleep. At the end of the day, the reverse will happen. You will be feeling more like waking up when everyone else is winding down for sleep.

As stated, it takes around seven to ten days for your circadian cycle to fully adjust to the time zone that you find yourself in. On returning to your regular time zone, you will have the same problem again, this time in reverse, until your body clock again readjusts and eventually settles in to the time zone where you find yourself.

If you have had a disrupted sleep pattern for a long period of time, it is very possible that despite following all the suggestions made above, you still wake up like clockwork at 2:00 a.m. This may simply be a problem of your circadian cycle having become well established in this unfortunate pattern. Your circadian cycle can become independent from the original reasons that caused this pattern to develop. For example, you may have been a night-shift worker for years and on retiring, find that you always become alert at 11:00 p.m., and start to feel tired at 8:00 a.m. Or the rebound effect of alcohol or cannabis may have woken you up for years at 2:00 a.m., and you find that this pattern remains despite no longer using these substances to help you sleep.

All of the suggestions so far in regard to sleep are likely to help change your circadian cycle. For example, engaging in vigorous exercise or having a hot bath three hours prior to going to bed and ensuring that you do not over-arouse yourself with exciting or frightening movies, TV programs or computer games before going to bed, etc.

An additional strategy to altering your circadian cycle is to work at forcing its timing into the pattern that you want. You can do this by setting your alarm (on the opposite side of your room, so you have to get out of bed to turn it off) at the time which you believe to be your ideal wake-up time, e.g. 7:00 a.m. While you are in a "vampire sleep pattern" (i.e. awake during the night and sleeping during the day), there is little chance of you waking up naturally at 7:00 a.m. Although you can't make yourself fall asleep at the desired time (e.g. 11:00 p.m.), you can *force* yourself to rise at 7:00 a.m., with the aid of your alarm. The discipline, of course, is to stay out of bed once you have risen to turn off the alarm. If you do so, you can guarantee that you will be more tired by 11:00 p.m. than you would be if you had have stuck to your pattern of staying asleep until mid-afternoon.

Another element of this strategy is to not give in to the urge to sleep during the day. If you do take a nap, you will have satisfied some of your need for sleep, and you will easily remain in the undesired sleep pattern. However, if you do manage to get up at 7:00 a.m., and remain awake for the entire day, you may very well have an uncomfortable day, but you will be naturally ready for sleep closer to the desired time, e.g. 11:00 p.m. This strategy, while usually effective, can take a matter of days to force a new pattern, so that the natural secretion of "go-to-sleep" and "wake-up" hormones occur at the desired times in the 24-hour cycle. You will need a willingness to tolerate a few uncomfortable days, but ultimately it will produce the desired results. If you find that your body clock is so deeply entrenched in an undesirable pattern, you may consider discussing with your GP the temporary use of melatonin in order to "manually" shift your circadian cycle.

Melatonin is the naturally occurring hormone, released by the brain, which promotes sleep. Taken in low doses, a melatonin supplement can help in creating changes in the sleep pattern. This is best used in conjunction with the other strategies suggested in this chapter so that a classical conditioning process can occur; i.e. the strategies (such as EFT) become associated with getting better sleep as a result of pairing them. There are fewer risks associated with melatonin compared to minor tranquilizers and sleeping tablets, however you will need to discuss the relative risks and benefits with your physician, as well as the appropriate dosage level.

The melatonin strategy is a temporary stepping stone to ultimately achieving better sleep. The potential advantage of this approach is that, like forcing yourself to wake up at 7:00 a.m., it can manually change your sleep pattern, so that your brain learns to associate the go-to-sleep hormones at the desired end of the day, and wake-up hormones at the beginning of the day. As such, a new circadian cycle can be created.

It is not uncommon for GPs to prescribe antidepressants to assist in sleep. Some current antidepressants are likely to have a sedating effect, and this will certainly help with getting more hours of sleep. The downside of course is all of the possible adverse side effects which can be associated with antidepressant use, including worsening depression, anxiety and panic, agitation (this can also occur in people who were not depressed or anxious to begin with), and for the most sedating antidepressants, feeling somewhat hung-over during the day. They can also interfere with your ability to get much needed REM sleep, even if they succeed in knocking you out.

Prior to considering any psychiatric drug, people should undergo a genetic test to establish whether their system is able to cope with the drug or not (see Chapter 15 under the section "Pharmacogenetics"). Unfortunately, these tests, while readily available, are still quite expensive. But this cost has to be weighed against the risk of consuming a drug which may make you feel worse, not better.

Sleeping tablets

These type of drugs are also increasingly prescribed to help with sleep, with a nearly 25% increase in prescription in the U.S. over the last few years.[4] The prescription of sleeping tablets are still the most common medical response to sleeping problems, despite what the evidence says about them. Research in Australia has recently shown that 95% of people complaining of sleep problems to their GPs are prescribed sleeping tablets.[5] As with many pharmaceutical drugs, there is often a downside which goes along with the potential upside.

All sleeping tablets and minor tranquillizers, such as Valium, have been demonstrated to interfere with various stages of sleep, including REM sleep.[6] While they may help you to spend more hours sleeping, you will usually wake up still feeling like you have not had enough sleep, as the drugs interfere with the normal sleep cycle. People will often respond to this increasing daytime fatigue by increasing the dosage level of the sleeping tablet that night, which further interferes with deep stage and REM sleep.

---

[4] Kripke, Langer, & Kline (2012). "Hypnotics' Association with Mortality or Cancer: A Matched Cohort Study." *BMJ Open.*
[5] *Melbourne Herald.* Sun. Sat 12th May, p5.
[6] Montgomery & Evans (1985). *You and Stress: A Guide to Successful Living.*

Keep in mind how important dreams are for our emotional well-being, so anything that interferes with your natural ability to dream can be considered potentially problematic. People who are relying on substances to increase the amount of hours spent asleep are running the risk of becoming REM-deprived. The result of this can be a worsening psychological state, lower mood and poorer mental functioning. Not what one generally hopes to get from a medicine.

People's central nervous systems will usually habituate to the 'hypnotic' sleeping tablets and minor tranquillizers (benzodiazepines), so an ever increasing amount is required to get the same result of sleeping more hours— this is a recipe for addiction. As such, rather than getting better, the sleep problem can just become worse, with the person feeling even more worn out and despairing. There is also the increased risk of accidental overdose with each new increase in dosage level.

When people have been using drugs for a long time to aid with sleeping, and then decide to cease using them, a rebound effect, as described with alcohol, can occur. This can go on for weeks, and may lead the person to feel even more agitated and unable to sleep, as well as increase the frequency of their nightmares. Some people also report odd and unusual experiences while taking hypnotic sleeping tablets.

Zolpidem, marketed Stilnox in Australia and Ambien in America, is the most prescribed hypnotic sleeping tablet in the world. It is also sold under generic drugs names such as Dormizol, Stildem, and Somidem. A recent review of violent or unexpected deaths of people who were taking Stilnox in the Australian state of New South Wales between 2001 and 2011 reported that in around a third of cases, zolpidem contributed to the deaths.[7] The study leader, Shane Darke from the National Drug and Alcohol Research Centre at the University of New South Wales, states that such a high prevalence of incidences render zolpidem an *unsafe* drug to take. It has been linked to bizarre and confusional behaviour, often with reports of no conscious awareness or memory, sleep walking, violence, and suicide. The evidence of such ill-effects are so strong that the study authors suggest that

---

[7] Stilnox sleeping drug considered unsafe by review—6th July 2012. http://www. smh.com.au/national/stilnox-sleeping-drug-considered-unsafe-by-review-20120705-21k8n.html#ixzz1zz7I8NWe

it should now be routinely tested for in all violent and unexpected deaths. GPs often prescribe zolpidem in the belief that the short-term inducement of sleep by hypnotics is better than no sleep at all. The effects of these drugs are particularly dangerous when taken in combination with alcohol, opiates and major tranquilisers; and when people take the drug but don't then go to bed. Obviously, the false perception of safety with hypnotic drugs needs to change.

In addition to these potential dangers, recent research has revealed that sleeping tablets are also associated with increased risk of death from cancer, heart disease and other serious ailments.[8] Researchers from San Diego studied a range of sleeping tablets on the market, including both zolpidem and temazepam (a benzodiazepine), which have been considered safer than older hypnotics because of their shorter duration of action. Their study matched 10,531 sleeping tablet users (average use time of 2.5 years) with 23,674 people who were not using the drugs, but were similar in other factors such as age, gender, and health status.

Even relatively low use of these tablets was found to be associated with higher mortality rates, with an overall 4.6 times greater chance of death for the tablet users. People who took only 1-18 tablets per year were still at 3.6 times more risk of death during the course of the study when compared to matched subjects who did not take the pills. For people who took up to 132 doses of the drug each year, their risk of contracting new cancers increased by 35% when compared to matched subjects not taking the pills. The *British Medical Journal Open* article, in which this research was reported, concludes with urging physicians to encourage their patients to use non-pharmaceutical and psychological approaches to address sleep problems.

If you decide that you would like to come off sleeping tablets, then discuss this with your doctor. If there is no compelling medical reason for you to remain on them, she may agree to assist you in working out a gradual withdrawal program. If not, then there is the chance that she has been overly influenced by the relentless marketing efforts of the drug companies that sell these products. Most physicians have not been trained in non-drug approaches to sleep problems or other psychological issues, such as

---

[8]   Kripke, Langer, & Kline (2012). "Hypnotics' Association with Mortality or Cancer: A Matched Cohort Study." *BMJ Open.*

depression and anxiety. As a consumer of health services, you are perfectly entitled to thank him/her for their advice, and then disagree if there is not sufficient reason to remain on the drugs. Although the attitudes of some will suggest that it is the other way around, *you* are actually employing the physician.

Each year, the old paternalistic attitude of medicine is changing a little, and more physicians are able to recognize that they are there to provide a service, not to impose their authority on their patients. They will often be in a good position to offer you advice on a range of health issues; however, you will be best served by becoming a well-informed health consumer who can do your own research. Sometimes, you may arrive at conclusions which are different from your physician.

Unfortunately, the quality of advice found on the Internet can vary widely. You will need to develop an ability to discriminate between various sources of information—a reasonable rule of thumb is to always look for research-based evidence in support of any health suggestion. If the health advice is just based on people's personal philosophy, or on their own unique experience, this may not suffice as a reasonable ground on which to accept their suggestions. Look for the evidence.

The same is true for selecting any health professional, or evaluating their advice. Some of the characteristics of a good health professional are the ability to listen to your concerns, and to respect your choices, even if this differs from their advice. Become a well-informed consumer of health services who expects accurate information and respect for your choices.

You will be more confident in taking yourself off sleeping tablets, either with or without your physician's support, if you have alternative strategies in place. This chapter has presented a range of strategies which work very well. Hold off with your gradual withdrawal program from sleeping tablets or minor tranquillizers until you are confident enough in these strategies. Ideally, you can become so confident with these strategies that you no longer believe that you need to use the drugs to assist with sleep. Then begin by reducing in small amounts. If you experience withdrawal effects, or a severe rebound effect which may make sleep a lot more difficult, then you have probably reduced by too much, and need to go back to your most recent dosage level in order to stabilize. Then recommence your withdrawal program, but at a lower rate of reduction. There is an amount of trial and error involved in finding the right withdrawal levels for you so that you do not experience withdrawal or rebound effects. If need be, seek open and knowledgeable health professionals who are willing to help and support you in this process. There is an increasing willingness amongst physicians to acknowledge the downsides of psychiatric drugs, and to help people successfully withdraw from them.

Herbal products which can aid with sleep also deserve a mention. There are often less toxicity problems associated with plant products than pharmaceuticals, however they are never entirely risk free. If any product induces a slower, more relaxed state in you, it is acting on your central nervous system. This settling effect may be just what is required to assist you with sleep, but it can also carry the same consequences in regards to rebound effects, and hampering of REM sleep as do pharmaceuticals. Some people's system may also be just as unable to metabolize natural products as herbs (see Chapter 15—pharmacogenetics). However, such products can be considered a viable short term option to manually "shift" your circadian cycle when used for no more than two weeks. Consult with a qualified herbalist, naturopath or herb-aware physician and stick with their dosage suggestions.

CHAPTER 14

EFT, Anxiety & Stress

Stress and anxiety are also highly relevant factors in regards to chronic pain in that these emotions diminish our ability to cope with challenges in general, and the challenge of chronic pain in particular. Our systems are well designed to be able to cope with moderate levels of stress; however, when the stress is extreme and/or sustained over a long period of time, a range of physiological and emotional problems can result. Amongst the results are likely to be a decreased ability to cope with pain, and a higher susceptibility to emotional pain. As pain is itself stressful, most sufferers of chronic pain experience anxiety to significantly higher levels than people not in pain. Stress and anxiety are part of our body's natural reaction to threat, with a range of typical responses being triggered by distressing situations.

Fight/Flight/Freeze response

The fight/flight/freeze response is our body's built-in survival process whereby we are physiologically and psychologically prepared to respond to a threatening circumstance. It is usually triggered by external events, but can also be triggered by the perception of pain, as this is often experienced as a highly threatening to one's well-being.[1]

When it comes to dealing with threats from the environment, the fight/flight/freeze response has served humans very well throughout history;

---

[1]   Grant (2009). *Change Your Brain, Change Your Pain.*

however, it is less useful when dealing with many contemporary threats (e.g. a critical boss rather than a hungry lion). It is also a less than helpful response to chronic pain.

In a threatening situation your brain has the capacity to decide if there is danger. In the initial stages of the stress response this is often done with little or no conscious processing by the thinking neo-cortex. The limbic system in concert with the brainstem prepares your body to take appropriate action and one of three options emerges: fight, flight or freeze. The amygdala is connected to the both the cortex and the lower brainstem and integrates sensory, cognitive and emotional information in order to facilitate a response to danger.

If either fight or flight increase your chance of survival, then your brainstem will mobilize your body's energy system to ensure that the physical activity necessary is actually possible. Almost immediately, we will recognize the threat and our limbic system will trigger a cascade of physiological changes that prepare us to take action required for survival, be it escaping to safety or fighting to defend ourselves.

In such a situation, our mind/brain will quickly become more alert in order to pick up on any cues that may be essential for survival. Adrenaline (epinephrine) will be released into the blood stream by the adrenal glands; our hearts will pump faster, shooting oxygen rich blood out to our arms and legs preparing our muscles to take action; our breathing capacity will increase with air passages in the lungs opening up more to allow a quicker intake of air; our digestive processes will slow down as digestion is less important during an emergency; our sphincter muscles contract to close the openings of the bladder and bowel; we may tremble and shake, have cold or clammy hands, and experience hot or cold flushes; blood clotting ability increases in case of a wound being incurred; sweating increases to cool the body; the mouth will become dryer with a decrease in saliva production; we may experience butterflies in the stomach and/or feel nauseous; and our body hair can stand on end to make us more sensitive to subtle environmental changes that may be associated with threat such as sudden movements nearby. All of these responses allow our body to better meet the physical and psychological challenges of the threatening situation in order that we survive.

If it increases your chances of survival by fleeing (the flight option) then your body has been physiologically prepared to take this action. If escape *was* an option for our hunter & gatherer ancestors when confronted by a saber-toothed tiger, then flight would increase their chances of living long enough to pass on their genes. The emotions which accompany the flight option are fear and anxiety. These feelings give us the motivation to take the action of fleeing and are the result of an evaluative processes of the limbic system in conjunction with the brainstem and nerve projections into the cortex.

If our ancestor was unable to escape the tiger by fleeing, then taking a stand and fighting may have increased their chance of surviving. Getting angry with the tiger may have been a useful strategy, with shouting and lashing out. Anger is the emotion which accompanies the fight option.

If neither fight nor flight is realistic, the final option is a freeze response. Where there is still a chance of survival, but neither fight or flight will increase the prospects of this outcome, stopping and listening intently may. The body's resources are still highly mobilized while we stop, wait and listen in anticipation of danger. This freeze response is used as our ancestor crouches still, remaining full of physical and psychological tension, searching for relevant threat cues and looking for a way to survive the experience.

The final option, if mobilization via fight, flight or freeze is unsuccessful, is to succumb to inevitable demise during an attack and simply give up trying to escape or fight. This is an *immobilization* of the body's resources, and in its extreme form in mammals can result in fainting and even death. Many of the body's systems close down during this immobilization, with decreases in heart rate and the reduced secretion of stress hormones.

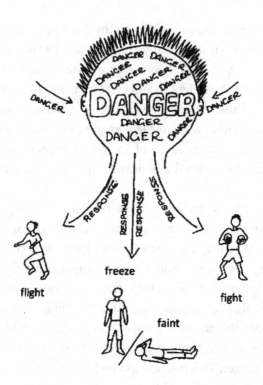

There may still be some adaptive qualities to this physiological and behavioral shut-down in that feigning death (with fainting) may cause a predator to lose interest in the hunt. However, such immobilization is not used as a survival strategy. Rather, it is a submission into a state of helplessness and hopelessness. When no *active* fight-or-flight options are available to humans in traumatic situations, leaving only this immobilization response of giving up, then PTSD and associated depression are more likely to ensue. A range of physical health problems are also associated with this immobilization.

It appears that energy psychology approaches are able to quiet the fight-or-flight alarm response when it is overactive or inappropriate to the threatening situation. In a scientific review of acupuncture, acupoint stimulation has been found to stimulate a range of brain chemical changes which signal the limbic system to *reduce* the fight-or-flight response.[2] The combined result of increased releases of calming neurotransmitters, and

---

2   Ulett (1992). *Beyond Yin and Yang: How Acupuncture Really Works.*

internally generated opioids which reduce pain, signals the limbic system to cease sounding the fight-or-flight alarm response, and instead activates a relaxation response. The release of endorphins not only inhibits pain triggers in the spinal cord and brain, but they directly reduce the heart's reaction to pain.

Research on the effect of acupoint stimulation has been conducted with people who were receiving first aid treatment from paramedics after being injured in an accident.[3] Three separate conditions were applied to the patients after medical treatment had been given and the patient was awaiting ambulance transportation to hospital. In the experimental condition, paramedics applied gentle pressure on a traditional acupuncture point for three minutes. In the second condition, fake acupuncture points were pressed for three minutes; and in the third condition, no point was held at all while the patient waited for three minutes. The results indicated a statistically significant improvement in pain, anxiety and heart rate levels for those who had pressure applied to their genuine acupuncture points, but not for the fake points. This is likely to be the result of the fight-or-flight response being dampened via the effects of the acupoint stimulation, and suggests that the points per se are important.

There is a very strong neural relationship between the experience of emotional pain and physical pain. Although it is a common assumption is that the brain must contain a specific "pain center" which specializes in experience of physical pain, in reality, there is no such structure. The areas of the brain that are involved with emotion and attention are as active when the person experiences pain as are the brain areas involved in just the perception of a non-pain sensation.[4]

As stated in Appendix 2, the ACC is the brain structure which straddles the space between the thinking neo-cortex and the emotional limbic system. It is particularly sensitive to information from the body, and is very active when a person feels pain resulting from physical sensations. However, not only does it light up when physical pain is perceived, it also lights up when emotional pain is experienced. The emotional pain of social rejection is

[3] Fenstein (2008). "Energy Psychology: A Review of the Preliminary Evidence." *Psychotherapy: Theory, Research, Practice, Training.*
[4] Grant (2009). *Change Your Brain.*

just as likely to create neural activity in the ACC as is the pain of stepping on a nail. Both situations can lead to the instigation of a flight-or-flight response.

Thoughts have emotional components that go along with them as part of the package. However, most of our conscious awareness tends to be on the thoughts with little awareness of their underlying emotional basis, which is the larger part of the process. The more rational and problem solving parts of the brain (the pre-frontal cortex) will often become inhibited during the fight/flight/freeze response as more blood and glucose are sent to the most active part of the brain, being the limbic system. As such, during threatening situations our ability to think our way out of the situation is compromised. Therapeutic interventions therefore often need to go deeper in the brain structure than the thinking neo-cortex, and approaches like EFT appear to do just that.

When your fight-or-flight response is triggered too often or too readily, it is common to feel anxious, stressed and ultimately depressed. Your body is repeatedly preparing you for actions required to survive the experience, even when a shouting boss or spouse is not actually threatening your life in the same way as a saber-toothed tiger. The response which served our ancestors very well throughout history can be inappropriately triggered by modern situations which are threatening in a very different way—usually psychologically challenging rather than physically challenging.

Stress/anxiety is usually associated with increased muscular tension in various parts of the body, and additional muscular tension can exacerbate the blood and oxygen deprivation associated with TMS, making the pain even worse. People suffering chronic pain are also much more likely than non-sufferers to experience depressed mood, and this can create just another vicious cycle with chronic pain. This negative impact on mood often follows on from being overwhelmed by unrelenting anxiety/stress.

Excessive levels of stress can cause a decrease, and ultimately depletion in the levels of neurotransmitters which are highly relevant to the experience of pain, such as gamma-aminobutyric acid (GABA) and dopamine. Changes in levels of these brain chemicals have flow-on effects to other neurotransmitters such as serotonin, as well as to hormones such as noradrenalin (norepinephrine) and the endorphins. Sleep and mood problems can follow on from a reduction in serotonin absorption, which can happen when GABA levels have become low. Poor sleep then leads to a weakening of the immune system, which can result in greater inflammation and subsequent pain.

Lower levels of dopamine will also result in a poorer mood. Extreme stress is associated with increases in a neurotransmitter referred to as substance P. This brain chemical *increases* your sensitivity to pain. As can be seen, a vicious cycle can be created between these different responses, such that the level of stress continues to increase as the ability to cope continues to decrease.[5] As such, it makes good sense for sufferers of chronic pain to develop strategies aimed at managing and minimizing both anxiety and stress, as this can create a positive cycle between improving ability to cope, better mood, and reductions in pain.

There are many anecdotal reports of the use of EFT in managing stress, anxiety and panic on the EFT universe webpage. It is worth looking these reports up to gain an idea of how ordinary people are using this approach to help. There is also research evidence that EFT works well with various forms of anxiety, including specific phobias, in addition to trauma anxiety and PTSD.[6] As an example, a study was conducted by Sezgin and Ozcan in which a sample of high school students were treated for test-taking anxiety.[7] Some of them were treated with EFT while others were treated with progressive muscle relaxation. Both groups showed a decrease in test-taking anxiety; however, the improvements for the EFT group were larger than for the progressive muscle relation group, with the difference being statistically significant. Benor and colleagues found that EFT was able to reduce exam-anxiety in students to the same extent as was CBT, but the results were obtained with only two sessions of EFT as opposed to five sessions of CBT.[8]

---

[5] Grant (2009). *Change Your Brain.*

[6] Fenstein (2010). "Rapid Treatment of PTSD." *Psychotherapy: Theory, Research, Practice, Training.*

[7] Sezgin & Ozcan (2009). The Effects of Progressive Muscle Relaxation and Emotional Freedom Techniques on Test Anxiety in High School Students." *Energy Psychology: Theory, Research and Treatment.*

[8] Benor et al (2009). "Pilot Study of Emotional Freedom Techniques, Holistic Hybrid Derived Eye Movement Desensitization and Reprocessing and Emotional Freedom Technique, and Cognitive Behavior Therapy." *Explore: the Journal of Science and Healing.*

EFT as exposure therapy

The EFT recital of the Set-up and Reminder Phrases, along with imagining the anxiety arousing situation can be viewed as a form of "exposure therapy."[9] This popular therapy was devised by behavioral psychiatrist Joseph Wolpe in the 1950s and has become the basic model of treatment to assist people in becoming less sensitized to anxiety arousing experiences, thoughts and environmental stimuli.

In the EFT procedure, a person is undertaking *psychological exposure* in that they are allowing themselves to think about, be aware of and experience the negative feelings in relatively short bursts. There is no effort to avoid these feelings, or to avoid thinking about them or the situations in which they arise. In fact, the opposite is attempted, thus the psychological "exposure" element of the procedure.

The ideal with exposure techniques is that the person experiences repeated exposure to the anxiety arousing stimuli; however, no adverse experience happens as a consequence. This is very similar to my experience with dental phobia. As a small child, I was terrified of the dentist as a result of him repeatedly hurting me with drilling (it seems that often he missed the nerve with pain killing injections that would have numbed my gum) and general rough handling. As an adult, I had the misfortune of requiring the lengthy procedure of root canal therapy. Perhaps perceiving my heightened level of anxiety in the dental chair, the dentist chose to perform the procedure over a couple of weeks with a series of twenty-minute sittings, with around two to three sittings each week.

The result of this repeated exposure was that I became desensitized to the environmental cues that would have ordinarily triggered my anxiety, such as the antiseptic smell of the clinic, the dental chair itself, having instruments put in my mouth, etc. During the root canal therapy, I experienced these cues several times a week over two weeks without a bad event occurring, such that my dental phobia began to naturally diminish. This was purely as a result of repeated exposure to the anxiety-arousing cues, and is a good example of exposure therapy. Unfortunately, I had not heard of EFT at the

---

[9] Lane (2010). Wolpe Not Woo Woo: A Biochemical Rationale for Using Acupressure Desensitization in Psychotherapy.

time as using it would have also helped me to eradicate what had been a persistent phobia.

In some forms of exposure therapy, a highly relaxed state is induced in the person through progressive muscle relaxation. This will create a state that is physiologically incompatible with anxiety, referred to as "reciprocal inhibition." Systematic desensitization, a technique devised by Wolpe, is an excellent example of using reciprocal inhibition to lessen an anxiety, as the relaxed state will inhibit the arousal of anxiety—you can't be both relaxed and anxious at the same time. A range of other forms of incompatible stimulation have been found effective as well, such as diaphragmatic breathing; relaxation techniques and biofeedback; and an "interoceptive" exposure technique of having people focus on their physical experience such as elevated heart rate, dizziness, hot flashes, etc.

Rather than working by reconditioning a person away from experiencing fear to spiders, for example, exposure is now thought to be working as a result of new learning experiences. Something new is happening in the mind/brain in the form of new associations that *override* the influence of old ones, rather than just old fears and anxieties becoming de-conditioned, extinguished or unlearned. The mind/brain can learn new information, such as that it is safe to be in the same vicinity as spiders.

Calming the amygdala with EFT

The part of the brain most involved in fear and anxiety is the amygdala of the limbic system. It can be thought of as the part of the brain which provides an emotional meaning of the experience (threatening or safe) by tying together all of the relevant information from the senses. While the limbic system generates the feeling state, it requires the pre-frontal cortex to consciously register the feelings—this is how we become aware that we are happy or sad. The limbic area is an alarm system which can react to incomplete or confusing signals from the senses in its efforts to scan the experience for danger. Within the limbic system, the amygdala is highly active in receiving and sending relevant information to other brain structures in order to mount an appropriate response, which is often the fight-or-flight response. At times, the response will be an entirely justifiable one to a genuine threat. At other times, the response is far out of proportion to the actual threat and is largely unwarranted.

The amygdala is in fact two almond-shaped clusters of brain cells sitting above the brainstem, one in each hemisphere. In the right brain hemisphere, the amygdala is connected to the hypothalamus (providing the outflow from the limbic system to automatic bodily functions as seen in the fight or flight response), the olfactory bulb (involved in the sense of smell), and the visceral nuclei in the brainstem (involved in nerve messages to and from internal organs such as the heart and the gut). The amygdala in the left hemisphere is connected with the thalamus (which is involved in relaying sensory and motor signals via its many nerve projections into the cortex, and is highly involved in alertness), and to the cortex directly.

Messages from the eyes, skin, mouth and ears go firstly to the thalamus and then to the amygdala; whereas messages from the nose go directly to the amygdala. The thalamus also sends these messages to the neo-cortex, where several layers of brain circuits are involved in 'mulling-over' the information before a thoughtful response is mounted. The amygdala receives the same messages from the senses and launches a response while the neo-cortex is still thinking about it, with the latter arriving at a conclusion around a quarter of a second later. Nerves from the hypothalamus (a limbic structure) stimulate the release of adrenaline (epinephrine) and noradrenaline (norepinephrine) from the adrenal gland, resulting in a heightened state of alertness and body preparedness for action. Judging things as good or bad in a simplistic sense, it is this limbic system and brainstem activity that allows us to immediately jump aside when we see a long slithery thing on the ground. And it is the actions of the neo-cortex which tells us a quarter of a second later that the slithery thing is a snake, and that moving away from it is a smart action to take.

In order to prevent an unnecessarily large response in light of the actual threat, other brain structures are activated to create a barrier that inhibits the threat response while the danger is still being assessed. The part of the brain behind the forehead, referred to as the dorsolateral pre-frontal cortex, plays the role of the brain's "damper switch," bringing a more thoughtful and perhaps appropriate response to the limbic system's emotional impulses. The pre-frontal cortex (the rational thinking part of our brain) is therefore able to instruct the amygdala to cease the entire sequence as a circuit-breaker if a false alarm is perceived. This circuit-breaker can be activated in light of new incoming information. The intruder coming in through the window turns out to be your teenage son who has lost his front door key. The emotional urge to run away screaming or to attack the intruder can be overridden by information processed by the dorsolateral prefrontal cortex: that it is actually your teenage son.

Psychological strategies that rely only on the thinking part of the brain to decrease the anxiety will often fall short because the amygdala's ability to control the higher brain centers is much stronger than the ability of the higher brain centers to control the amygdala.[10] A heavy input from the limbic and brainstem areas can inhibit activity in the neo-cortex. This explains the sometimes limited use of purely talk therapy, cognitive restructuring and other interventions that rely mostly on higher brain structures to eradicate anxiety. People can engage in a large amount of challenging their anxiety arousing irrational thoughts, but the anxiety may persevere simply because an alarmed amygdala is much more powerful than the more cognitive parts of the brain. Despite this, cognitive strategies such as reciting coping statements while in a stressful situation are likely to be of some help, and people will usually appreciate any help they can get.

Due to the power of the amygdala, emotional distress is not easily altered without using approaches that directly address these deeper brain structures. It appears that procedures such as acupuncture and tapping on acupoints can work on these deeper brain areas (as does the psychological therapy EMDR, described in Chapter 16). Research conducted at the Harvard Medical School using fMRI readings has demonstrated that the needling of a particular hand acupoint produces significant activation decreases in the amygdala, hippocampus and other brain structures associated with fear and pain.[11] Other research using EEG readings of brain activity examined the neurological effects of acupoint tapping and showed normalized brain wave patterns of anxiety arousing memories when the tapping was used.

It appears that EFT for anxiety states works by combining psychological exposure (via the Set-up and Reminder phrases) with physical stimulation

---

[10] Fenstein (2010). "Rapid Treatment of PTSD." *Psychotherapy: Theory, Research, Practice, Training.*

[11] Fenstein (2008). "Energy Psychology." *Psychotherapy: Theory, Research, Practice, Training.*

of acupoints. This sends signals to the exposure-aroused limbic system (the location of the excited neural pathways) that reduce the limbic hyper-arousal, leading to inhibition of the typical anxiety response. As such, it can also be thought of as a method of creating reciprocal inhibition, and is thus training a person to recondition themselves so as to remain calm in the face of particular stimuli, rather than remain anxious.

Does any type of physical stimulation have the same effect? Several random control trials have shown the stimulation of traditional acupuncture points to be superior to otherwise identical procedures that instead used "sham" points for reducing anxiety and pain.[12] Other studies have been undertaken to rule out a possible placebo effect to explain the results. One such study used control groups, double blind procedures and placebo controls to investigate the effectiveness of Callaghan's TFT in the treatment of fear of heights. One group was instructed to tap fake points, while the TFT group tapped legitimate acupoints. Both groups showed some improvement, with the TFT subjects showing significantly more improvement than the people tapping fake points. Upon review of the study, some of the fake points were observed to have actually been legitimate acupoints, tapped by mistake.

Rather than just being random locations to tap, the actual acupoints do seem to matter. It appears that the stimulation of specific acupoints sends more signals directly to the amygdala which deactivate the level of arousal that has been caused by memories or cues relating to the anxiety arousing events or situations. Reciprocal inhibition occurs as stimulation of the points reduces the arousal level of the amygdala, and an extinction of the fear or anxiety response follows. With this, a new response can then be learnt.

Pre-emptive use
In using EFT for anxiety, the instruction is similar to when using it for sleep. That is, you should do the procedure in anticipation when you are not anxious; and then do it when you are anxious. The purpose of doing it when not anxious is that you are giving your brain a range of different neural pathways which can act as alternate channels for the electrical activity to travel down when an anxiety arousing situation is present. The more

---

[12] Fenstein (2010). "Rapid Treatment of PTSD." *Psychotherapy: Theory, Research, Practice, Training.*

activation these alternate pathways get prior to feeling anxious, the more likely is the electro-chemical activity to utilize these alternate channels when the anxiety arousing situation is present. As such, your brain will have more practice in a different response, and therefore be more likely to not resort automatically to the same stress response in the situation which usually triggers it.

It is important to get the Set-up and Reminder Phrases right so as to maximize the effect. If you are always anxious about giving presentations at work, you may focus on *"Even though I feel anxious when giving presentations . . .";* however, the real underlying emotion may be a lack of belief in your own ability and/or worth. As such, if you are focusing on a more surface level feeling, the procedure may be less effective. If you are able to peel more layers off the onion, going deeper to get to the core issues, then the chances of EFT working increases. You may therefore decide to use the following Set-up Phrase:

> *"Even though I feel unworthy and inadequate when giving presentations at work, I deeply and completely accept myself."*

In this example, the Reminder Phrase would be: *"Feeling inadequate and unworthy,"* alternating with *"Feeling anxious about the presentation."*

It can be seen that some thought needs to go into the wording of these phrases—your deeper mind/brain knows what the issue is about, even if your conscious mind wants to skirt around it. It is best to go with the deeper implications, even if it is only vaguely known. Keep on persevering with this until the real core issues become evident. It is not unusual for people to develop a sense of the core issues while they are engaging in the procedure. This may present itself in a new awareness, or a word, phrase or feeling that just presents itself to the consciousness. It is important to just "go with" whatever material comes up and see where it leads you.

When anxious

In addition to doing the EFT procedure pre-emptively, you will also need to do it while you are feeling anxious. However, you will most likely find that when the anxiety arousing situation or thoughts are upon you again, your mind/brain will naturally revert back to the old neural pathways of intensifying anxiety. After much practice at being anxious, this is natural and to be expected—you will need to persevere to make a significant impact on this problem.

When doing EFT whilst experiencing anxiety, begin with rating the strength of the anxiety from 0-10, with 10 being the most anxious you can possibly feel. After going through the entire procedure once, go back to the rating scale and give your anxiety another score. In doing the procedure, you will be exercising the alternate neural pathways that you have already created in your pre-emptive procedures, and thereby strengthening them.

Remember, neural pathways work on a "use it or lose it" principle, so the more you use particular pathways the more accessible they will be when the pressure is on. You will most likely notice that you are feeling less anxious after doing the procedure, and this will be reflected in your score from 0-10. You will probably want to do it again in order to bring the level of anxiety down to a score that you are comfortable with, which may be a few points on the scale, or zero.

When doing the procedure again for the second and subsequent times, you need to build into your Set-up and Reminder Phrases an acknowledgement that the level of anxiety has gone down. For example, you may say:

> *"Even though there is still some residual anxiety/ or some remaining anxiety, I deeply and completely accept myself."*

Also, add this acknowledgement into your Reminder Phrase with *'still some residual anxiety'* or *'some remaining anxiety.'*

If you persevere with this approach, with each time you do it, either pre-emptively and whilst anxious, you are giving your mind/brain a new learning experience and strengthening an alternative to the pathways of increasing anxiety. In our plasma ball model, you are repeatedly flattening the battery; and in the dirt road model, you are constantly digging feather drains to allow the rain water to dissipate in different directions away from the main channel.

How effective is EFT in dealing with anxiety? Psychologist Dr. David Feinstein and medical doctor, Joaquín Andrade conducted large scale research in South America in order to gather masses of data relating to its effectiveness.[13] Over a fourteen-year period, they collected data from around 29,000 people who received services in eleven health treatment centers in which EFT was being used. A variety of research techniques were used in the data collection, including a randomized controlled study with a sample of around five thousand people conducted over five years. These patients were assessed as suffering from anxiety disorders and were randomly allocated to either an EFT treatment group or a control group in which they received CBT/medication (the usual treatments). The drug used was a benzodiazepine such as Valium. On average, people had around three sessions of EFT and around fifteen sessions of CBT/medication.

The outcomes were rated by independent clinicians who assessed the patients at one month after conclusion of treatment, as well as three months, six months and twelve months later. The raters assessed whether the patient had shown a complete remission of symptoms, partial remission, or no recovery at all. Importantly, the raters did not know which treatment the person had received—only their initial diagnosis and severity of symptoms as judged by the intake staff when the person first presented for treatment.

At the close of therapy, 90% of the EFT group were assessed as having improved, while 63% of the CBT/medication group were assessed as having improved (around the level that placebo treatments are usually seen to produce). Further, 76% of the EFT group were assessed as having no symptoms of an anxiety disorder, where 51% of the CBT/medication group were judged as being symptom-free. At the one-year follow-up, the gains observed with the acupoint tapping treatments were less prone to relapse than those with CBT/medication, as indicated by the independent raters' assessments.

Rather than being definitive, the researchers viewed this as an extremely important preliminary study, as it indicates the potential which this approach obviously has. As part of the research, a small sample of subjects were assessed for biochemical measures of change. The EFT group showed more normalization of brain wave activity on EEGs compared to the CBT/drug treatment group. In terms of measures of neurotransmitters (the chemicals which brain cells communicate to each other with), the EFT group showed

---

[13] Andrade & Fenstein (2003). *Preliminary Report of the First Large-Scale Study of Energy Psychology.*

lower levels of noradrenaline (norepinephrine). A third sub-study of seventy-eight subjects compared the efficacy of acupuncture needling with acupoint tapping. The results indicated that tapping was more effective in reducing anxiety symptoms (positive response in 78.5%) than using acupuncture needles on the same points (positive response of 50%). This suggests a greater effect of tapping for emotional issues than the insertion of needles for this issue.

There are many applications of EFT, and many reports of it being effective with a wide range of health and psychological issues. In this chapter, I have presented the applications of EFT to stress and anxiety; however, I encourage you to explore the full range of possible applications for yourself via the EFT universe webpage.

Only a minority of people require a referral to psychologists for depth-psychology therapy due to not being responsive enough to the provision of information or self-help approaches. These people tend to be the most anxious and cautious, guarded and hyper-vigilant, perhaps as a result of their traumatic experiences in life. The next chapter will discuss psychotherapy options for those who find that information and self-help alone are not enough to assist them in becoming pain-free.

CHAPTER 15

Psychotherapy for Pain

Hopefully, after having digested the information presented in this book so far, you will not think the notion of receiving psychotherapy for physical pain such an odd idea. As already stated, *The Hidden Psychology of Pain* is not about abnormal psychology or psychopathology. It is a common and relatively normal experience to have chronic pain generated by psychological factors, even if the prevailing culture is largely unaware of it's true causes.

You might like to explore psychotherapy as an option if the presentation of information and the self-help exercises of previous chapters have not created the desired results. A particular approach to psychotherapy which can help with both trauma and associated chronic pain, Eye Movement Desensitization and Reprocessing (EMDR) will be presented in the next chapter, however, this is just one of several viable options. The types of services which mental health professionals are able to provide are presented in this chapter so that you can be realistic about what to expect from different professionals. Mental health services present a plethora of options and possible treatment approaches. As a potential consumer of such services, you need to be well informed so as to able to provide informed consent to any of them. The information provided in this chapter will help you to decide which are the best choices for you.

In my own practice, I give my clients individually tailored information about The Hidden Psychology of Pain. Beyond this, I am able to embark with them on a journey of discovery, attempting to ascertain with them what purpose the chronic pain could be playing in their lives. The main treatment John Sarno gave his patients was information. He did this in the form of two group seminar presentations where people were introduced to these ideas, and where they got to ask specific questions. The opportunity to discuss and openly raise questions and objections is a valuable part of the process. Obviously, no book will allow you to do this. You can, however purchase Sarno's DVD off the Internet, which shows the two seminar presentations, and includes people giving their own accounts of their pain and the difference which the information made to them. You will also see them asking questions and raising objections similar to what may be going on in your mind. In addition, there are discussion groups dedicated to The MindBody Syndrome, or TMS, on the Internet, which you may find helpful. These will give you the opportunity to toss around ideas, as well as gauge and deepen your own level of understanding. TMS wiki (http://tmswiki. org/) is one such Internet site with a range of valuable resources. On this website, you will read many stories that have a positive outcome, posted by the people who underwent the healing process.

Many people are able to have a positive impact on their pain simply by learning of this approach and applying the information to themselves. But ultimately, you may be one of the people who need more than just information to get better. If you have not found the relief you desire with the self-help strategies provided, you may need to see a well-informed psychologist or physician so as to verbalize your queries and discuss the range of possibilities. Or you may be a person who is able to eliminate their pain quite successfully with simply using ideas, but you would *also* like to address the emotional material underlying the pain. I see my job as a psychologist as being to help people overcome their physical and their emotional pain. People will often consult with me for the emotional pain after their physical pain as abated, considering that the job is not yet over until they have resolved some deep psychological issues as well.

If the role of chronic pain is to deflect and monopolize attention so that unconscious distress can remain unconscious, when armed with accurate information, you have a choice: you can choose to comply with your mind/ brain's strategy and remain in chronic pain, or you can choose to bring the unconscious material into your conscious awareness, rendering the pain a pointless and unnecessary defense mechanism.

It is not always easy to make unconscious emotions become conscious on your own. In fact, unless it feels safe to do so, our mind/brain may do all it can to ensure that we don't become conscious of this material, thus the use of elaborate defense mechanisms. There is a slippery quality to unconscious feelings- are they *really* there? Is that what they *really* are, or am I just kidding myself? Have I hit upon some genuine unconscious material, or is it just yet another defense mechanism? These are very hard questions to have to answer for anyone, so having the guidance of a skilled psychotherapist can be invaluable. It may not feel safe to allow this unconscious material to surface unless it is in the context of the support provided by a psychotherapist.

However, please note that many, if not most psychologists and physicians are simply unaware of these notions. You will need to be selective to either find one who is familiar with The Hidden Psychology of Pain (although they may refer to it with another term), or one who is at least open minded enough to be willing to learn. Give your health professional the opportunity to learn of these ideas, and you will find that many may actually be open to them. They are, after all, genuinely wanting to see you get better.

Psychotherapists will often mistakenly accept and support their client's view that the pain is purely physical and therefore needs to just be endured.[1] As such, it is important that you are well-informed about chronic pain in advance of meeting with them, so that you are able to do more than just reinforce erroneous messages. People, including many psychotherapists, will often mistake minor degenerative changes that show up in scans as evidence of serious physical disorder. Being ignorant of the emotion/pain nexus is no crime, even for health professionals. But being willfully ignorant or even arrogant, believing there is no need to learn new information and approaches, is a more serious problem. If this attitude is displayed by your health profession, it should serve as a warning that you may have chosen the wrong person to work with. They may be excellent service providers on other issues, but at least on this issue, you may need to keep looking.

Being trained in science, most health professionals tend towards skepticism, which is often misunderstood as being closed minded. It is actually a preference for withholding judgment until the data is in, rather

---

[1] Streltzer et al (2000). "Chronic Pain Disorder Following Physical Injury." *Psychosomatics.*

than deciding in advance to believe or disbelieve in something. As such, skepticism is more aligned with being open minded rather than closed-minded. Close-minded people will dismiss possibilities *prior* to examining the evidence. Unfortunately, the closed-minded version of skepticism seems to be quite prevalent in the treating professions.

If you can't find a psychologist or physician who is well-informed about these issues, at least try and find one who is willing to suspend judgment until the evidence about you is in. Such a health professional may also be willing to locate and review the evidence regarding The Hidden Psychology of Pain. *The Divided Mind,* edited by John Sarno, with contributions from other medical experts, is an excellent book aimed at educating health professionals about these issues. This book will also be a useful learning tool, so consider sharing it with your health professional.

If a particular psychotherapist helps you to understand the nexus between unacceptable emotions and physical pain; helps you to learn to tolerate your own feelings and wishes, even the negative and unflattering ones; helps you to moderate your own hyper-vigilance about both physical and emotional pain; helps you to learn to accept yourself, regardless of any negative aspects; helps you to recognize your own worthiness, even if not everything about you feels "alright"; helps you to stop overly scrutinizing your own physical symptoms; and finally, helps you to question your own rigid standards of perfectionism, then there is an excellent chance that you will be helped by this person to become pain-free. As Sarno & Coen state,

> The capacity to tolerate one's affective (i.e. emotional) life seems, in effect to preclude the back pain syndrome. We believe that the more able patients are to tolerate what they feel, including their anxiety, vigilance, mistrust, anger and depressive feelings, the less troubled they will be by back pain.[2]

A capable psychotherapist should be able to help you with all of these psychological challenges; however, the reduction of chronic pain is most

---

[2] Sarno & Coen (1989). "Psychosomatic Avoidance of Conflict in Back Pain." *Journal of the American Academy of Psychoanalysis.*

likely to result from therapy informed by an awareness of the connection between psychology and physiology.

The type of psychotherapy most likely to help you overcome chronic pain is "depth-psychology". This term is based on the German word *tiefenpsychologie*, so named by one of Freud's predecessors, Eugene Bleuler. Typically, it refers to psychoanalytic approaches to therapy that take the unconscious mind into account. The term has also come to refer to the theories and therapies pioneered by Janet (another one of Freud's predecessors), William James (the founder of psychology in America), and many of Freud's "students," such as Jung, Adler, Rank, Alexander, etc. As such, the contemporary use of the term depth-psychology refers to more approaches than just Freud's model of psychoanalysis.

A corner stone of depth-psychology is its exploration of the relationship between the conscious and the unconscious mind, conceptualizing the unconscious as operating at a deeper level than the conscious mind. It is the conscious mind which is the place of the surface level cognitions—these are the focus of psychological approaches such as CBT. The common assumption to depth-psychology is that the uncovering of underlying motives will be intrinsically healing.

As depth-psychology became associated with the ideas that Freud became famous for, does this mean that you will need to see a Freudian psychotherapist to eliminate pain? The answer is no. Very few people, myself included, practice psychotherapy which could be called "Freudian" in any meaningful sense.

Freud was a pioneer in this field, however there has been over a hundred years of evolution in psychotherapy since he developed his ground-breaking approach. There are many depth-psychology approaches that have evolved to look very different to what Freud was doing at the turn of the 20th century: however many of them can trace their lineage back to some of Freud's original ideas as well as to other influences, such as William James. The more distance from Freud's original concepts a depth psychology approach has, the more it is likely to be referred to as *neo*-psychoanalytic, meaning "new" psychoanalysis. Franz Alexander, and following him, Sarno's psychologist colleague Stanley Coen, can be thought as neo-psychoanalysts, as they reformulate Freud's original ideas into new approaches. With increasingly sophisticated brain imaging technology and well thought out study designs, many aspects of depth-psychology are obtaining a solid research evidence base which was only hypothesized in past decades. As such, the old criticism of psychoanalysis, or more broadly depth-psychology, being unscientific is becoming harder to maintain. Elements of modern neuroscience are blending well with elements of psychoanalysis, and confirming many of depth-psychology's foundational assumptions.

The overall aim of a depth-psychology approach is to heal damage which has been inflicted in the past, but which continues to "reverberate" within the person. Freud's notion was that "The only way to forget is to remember," and this is the general aim of depth psychotherapy—to help the person resolve emotional issues which have arisen from past events by revisiting them.

Coherence Therapy, initially called Depth Oriented Brief Therapy, is an example of a contemporary depth-psychology approach which is utilising current neuroscience to initiate transformative change in sufferers of problems such as chronic pain, depression, anxiety, grief, etc.[3] This approach seeks to work directly at discovering the unconscious psychological wounds, associated emotional patterns and schemas, bringing these into the person's conscious awareness for the ultimate purpose of transformation. If chronic pain is serving a psychological purpose, Coherence Therapy aims to discover and bring this purpose to conscious attention through a highly experiential and emotional approach. It presumes that in addition to a sufferer having an 'anti-symptom' position (the reasons why you would prefer to not have the symptom), we also have an unconscious 'pro-symptom' position- this is what makes the symptom, from a certain perspective, more important to have than not to have, be it chronic pain or depression. The pro-symptom position is generally unknown to the sufferer, but is responsible for creating and maintaining the symptom for reasons that do make sense, usually in relation to a psychological wound and associated distressed emotions and schema. It was my unconscious pro-symptom position which created and maintained my groin pain for eighteen years in preference to having me crushed by ongoing psychological trauma. The 'emotional truth' which I was being protected from, derived from my car accident experience, involved a knowledge that life-threatening trauma can happen at any moment- none

---

[3]   Ecker, Hulley & Ticic (2012) *Unlocking The Emotional Brain.*

of us are actually safe and life is not guaranteed. There was an extreme emotional wound which went with this insecurity schema, all of which threatened to not only derail me as an eighteen year old, but to keep me derailed for life. Instead of submitting to this fate, an unconscious part of me considered chronic physical pain a better option for me to focus on than the emotional pain and insecurity schema. This is usually the case with chronic pain- a part of us views it as much more important, for an emotionally compelling reason, to be in physical pain than to have to confront or live with emotional pain. Coherence Therapy is a process of discovering what this compelling reason could be, followed by transformative experiences which render this pain producing reason obsolete.

The term "psychotherapist" traditionally meant psychologists, psychiatrists or clinical social workers who were trained in depth-psychology approaches to helping people with emotional issues. Although they are less embracing of the term as a whole, some CBT practitioners will also refer to themselves as psychotherapists. Some psychotherapists may not be registered health practitioners such as psychologists, psychiatrists and mental health social workers, and in fact may have bypassed all of this education and training in preference to their own non-academic training. In most jurisdictions, the terms psychologist, psychiatrist and social worker are legally restricted, meaning that you must be registered with governing bodies in order to refer to yourself with these terms. And you must have undergone specified training in order to be registered with these legal bodies.

The term psychotherapist, however, has no such restrictions. The problem this creates is that there are few quality controls with the unrestricted use of this term. Under the banner of "psychotherapist" can be both people who are highly trained, skilled and ethical, as well as people who are lacking all of these qualities. Of course, there can be unskilled and unethical people in regulated professions as well, so belonging to one is not necessarily a guarantee that a practitioner is of high quality. State registration does, however, increase the chance of quality-control.

People need to be realistic about what to expect in seeking help from different types of professionals, so the various options will be presented here. There still is widespread confusion about the different professions, and about what to reasonably expect from them.

Psychologists

Psychologists are mental health professionals who have focused on studying the academic discipline of psychology over many years. Each jurisdiction has a different education and training system, however most will require psychologists to have focused primarily on studying psychology for at least four or five years at university. This is generally followed up with internships of one form or another, usually amounting to two years of post-graduate on the job training. As such, psychologists have undergone a rigorous academic education in behavioral science, usually taking in some scientific research at the higher levels, as well as skills development in an internship. This training, in some parts of the world, will result in a doctorate or PhD in psychology; whereas in other places, it will simply result in registration, allowing them a license to practice as a fully qualified psychologist. What all psychologists share is a background of six to eight years of education and training specifically in psychology, the science of human experience and behavior.

Many psychologists will simply not be able to provide the type of service I would recommend as useful in helping you to eliminate pain, simply because they have focused on a purely cognitive-behavioral approach to psychology and remain unaware of the ideas presented here. Psychologists who are able to combine both a cognitive-behavioral (as seen in the informational components of this book) and a depth-psychology approach (as seen in particular approaches to psychotherapy) have the best chance of helping you with chronic pain.

Research demonstrates that on average, there are very few differences in the effectiveness of various forms of psychotherapy. Most forms of psychotherapy, from brief psycho-dynamic therapy through to CBT and forms of interpersonal psychotherapy, will generally produce positive changes in psychological issues to much the same degree. People who receive psychotherapy of any type are psychologically better off than 80% of people with the same problems who do not receive psychotherapy.[4]

---

[4]   Miller et al (2008). "Supershrinks: What Is the Secret of Their Success?" *Psychotherapy in Australia.*

As such, it essentially comes down to a personal choice in regards to which approach best suits which person. Some people will have a clear preference for delving into their past and making sense of the overall meaning of their lives, while others will prefer to just stick to focusing on their current thinking styles and behaviors. However, when it comes to a specific problem like chronic pain, there is evidence that a strict cognitive-behavioral approach, such as CBT, will at best result in an adjustment to the reality of the pain, rather than an eradication of it.

As detailed in this book, psychologists with a depth-psychology approach are aiming for much more than mere acceptance. The irony is that a cognitive approach, such as the ideas presented in this book, will be highly effective in regards to chronic pain when it is using depth-psychology notions. These two approaches, cognitive-behavioral and depth-psychology, usually do not go together. However, *The Hidden Psychology of Pain* can reasonably be viewed as a cognitive-depth psychology approach. It just is not the type of cognitive approach most psychologists are familiar with.

Within psychology, some will refer to themselves as "clinical psychologists," some as "counseling psychologists," and some as "health psychologists," to name just a few. Most clinical psychology training programs in Western countries are heavily biased towards training in an almost exclusive focus on CBT, whereas counseling psychology programs tend to teach their students a broader range of approaches. There are also some clinical psychologists who do not feel beholden to a purely CBT approach, but instead are willing to venture into depth-psychology as well. You will need to assess the orientation of any psychologist, regardless of his or her academic training. Their educational background is no guarantee of either their orientation or quality as a psychologist, as there is simply no evidence of superiority of any one type over another. The effectiveness of the psychologist is really more a matter of their orientation as individuals, rather than their academic training, and this has more to do with the type of person they are. Some personal characteristics of effective psychologists have been repeatedly demonstrated in decades of research, and there is no evidence that these qualities can be taught—they seem to be qualities inherent to the person. As such, you need to judge the quality of psychologists individually, and look for a good fit between the type of person you are, and the type of person they are.

Psychiatrists, psychotherapy & drugs

Our culture still has a particular impression of psychiatry as a profession, although this view is now more an aspect of popular imagination and very old films in which we see psychiatrists conducting psychoanalysis, often complete with the traditional couch. Contemporary movies still perpetuate this stereotype as well. This image of psychiatry is maintained, in part, because while very few psychiatrists are *also* psychoanalysts, most psychoanalysts *are* psychiatrists. Despite the stereotype, the current reality is that psychoanalytic psychiatrists (those following Freud's psychological approach) constitute only very small proportion of contemporary psychiatry.[5]

Psychiatrists are mental health professionals who have undergone firstly a medical degree, followed by specialist training in psychiatry. As with psychology, different parts of the world have different pathways to becoming a psychiatrist, however, they all begin their careers with a medical degree.

While the situation is slowly changing, there is still very little psychology taught in most medical degrees. This is understandable as the amount of information required to educate a student about the physical functioning of the body alone is phenomenal. As such, an aspiring psychiatrist has very little exposure to psychology until she or he is undertaking their training in psychiatry following the completion of their medical degree. In the past, this may have been an opportunity for them to learn about psychology. However, in recent decades, this training in psychiatry has become primarily focused on learning the psychiatric classification system of mental disorders, and which drugs to apply to which label. This is not a psychological enterprise, nor is it informed by psychological science. As such, it has become the norm for contemporary psychiatrists to have little training in or awareness of psychology, Freudian or otherwise. As the originator of CBT, Aaron Beck is a psychiatrist, if contemporary psychiatrists show an interest in psychotherapy at all, it is often CBT.

If you consult a psychiatrist, he or she is more likely to be interested in prescribing drugs for you than delving into your background. There are some notable exceptions to this, with some psychiatrists seeking out a

---

[5] Moncrieff (2009). *The Myth of the Chemical Cure.*

thorough training in psychology, but by and large, contemporary psychiatry is essentially a biochemical enterprise. As such, most contemporary psychiatrists are not interested in psychology, and view it as subservient to biological theories of mental disorders. As an example, some psychiatrists proudly boast that they have no interest in their patient's thoughts, feelings or experiences, as these are all irrelevant to their biochemistry and the endeavor to change it with drugs.

Amongst the psychiatrists who have rejected this overwhelming redefinition of their own profession, from being psychology focused to biochemistry focused, are those mentioned throughout this book, such as Daniel Siegel, Bessel van der Kalk, Norman Doidge, and Allan House. Brian Broom, Professor of Immunology at Auckland University in New Zealand, is another notable exception.[6] Recognising the limited role of a bio-chemical approach to patients with immunological disorders, and seeing the importance of psychological factors, he decided to undergo the training to become a psychiatrist so as to add a depth-psychology approach to his therapeutic work. His illuminating books describe many therapeutic successes with symptoms broader than just immunological disorders, extending to cancers and chronic pain syndromes.

Such notable practitioners and psychiatric authors have aroused great interest in the public because of their sophisticated theories and approaches-usually quite different to the simplistic biochemical theories espoused by drug companies and the psychiatrists they employ for marketing.

As well as having an interest in psychology, they often also practice an authentic neuro-psychiatry, exploring the role of brain functions in human problems. Such notable practitioners and authors have aroused great interest in the public because of their sophisticated theories and approaches— usually quite different to the simplistic biochemical theories espoused by drug companies and the psychiatrists they employ for marketing.

Biochemical theories of psychological problems, like any other, are valid as theories. The problem is that these psychiatric theories have been promoted to the status of established fact, especially where the pharmaceutical industry has developed a drug treatment which follows on from the theory. If human

---

[6]   Broom (2007) *Meaningful Disease: how personal experience and meanings cause and maintain physical illness.*

problems in living prove one day to be reducible to aberrant brain chemicals, then they would be added to the list of neurological disorders, and as a result, the list of psychiatric disorders would decrease. Where neurology investigates actual brain conditions, such as neurological illnesses and injuries, psychiatry studies presumed brain conditions, for which there is often little neurological evidence.[7]

There is no doubt that depressed emotion and delusional beliefs exist, and that these can reach an extreme level in some people. However, it is another thing again to suggest that such conditions exist because of a chemical imbalance in the brain.

In his magnificent book on stress, *Why Zebras Don't Get Ulcers*, renowned biologist Robert Sapolsky presents what must be one of the most thorough discussions of the possible biology of depression. It could leave even intelligent readers dazed and confused by all the biological and neurological factors which research suggests *may* play a role in depression. However, even Sapolsky's brilliant account simply raises more questions than it answers. I can't help but feel that it is yet another example of reductionism in life sciences, with the hope that if we reduce a complex phenomenon down to its basic building blocks, we may be able to explain it. Apart from being a collection of speculations, such reductionism leaves little trace of the human experiencing the problem, and also eliminates awareness of higher order issues such as psychology, social and political considerations. As an example, such a biological reductionist approach ignores the fact that living in poverty is extremely stressful, and will often result in anxiety and depression.

The biological reductionist approach is akin to watching *The Titanic* and explaining the emotional impact of it in terms of the actions of various brain chemicals. No doubt, watching this film will have a different biological impact than watching a comedy—there are likely to be more stress hormones in your blood supply after watching *The Titanic*, for instance. But, does it actually explain anything to refer to the different actions of chemicals as a way of making sense of the experience of watching the different movies? Does the increase of stress hormones cause the emotional impact of watching *The Titanic*; or does the movie itself produce the emotional impact as well as the change in brain chemicals? Are the changes in brain chemistry causing

---

[7] Moncrieff (2009). *The Myth of the Chemical Cure.*

the emotional response, or are they merely correlated to the emotional response?

Different life experiences will result in different biological realities in our bodies. These are perhaps best viewed as facts that simply go together (correlates), rather than as relationships of A causing B. The evidence which Sapolsky provides of biological possibilities in depression is really just a collection of working hypotheses. The research is inconsistent and inconclusive, with much of it contradicting other findings. Yes, we are biological beings as much as we are psychological and social beings. There are no doubt biological correlates for all of our experiences, including depressed mood. However, with the current state of scientific knowledge, these observed correlations do not establish causal relationships. From both philosophical and common sense perspectives, it is doubtful whether they ever will.

Commenting on the failure of psychiatric drugs to successfully treat many conditions, medical genetic researcher Kirchheiner states that, "Despite the availability of a wide range of different drug classes, about 30-50% of patients will not respond sufficiently to acute treatment, regardless of the initial choice of standard psychiatric medication." When people report that drugs such as antidepressants have helped them, they are no doubt being entirely honest, but research suggests that the improvement may also be due to a placebo effect.[8]

Pharmacogenetics

Some people enthusiastically report that going on to an antidepressant has been the best thing for them, while others report that their depression radically worsened as a result, bringing them to the point on suicidal despair. These widely different responses to psychiatric drugs are in some part attributable to differences in liver enzymes which are now detectable with genetic testing. All substances which we put in our body need to be metabolized in order that the chemicals be expelled from our system. If

---

[8] Kirchheiner et al (2004 p.442). "Pharmacogenetics of Antidepressants and Antipsychotics." *Molecular Psychiatry.*

this process does not occur, we become poisoned by an accumulation of the chemicals. Many drugs also require bioactivation to form the active compound and desired effect within our body. Pharmacogenetics is the scientific study of inherited variations in the ability to metabolize different drugs via specific liver enzymes.

One family of liver enzymes play a large role in the metabolizing of antidepressants: the CYPs. The existence and amount of these particular liver enzymes in any individual, seen in the cytochrome CYP450, derives from our genetic inheritance. We usually have two copies of each gene, but if one or both copies of the gene don't function properly, then the drug will be processed too slowly. The blood concentration will then be higher than normal, as the rate of excretion from the body is too slow. With antidepressants, this can lead to side effects such as worsening depression; increased anxiety, panic and agitation; increased suicidal ideation; and a raft of physical adverse effects.

If a person has both CYP450 genes that do not work properly, s/he is referred to as a *poor metabolizer*. The person who only has one of the genes working for that enzyme (referred to as an *intermediate metabolizer*) processes the drug more slowly than normal, but not as slowly as a poor metabolizer. A person who has both genes working is called an *extensive metabolizer* (i.e. "normal"). And people who have more than two relevant genes are referred to as *ultrarapid metabolizers*.[9]

These genetic differences have a very large role to play in how our body reacts to drugs, however they do not explain everything—there are other relevant factors. People who are lacking in the cytochrome CYP450 system are likely to be the ones who experience the most adverse side effects from antidepressants currently being prescribed. A poor metabolizer is likely to experience the onset of adverse side effects soon after taking the antidepressant, whereas an intermediate metabolizer may experience side effects over a period of time, as the chemicals from the antidepressant slowly accumulate in their system—this may take months or even years. Extensive metabolizers are less likely to experience problems with antidepressants at

---

[9]   Lucire & Crotty (2011) "Antidepressant-induced akathisia-related homicides associated with diminishing mutations in metabolizing genes of the CYP450 family. *Pharmacogenomics and Personalized Medicine* 2011:4 65-81

the recommended dosage levels; and ultrarapid metabolizers are the least likely to experience side effects, as their system is able to quickly metabolize and expel the chemicals.

These differences in genetic inheritance go a long way to explain the wide range of responses that people can have to antidepressants. In fact, these genetic differences can explain about 75% of the variations in responses to the drugs. As the cytochrome CYP450 system is also responsible for the metabolism of alcohol, cannabis, nicotine and amphetamines, the combined use of these substances with antidepressants or other psychiatric drugs can cause additional problems. This is due to the metabolic pathway already being busy with the psychiatric drug when the additional substances are added. The body becomes even less able to expel the chemicals, due to the pathway being overloaded, and more problematic side-effects can be experienced.

Many other drugs will also increase or decrease the activity levels of various CYP enzymes, either by directly inhibiting the activity of the enzyme, or inducing the biosynthesis of enzymes. This can cause dangerous interaction effects between drugs as changes in the CYP enzyme activity may affect the metabolism and clearance of other drugs. As such, if one drug inhibits the metabolism of another drug, the latter drug may accumulate in the body and reach toxic levels. This is particularly relevant for people who are taking both antidepressants and pain killers, as many analgesics are metabolized by the same enzymes as are antidepressants (e.g. CYP 2D6). Some high profile celebrity drug deaths in the last few years could be explained by this phenomenon. Sudden changes in dosage levels of one of the drugs can lead to unanticipated problems in metabolizing and clearing the other drugs.

Another example of a contributing substance is the herbal depression remedy, St. John's Wort, which acts as an inducer of CYP3A4, but as an inhibitor of CYPA1, CYP1B1, CYP2D6 and CYP3A4. Bioactive compounds in seemingly innocuous grapefruit juice can also inhibit CYP3A4 mediated metabolism of certain medications, leading to an increased possibility of overdosing because of the increased bio-availability of the substance which the juice creates.

For these reasons, it is advisable that people on combinations of medical and recreational drugs consult with a pharmacist who is aware of the role of liver enzymes and different interaction effects, prior to making any changes in dosage levels.

If you decide that you would like to withdraw from psychiatric drugs, a very useful resource is the *Harm Reduction Guide to Coming off Psychiatric Drugs*, published by the Icarus Project and the Freedom Center. This extensive manual is available via a free download from the webpage comingoff.com, and is recommended by a range of services, including the British Department of Health.

In terms of how long one should take in withdrawing from medical drugs, the question is similar to "How long is a piece of string?" The answer is "As long as it takes." Most GPs are informed about withdrawal time frames by the pharmaceutical companies. A cynic might suggest that these companies deliberately mislead them to underestimate how long it takes in order that people fail in their withdrawal attempts (the recent $3 billion fine against pharmaceutical giant, GlaxoSmithKline, would indicate that big-pharma is not above illegal and unethical practices in order to sell their products). Such people can then mistakenly conclude that they need to be on the drugs for life.

On average, most people will be able to successfully withdraw over a three-month period, but there are exceptions at either end of the continuum to this general time frame. Some people may reduce quickly with no or few complications, and others will take much longer than three months. It is not worth you trying to find out your response to rapid withdrawal the hard way.

The length of time required is possibly related to a range of physiological and biological factors, and is not a moral failing. The best rule of thumb is to undertake any withdrawal very slowly so as to not invite unwanted withdrawal effects. It is important that you feel well informed about the pros and cons of withdrawal so as to be able to exercise informed consent. Your GP may advise you against withdrawal altogether, however unless you are legally required to take the drugs, you are entitled to listen to your GP's advice, and still exercise your own decision making rights. Such exercise of informed consent is predicated on the notion that you are actually well informed about the medication and its potential benefits as well as risks. As such, it is important that you *are* well informed of these. Some pharmacists have studied such drugs and withdrawal effects and can be another source of valuable information.

Pharmacogenetics is a relatively new area of research. However, there are pathology labs that can perform a simple genetic test to assess for people's ability to metabolize many medical drugs, including antidepressants. Predictions are that this trend towards individually tailored medication will see pharmacogenetic tests becoming a regular part of medical practice over the next decade, such that drugs will not be prescribed until it is established whether your system can actually cope with the substance.

I have sometimes been misperceived at times as simply "anti-drugs," but in reality, I am merely pro-informed consent and choice. From a civil libertarian point of view, I respect people's choices to do whatever they want with their bodies as long as it harms no one else. This value extends to the voluntary use of both prescription and illicit drugs. As long as people are exercising informed consent, I have no problem with them choosing to use any substances to the extent that it affects no one else. In order for people to be able to exercise informed consent, however, they need firstly to be well informed.

Unless a psychiatrist is personally recommended to you as a practicing psychotherapist (rather than simply a prescriber of drugs) there is simply no reason to assume that he or she will have any awareness of or interest in depth-psychology in general, or The Hidden Psychology of Pain in particular. If you are seeking a "drug solution" to your problem, then most psychiatrists will be willing and able to treat you with prescription drugs. You need to be aware, however, that no drugs have been proven an effective treatment of chronic pain, and most have adverse side effects associated as already detailed.

If, instead, you are seeking to explore a psychological solution to your problems, then most psychiatrists will be in equal measures both unwilling and unable to help. You will have to actively and persistently search to find a psychiatrist who is more interested in psychology than theories of aberrant brain chemistry, and a personal recommendation will be your best chance of finding one. Some psychiatrists, who work primarily as psychoanalysts rather than as drug prescribers, will be much more open to *The Hidden Psychology of Pain*.

Social workers and counselors

Like the word "psychologist," the term "social worker" is legally restricted to those people who have done accredited university training as it is also a regulated term. Some social workers will be highly trained in psychotherapeutic approaches, and some will not be. Traditionally, "clinical social workers" often had a good background in depth-psychology training, however this has somewhat fallen by the wayside as such approaches have lost ground to the cognitive-behavioral revolution of the last couple of decades. Like some psychologists, some social workers will be in an excellent position to provide psychotherapy that could prove helpful, and others will not be. Again, as with any other mental health professional, in the absence of a personal recommendation there is no reason to assume in advance that either a social worker will be familiar with the ideas presented in this book.

And finally, we have a plethora of people calling themselves counselors. Some of these people are well trained and capable, and others are not. Like the term psychotherapist, the word "counselor" is not a regulated term, so anyone can give themselves this title. Unfortunately, the use of the word counselor does not guarantee any level of quality or ethical standards. The exception to this is rehabilitation counselors who have done university degrees in this field so as to work with people who are seeking help in overcoming a range of problems associated with disabilities. Few, if any of these people will call themselves psychotherapists, or offer depth-psychology approaches. There are also some university trained people who receive degrees with a major in counseling, but the quality of this is quite variable, and very few will be trained in depth-psychology.

While most medical doctors are unfamiliar with The Hidden Psychology of Pain, I am aware of some physicians who are either highly accepting of this approach (perhaps under different terms), or are excellent psychotherapists. Some are both, and no doubt can provide very helpful care to their patients. They are a rare breed but they do exist, albeit in too few numbers. Again, only luck or a personal recommendation is likely to take you in their direction.

In finding a suitable psychotherapist to help you, the bottom line is to make no assumptions based on the membership of any particular profession; and to adequately assess the person's general orientation at the outset. You are looking for a good 'fit' between who you are and what you want from them, and what they have to offer.

There are many approaches to depth-psychotherapy currently in use which can be helpful in addressing the psychological factors behind chronic pain, especially when joined with a recognition of the nexus between physical and emotional pain. As stated earlier, I find Coherence Therapy an excellent approach to working with this and other issues. Practitioners trained in Coherence Therapy are still a relatively rare breed, however you can learn more about this approach and see if there is a practitioner near you via http://www.coherencetherapy.org Another psychotherapy which I am very familiar with, Eye Movement Desensitization & Reprocessing, or EMDR for short, is very able to work with psychological factors producing chronic pain, especially when emotional trauma is part of the mix- this approach will be described in the next chapter.

Many people will not need to see a psychotherapist for help. Humans appear to have a very good ability to adaptively resolve distress as an innate capacity. However, there are people who have been so damaged by their experiences that they would benefit from some competent psychotherapy, and chronic pain that is not relieved by the processing of essential information may be an indicator of this need.

From the perspective of The Hidden Psychology of Pain, when your mind/brain recognizes that there is no longer a need to protect you from what had seemed unsolvable emotional problems, there is no further need to distract your conscious attention with physical pain. When the mind/brain learns that something can be done to resolve these issues—that relief, answers and perspective can arise where there had only been pain and confusion—it can relinquish the need to generate pain. Without unresolved emotional pain, the defense mechanism of chronic physical pain becomes a pointless exercise. The next chapter will explore EMDR, an approach to psychotherapy which is getting excellent results with both emotional trauma and associated chronic pain.

CHAPTER 16

Eye Movement Desensitization
& Reprocessing

"The most exciting phrase to hear in science, the one that heralds new discoveries, is not 'Eureka!' but 'That's funny ....'"[1]

PSYCHOTHERAPY IS A RICH AND varied application of psychology to human problems, with more than a hundred different variations at this time. As stated, many forms of depth psychotherapy can assist with the healing of chronic pain and health conditions. Brief psychoanalytic therapy is used effectively to treat chronic pain and health conditions by the psychologists who worked with John Sarno at the New York University Medical Center. As long as the psychotherapy is informed by depth-psychology notions, and an awareness of how unconscious emotions can result in chronic pain, then there is an excellent chance of it being helpful with this problem.

In her informative book *Mapping the Mind,* neuroscientist Rita Carter bemoans the fact that we are unable to overcome trauma by simply isolating the offending memories and stripping them of their harmful content. While nothing to do with human suffering is that simple, it is apparent that Carter has never heard of EMDR.

---

[1]   Isaac Asimov—http://www.americanscientist.org/issues/pub/thats-funny/1

A chance observation

EMDR is an innovative form of psychotherapy, and in combination with *The Hidden Psychology of Pain*, can achieve a great deal for sufferers. It was developed by the brilliant American psychologist, Francine Shapiro, in 1987 after an odd but fortuitous personal experience. Shapiro reports that whilst undertaking postgraduate studies in English literature in 1979, she was diagnosed with cancer and was given a very poor prognosis. Recognizing that studying English literature was not likely to help her meet this challenge, she switched over to studying psychology in the hope of learning all she could about mind/body medicine. She read widely, and attended as many workshops as possible in the hope of finding something in psychology and mind/body medicine that would help her to prevail over the cancer.

Shapiro reports that while searching for a topic for her doctoral dissertation in psychology during 1987, she had an extraordinary experience which led to a serendipitous finding. She recounts that while walking in a park in an emotionally distressed state, she noticed that the upsetting thoughts disappeared without any conscious effort on her part. When she brought the thoughts back into her mind, they no longer held the same emotional "charge," i.e. they were no longer so upsetting. She recognized that while she had been walking, during the time in which the upsetting thoughts were losing their emotional charge, her eyes were moving back and forth. Shapiro experimented further and noticed that when she brought up distressing thoughts, her eyes spontaneously moved back and forth in a rapid manner. She was already aware of research which demonstrated the effects of eye movements on higher cognitive and brain functions, so she was able to make some kind of immediate sense of this experience.

Fascinated, she began to deliberately bring up distressing thoughts and noticing the effect when she moved her eyes. Again, the emotional charge of the thoughts dissipated, and the negative thoughts seemed to lose something of their previous power. Shapiro took these observations and began experimenting with friends, colleagues and other participants in workshops which she was attending. She instructed them to bring up thoughts of current and past problems and taught them how to move their eyes rapidly, following the movement of her hand while keeping their problems in mind. Many people reported the same finding: emotional distress decreased.

Over the course of the next six months, Shapiro experimented with about seventy people and developed a treatment protocol which she tested on a sample of traumatized people. This sample consisted of twenty-two subjects who met the diagnostic criteria of PTSD, and included Vietnam veterans, as well as rape and molestation victims. This was the first scientific study of EMDR. The subjects who received this treatment showed marked changes in their anxiety levels, as well as an increase in their positive beliefs about themselves. Prior to the treatment, they were highly anxious and held mostly negative self-beliefs. Overall, it was seen that people who received the EMDR became "desensitized" to the memories which had previously caused them a great deal of distress. This meant that they could be in touch with the memory of a negative event, but the memory no longer triggered the same level of upset.

These positive results were seen to hold over time, rather than just being a flash-in-the-pan finding. The research was reported in *The Journal of Traumatic Stress* in 1989, and caused an instant controversy in psychology due to its highly novel nature and remarkable outcomes. The only other published studies, using psychological or pharmacological approaches, had reported much more modest findings than Shapiro.

I remember reading about the EMDR controversy in the literature as a relatively new psychologist during the late 1980s. Like many others, I thought it simply sounded too good to be true, and was highly suspect of the value of anyone waving their hand back and forth before someone's eyes. Without investigating it properly, the whole proposition seemed very easy to dismiss at the time, which is exactly what I did. Consequently, I did not look further into EMDR until well into my career, by which time psychologists other than Shapiro (who wanted to stand apart from the accumulation of evidence) had conducted a great deal of controlled experimental research on its efficacy in treating trauma.

As it now stands, EMDR has undergone more research than any other approach dealing with trauma, and also has more evidence of its effectiveness than anything else that psychology has come up with in the last 120 years. The score is well and truly on the board. In recognition of its evidence base, EMDR is now accepted by most of the world's psychological and psychiatric associations as a treatment of choice for trauma, including the World Health Organisation which recently recommended it as a treatment of choice for psychological trauma.

Comparison with antidepressants & CBT

Bessel van der Kolk, an eminent neuropsychiatrist and Professor of Psychiatry at Boston University Medical School, has compared the results of EMDR for PTSD with the results obtained from antidepressant drug treatment, and a placebo drug treatment. In this study, reported in a 2007 edition of the *Journal of Clinical Psychiatry*, EMDR was compared with the antidepressant drug fluoextine (marketed as Prozac) for its ability to reduce depression, as measured by the Beck Depression Inventory (BDI) which gives people's symptoms a score out of 20. Immediately after a course of either treatment, people who received EMDR were slightly less depressed than those who received fluoxetine. At the follow up some time later, those who had received EMDR had reduced their level of depression from 16 on the BDI at the beginning of the study, down to a score of slightly over 5 on the BDI. Those who had received fluoxetine had reduced from around 18 on the BDI down to only 13. At the completion of the treatment, the recipients of EMDR were only half as depressed as those who had received the popular antidepressant.[2]

---

[2] van der Kolk et al (2007). "A Randomized Clinical Trial of Eye Movement Desensitization and Reprocessing (EMDR), Fluoxetine, and Pill Placebo in the Treatment of Posttraumatic Stress Disorder." *Journal of Clinical Psychiatry.*

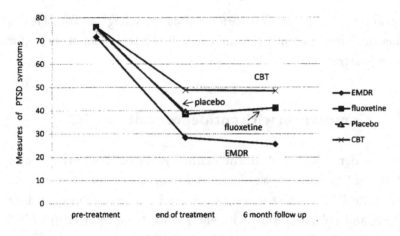

Outcome data derived from Van der Kolk and Schnurr et al's studies, comparing the treatment effects of EMDR, fluoxetine (SSRI antidepressant), placebo tablet, and CBT on measures of PTSD taken before treatment, at the end of treatment, and six months later (note: It is difficult to distinguish on the graph between the effects of fluoxetine and the placebo tablet, as there was virtually no difference in their level of effectiveness in reducing PTSD symptoms. There was no 6 month follow-up of the placebo).

The antidepressant treatment performed only 2% better than did a placebo tablet (which has no inherent therapeutic value at all) in reducing the PTSD symptoms of distress, with the placebo reducing symptoms by 44% and the antidepressant reducing them by 46%. Such a decrease is not enough to be considered clinically significant in people's lives. The EMDR treatment decreased the symptoms by 59%, which does represent an improvement of both statistical and clinical significance. Where the PTSD symptoms of the antidepressant group *got worse* over time (after the completion of treatment), the symptoms of the EMDR group *improved* over time as measured at two—and six-month follow ups. [3]

When comparing the benefits of EMDR with CBT for post-traumatic stress, Schnurr and colleagues found that the effect of CBT was even less than the effect of antidepressant drugs found in van der Kolk's study (and performed worse than the placebo drug). Where the drug treatment saw an increase of symptoms again at the six month mark after treatment ended, CBT showed no real change.[4] In contrast, EMDR produced the greatest

---

[3]   Ibid.

[4]   Schnurr et al (2007). "Cognitive Behavioral Therapy for Post-traumatic Stress Disorder in Women." *Journal of American Medical Association.*

drop in symptoms at around a 60% decrease in distress, and the gains from EMDR again improved as time went on from the cessation of treatment. This continuation of improvement with time is regularly seen by EMDR practitioners.

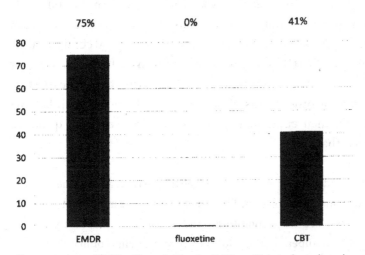

The percentage of PTSD sufferers in Van der Kolk's and Schnurr's studies who recovered so well from the treatment provided (EMDR, SSRI antidepressant-fluoxetine, or CBT) that they no longer qualified as suffering from PTSD.

It is estimated that there are around 70,000 therapists in the world trained in this procedure, and well over three million people have benefited from it in the last two decades. Since the first article appeared about EMDR in 1989 in the *Journal of Traumatic Stress*, there have been over three hundred research papers written, and around twenty randomized controlled trails which testify to its effectiveness. Francine Shapiro is the recipient of the American Psychological Association Division 56 Award for Outstanding Contributions to Practice in Trauma Psychology (2009), and the International Sigmund Freud Award for distinguished contribution to psychotherapy.

Bilateral stimulation

The desensitization phase of the EMDR process has clients focusing internally on a traumatic memory while they are watching the therapist's hand move back and forth across their visual field (other forms of "bilateral" stimulation can be used as well, such as sounds alternating between each ear, and even tapping on each knee in turn). Some psychological commentators question whether EMDR introduces anything new to psychology, or whether it is just another therapy fad. In particular, they query the role that eye movements (or other forms of bilateral stimulation) play in helping people to resolve their emotional problems. In response to this question, Shapiro reports that,

> In the past decade, about 20 randomized trials have evaluated the eye movements in isolation. They compared the eye movements with exposure-only conditions and consistently reported significantly superior effects for the eye movements compared to the no-eye-movement groups."[5]

These research studies are presented on the EMDR Institute website. Together, they demonstrate that bilateral stimulation is an essential and key component of EMDR in helping people to overcome trauma. In addition to the demonstrated value of bilateral stimulation, EMDR incorporates the most useful elements of psychology that have evolved to date. Shapiro has managed to cherry-pick the best aspects of different schools of psychology from a hundred years of its evolution (see Appendix 6), and amalgamate them with her own novel approach into a coherent and extremely effective approach to psychotherapy. As such, it does not stand apart from other developments in psychology. When combined with the other aspects of the EMDR process, bilateral stimulation regularly produces extraordinary results.

Clearly, early traumatization creates physiological changes in the mind/brain and body. Traditional neurological wisdom was that once these changes are created, we are stuck with their effects on the brain. More recent evidence

---

[5] Shapiro (2012b). "The Evidence on EMDR". *The New York Times—Health*

from neurology has demonstrated the ability of the brain to change itself in response to therapeutic and rehabilitative experiences.[6] [7] This observed fact is referred to as *neuroplasticity*, and EMDR is a process that enables such changes to occur at both a mind/brain and physiological level.

When EMDR has been effective, people typically report that while they still have the memory, they are no longer emotionally distressed by it; they have more self-enhancing beliefs rather than self deprecating beliefs; and their bodies show no signs of stress or tension when they are in touch with the memory. As EMDR allows people to retain memories, none of the potential problems of "forgetting pills" (currently being researched) are relevant to it. We do need to have our memories, but we don't need to be forever crushed by them.

I would suggest that EMDR be conceived of as a neuro-psychological approach, as it works on both neurological as well as psychological levels. There are around a dozen studies which have documented how EMDR changes brain functioning, via brain imaging techniques like Single Photon Emission Computed Tomography (SPECT) brain scans. An example of the effects of EMDR on the brain can be seen in the SPECT scans of PTSD sufferers, both before and after therapy, on http://www.emdrtraining.com/ files/EMDR_AmenScans.pdf

Although reading about EMDR is not the same thing as receiving the actual treatment, and no book or pure information will be able to replicate what the treatment itself can do, it is important to present this information. I believe that EMDR is possibly the most beneficial approach that psychology has come up with in the last 100 years, so the more people know about it, the more they will seek it out. This increases the chance that they will subsequently recover from their traumas and chronic pain.

The basic contention of *The Hidden Psychology of Pain* is that your mind/ brain is creating a physical symptom in order to prevent you from becoming consciously aware of unacceptable emotions, unsolvable dilemmas and extreme upsets which are stored in your unconscious mind. Much of this unconscious emotional material would have been inflicted upon you in the context of traumatic situations.

---

[6] Doidge (2007). *The Brain That Changes Itself.*
[7] Arden (2010) *Rewire Your Brain.*

Remember Max, who was repeatedly sexually abused by his brother. It is easy to view his distress as fitting the criteria for trauma as the violation was extreme and sustained. Joanne, who suffered social abuse from her peers due to her malformed spine, also suffered trauma even though it was not life-threatening or as extreme as Max's. Experiences of humiliation, invalidation and conflict as children are also likely candidates as causes of ongoing problems. In the trauma literature, these are often referred to as "life events," or "small-t" traumas rather than as traumatic events.

Research indicates that the accumulation of many small-t traumas can reach such a level of distress as to affect a person as much as "big-T" traumas, like combat experience. Social humiliation and exclusion of children can be so damaging as it relates to our evolutionary history, where to be left out of the tribe meant to die. Symbolic death through social exclusion, through maltreatment by parents, or through violence and combat still amounts to much the same thing—a lack of viability in living. Studies have recently demonstrated that children who are maltreated by their caregivers show the same pattern of traumatized brain activity as do combat soldiers.[8]

There are not too many people who have had completely blessed childhoods in which they were free from any type of upset. Life has a tendency of ensuring that most people emerge from their early years with some kind of emotional burden in varying degrees. Some people carry more of this burden than others—it can range from negligible to the extreme. These type of upsetting experiences, along with the big-T traumas, such as war or being a victim of violent crime, create the type of emotional distress from which our mind/brain may try to protect us.

Families in which there is a lot of overt anger expressed, contempt and hostility between members, extreme conflict between parents, maternal depression, frequent episodes of sulking and crying, and harsh and overly restrictive parenting are all examples of life events which can have deleterious effects on a child's psychological and brain development. In addition, humiliation within one's peer group and large failure experiences can also have very negative psychological impacts on children. Sadly, the sexual, emotional or physical abuse of children is not uncommon either and will

---

[8]   McCrory et al (2011). "Heightened Neural Reactivity to Threat in Child Victims of Family Violence." *Current Biology.*

often result in deep emotional distress. Each of these types of experiences carries with them a range of negative consequences in terms of not only the distressed emotion, but also extremely negative views of the self.

In The Hidden Psychology of Pain, the unconscious fear is that we may not be able to psychologically and emotionally cope if the distressing material wants to erupt into our conscious awareness. For some *few* people, this fear may be well founded. I have worked with people who have experienced such eruptions of distress which their mind had been suppressing for many years. It can feel like they have gone totally insane, and if viewed with a lack of understanding it can appear this way to others as well. People often refer to these experiences as nervous breakdowns. However, it is reasonable to view them as suffering more from an eruption of previously repressed emotions that were generated in a context of extreme trauma.

Most people will not have this reaction and will be able to cope with whatever material their mind/brain would prefer remains hidden. Now as adults, they will be able to make a better sense of their experience, often with the help of good friends or supportive family members, and/or a psychotherapist who is familiar with such occurrences. Trauma is often at the heart of repressed emotional distress, and EMDR is particularly good at treating trauma—in fact, better at it than anything else psychology has come up with so far. An increasing number of studies are also indicating the usefulness of EMDR in treating trauma-related pain.[9]

During a typical EMDR session, specific memories are targeted for reprocessing as they contain the emotional, mental and physiological components of the distressing experience. Where heightened distress remains for years after the event, it is apparent that information relating to the experience, including its emotional impact, has been insufficiently processed and stored in the nervous system. Inadequately processed memories contain the emotions, thoughts, sensations and behavioral responses that were active in the mind/body during the negative experience. We have a natural capacity to process information in a manner which is adaptive, meaning that our mind/brain has an innate ability to let the distressing aspects of our experience go. However, this ability can become blocked, often just by virtue of the trauma itself.

---

[9] Grant (2009) *Change Your Brain, Change Your Pain.*

Possible therapeutic mechanism

How does EMDR achieve the remarkable results which research has demonstrated? The process appears to replicate the neurological activity which occurs when our brains are the most active at processing our experiences: while we are dreaming. After having distressing experiences, over a matter of days to months, our mind/brains normally reduce both the intrusiveness of the memory as well its emotional impact. Memories of the events are transformed and encoded by our mind/brain in such a way that allows them to be integrated with pre-existing and related memory networks, which include positive experiences and memories as well. This allows us to develop a meaningful and accurate understanding of the experience, to see it in the context of our overall lives, to develop perspective, and to gain an understanding of its implications for our future in the form of learning important lessons.

This natural digestive process, however, does not always work in the intended manner, and various forms of psychological distress can result. This includes PTSD, wherein the innate ability to process distress is simply overwhelmed by the enormity of the bad experience. Some people are simply born more sensitive than others, and this poses a possible genetic predisposition to being overwhelmed. And sometimes the accumulative effect of many bad experiences in childhood can make people more prone to being overwhelmed by a distressing experience as an adult—a threshold has simply been reached.

Where the natural digestive process appears to not be helping a person overcome the trauma, EMDR is able to replicate the brain activity typical of the dream state, and thereby can replicate (and bolster) the natural psychological healing that dreams can produce. The rapid eye movements of EMDR appear to push-start the mind/brain activity associated with the rapid eye movements that occur while we are dreaming. As these movements are associated with the digestion or processing of memories, the therapeutic "pushing" of the eyes, while in touch with the distressing memory, can lead to remarkable results.

The scanning of the environment for potential dangers is the job of the brainstem, in conjunction with the limbic system and areas within the cortex. This is done in a largely unconscious manner, and will be active, for example, when a person is walking in countryside where dangers such as snakes are present. The brainstem is governing the constant scanning of the ground ahead, highly sensitive to potentially dangerous objects that are moving. This powerful function of the brainstem can be seen even when a person is "brain dead" (all parts of the brain other than the brainstem, which is keeping the heart pumping and respiration happening, are no longer functioning). Such a person has no conscious awareness at all, and if their eyes remain open, they will stare blankly ahead of them. However, if a person enters their hospital room from a door at the side, their eyes will move and follow the person across the room—all with no conscious awareness.[10] The brainstem is able to still undertake this scanning-for-danger function even though the rest of the brain is essentially dead.

In conjunction with the limbic system, the brainstem is responsible for our fight/flight/freeze response (see Chapter 14). EMDR, with the crossing back and forth of an object in the person's visual field (the therapist's hand) engages and occupies the scanning-for-danger function of the brain stem. This prevents it from becoming fully engaged with the traumatic memory which the person is connecting with. As such, the brainstem is prevented from going into the fight/flight/freeze mode which it usually does when in touch with the difficult memory. This, in turn, allows the emotional limbic system to reprocess the memory without the normal panic (from the brainstem) becoming activated. The person's mind/brain is therefore able to bring up the memory again, but this time without being overwhelmed by the emotional distress that usually goes with it. Consequently, the mind/brain is able to review and digest the memory without the overwhelm of the brainstem's panic, as this is being engaged by the movement of the therapists hand.

The psychological digestion of experience involves the mind/brain undertaking a process whereby useful aspects of the experience are extracted and stored away in the memory network, and aspects of the experience which no longer serve us are discarded. Such discarded elements may include distressed emotions, unhelpful thoughts and beliefs, unnecessary sensory data and physiological reactions which are not adaptive to the ongoing circumstances. Many of these aspects of the experience will be felt by the

---

[10] Carter (2010) *Mapping the Mind.*

person as "toxic." Healing is the process of eliminating the toxic elements of the memory from the person's mind/brain/body, to such an extent that the memory no longer elicits emotional distress, negative views of the self, or bodily indicators of stress or tension. EMDR is aimed at deliberately initiating this healing capacity of the mind/brain.

This clearing process of EMDR is continued with a range of memories which have added to the person's burden of emotional distress. Just clearing one memory is unlikely to make a great deal of difference, so the process is repeated with many of the stand-out memories of upsetting events which people carry. In doing so, we are effectively reducing a person's reservoir of distress, memory by memory.

The therapist does not need to work with all the memories of distressing events, as these tend to be related in the memory system by themes. For example, if a person was humiliated by an angry parent two hundred times, we need to only work with the stand-out memories of this "theme" in order to affect all of the related memories. This allows a clearing of the distress associated with each experience in a ripple effect, with such related memories being more likely to feel resolved as well. As a result, humiliation experiences at the hands of teachers may also lose much of their emotional sting.

When we have done this with enough memories, the person is generally able to review all of their bad experiences and not feel distressed by them. They are likely to feel unburdened by this emptying out of distress, and therefore find a new freedom in terms of how to feel about themselves and their life in general. New positive perceptions of themselves usually arise naturally, and people will not be weighed down by the forms of distress which had been ever-present for them, e.g. anger, anxiety, shock, confusion, fear, frustration, etc. As you would expect, when this has been successful, people often feel that they have a new lease on life, or at least a fresh psychological start (see the final paragraph of Rebecca's story in Appendix 10).

The material that we typically address with EMDR is often the type of distress which can be operating at a less than conscious level within the person. *The Hidden Psychology of Pain* posits that our mind/brain is producing real physical pain in order to distract our conscious attention away from an awareness of deep emotional distress and dilemmas which it figures are unsolvable. If this material was in fact unsolvable, then we may agree with the logic of the mind/brain in producing the pain. However, the fact that many people are able to overcome their chronic pain using the methods suggested in this book indicates that this material is not so unsolvable after all. Clearly, their mind/brain is able to learn that they can cope with this material becoming conscious, and learn that something constructive can be done with such material. My personal preference is to treat such people with EMDR as this is proven to be a most effective approach to resolving trauma, however other approaches, such as brief psychoanalytic therapy, are obviously effective as well.

Some therapists are combining EMDR and EFT in what they refer to as a hybrid therapy. This involves performing various forms of bilateral stimulation on oneself while repeating the Set-up and Reminder Phrases. The tapping procedure can be turned into a self-administered form of bilateral stimulation, tapping on the opposite side of the body to the hand being used. "Butterfly taps" are another forms of self-administered bilateral stimulation—crossing ones arms (as though hugging yourself) and tapping on each upper-arm in turn. This can prove very effective for many people in self-calming, especially in regards to problems like anxiety.

The only caution I would add with doing this on your own is that if you are wanting to address past trauma experiences, then it can be risky to "open-up" these hurts unaided. Attempting to perform the therapy on yourself, at the same time as you may be having a large emotional response, would be difficult for anyone. Often, we don't actually know the strength of the distressed emotions until we tap into them. It is a common experience when doing EMDR that people learn of the intensity and depth of the distressed emotions for the first time when we begin the bilateral stimulation. Prior to this, they often assume that there is no undigested distress within them relating to the bad experience of many years ago, as none is apparent on a conscious level (although there may be other indicators such as emotional patterns and bodily sensations).

The benefit in doing this with a therapist is, of course, that you can simply "go with" the experience rather than trying to guide it at the same time. In so doing, you can be confident that the therapist is gently supporting you and facilitating the process. This can be very difficult to do on your own. EMDR practitioners will often teach people how to do butterfly taps *after* it is evident that all or most of the historical distress has been successfully dealt with and cleared. At that point in time, there is a far less chance of you hitting upon a pocket of undigested distress whilst self-administering bilateral stimulation. As such, I would advise against using either EFT, or other forms of therapeutic bilateral stimulation on yourself with un-processed trauma which is obviously of a serious nature. As stated, it is best to seek professional help with this. This is not a problem with lesser forms of emotional distress, and you can safely self-administer the procedures presented.

Other forms of bilateral stimulation are naturally occurring, and tend to go with activities which we enjoy. Such physical actions as walking, running and swimming are all examples of bilateral stimulation as per the required body movements of left-right-left, etc. These activities require that the two sides of the body, and therefore both hemispheres of the brain are being used in an alternating pattern. It is common for people to report that they feel emotionally better after engaging in these types of activities. Even more sedentary activities such as knitting would qualify as bilateral stimulation, as regular right/left movements are being made in the process. As such, doing these actions will often allow you to feel like your head has cleared afterwards, making it easier to hold some perspective on a challenging situation. These are often very calming activities, and therefore worth engaging in.

My Bi-lateral stimulation & Relaxing Nature Sounds CD can be helpful in assisting you to emotionally settle after a distressing event, or even just for pleasant self-soothing. It can be obtained as an MP3 download from my website, www.drjamesalexander-psychologist.com It has bilateral stimulation sounds combined with a range of nature sounds which most people find very pleasant. You may also use it in twenty—to thirty-second sets to self-administer bilateral stimulation in regards to emotional issues of a less serious nature.

EMDR, along with an awareness of what produces chronic pain is the perfect combination to make the pain redundant. Not only does it result in a lessened burden of distress, but EMDR teaches your brain that you can in fact do something constructive with the burden—that you will not have a nervous breakdown as a result of processing the distress in a constructive and healing manner. As a result, your brain can recognize that there is less point in generating a chronic pain. This combined approach, of joining EMDR with The Hidden Psychology of Pain, represents "holistic" healing, in that both the psychological and the physical pain can be addressed and resolved.

You will be able to locate an EMDR practitioner by looking up the EMDR Institute webpage, clicking on the "Find an EMDR Clinician" and searching for a therapist in your part of the world. Psychologists, psychiatrists, GPs, and social workers are amongst those who have undergone this training and can provide the therapy. If seeking EMDR, make sure that you work with a person who has done the required training. A credible therapist will have no problem with you asking them about their training background and experience. Be wary of people who offer therapy that is "like EMDR," in that it also utilizes eye movements; or therapy that has been "inspired" by EMDR. Many of these variations may also be useful, however relatively un-trained people may be offering them. The only way to ensure that what you get is genuine EMDR is to seek it from a therapist who has done the required training, and who sticks to the eight-stage process as devised by Francine Shapiro.

CHAPTER 17

Mindful Awareness of the Present Moment

T HE TOPIC OF THIS CHAPTER has very deliberately been left for the end of the book. Other books may either focus purely on the themes of this chapter, or at least have them prominent at the beginning. You will read in this chapter that it is possible to develop a higher level of acceptance of being in pain, and that this can paradoxically decrease the experience of pain and/ or increase your ability to cope with it.

If your experience is that you have tried all the interventions suggested in this book, from gaining a better understanding of what chronic pain is about to clearing yourself of past traumas with the self-help strategies and EMDR, to managing anxiety and sleep problems better with EFT, and you are *still* in chronic pain, then you will find useful pointers in this chapter and suggestions for a way forward.

The standard medical and psychological responses to chronic pain resort to the fall-back position of "learn to adjust to being in pain" way too quickly. Pain management programs that are currently popular in our clinics, such as ADAPT, present strategies to help an adjustment *to* pain, not an elimination of pain. The information provided by a prominent pain clinic in Sydney states that ADAPT is for "When no effective or curative treatments are available." This is promoted after the pain has been there for three months. As such, no time is spent in actually establishing if "effective or curative treatments" of the chronic pain are available *before* people are urged to accept being in pain.

In the absence of more useful interventions and poor outcomes with conventional treatments, adaptation to chronic pain is pretty well all that they can offer. On the advice of programs like this, the person in pain then needs to shift their focus from seeking pain-relief to mere adaptation to it. I suspect that programs like ADAPT are very good, however the very notion of offering a pain management program rather than a pain eradication program is unduly pessimistic in regards to what is actually possible for most people. We all pick up on the cues offered, and the sense made of pain is a very powerful contributor to its continuation.

By contrast, I do not want to suggest that "getting used to it" is either a good or necessary choice for most people. In conventional treatment, the psychological causes of chronic pain are not addressed. As a result, the person often does not improve and the health professional usually resorts to "getting used to it" as the default position.

Unfortunately, this is such a common message given to people in pain that it can barely be called the *last* option—it is usually suggested to people at the *beginning* of their chronic pain journey, and not after other psychological approaches have been tried. Keep in mind that this advice is given by conventional pain management programs not because chronic pain is untreatable, but because most of the treaters have no awareness of the psychological causes.

So, it is with a tinge of caution that I offer this chapter and deliberately do so at the end of the book. The risk is that if you have tried all the suggestions in this book to no avail, you may conclude that your pain can't be successfully treated and you may simply give up in a state of helplessness. An unconscious part of you is still believing that it is more important for you to be in pain than to not be- you have more 'discovery work' to do, and perhaps a skilled psychotherapist can help you with this process. My advice is to seek symptom control through whatever means work best for you (which could be pharmacological, or psychological programs like ADAPT), however continue thinking psychologically about your pain regardless. It may mean that this is simply not the right time for you to eliminate your pain with psychological methods. However, these reasons are likely to change over time and you may be able to revisit *The Hidden Psychology of Pain* at a later point in your life. Please do not dismiss the psychological possibility for all time just because it may have not produced results for you at this time.

Acceptance of what is

Acceptance does not mean either liking or doing nothing about pain. It merely means accepting the reality that in this moment there is pain. The Hidden Psychology of Pain never suggests that people need to deny their reality and kid themselves that they aren't in pain when clearly they are. You can learn to accept the reality of pain while at the same time being aware of the unconscious factors that may be causing it. There is no inherent contradiction here, as acceptance can lead to action to remedy a bad situation. The attitude of acceptance will simply create a different quality to your efforts at creating change. You can work on the strategies suggested in this book while fostering an acceptance of whatever the present moment brings you, even if this includes pain.

Ever since celebrities such as the Beatles developed an interest in Eastern forms of mysticism in the 1960s and 70s, a steadily growing influence of Asian psychological/spiritual philosophy has been evident in the West. In fact, this interest did not actually begin with the Beatles, but came on the back of the Beat Generation's having an interest in existential issues and an openness to different ways of viewing reality.

Part of this may be due to the ingestion of mind-altering substances that were part of the cultural milieu of beatniks, musicians, poets and authors at the time. In part, it was also due to the influence of Alan Watts, an English spiritual philosopher who was adopted by and ultimately came to be viewed as the godfather of the beatniks, as well as of the "flower-children" a decade later.

Watts was a child prodigy, born in a small village in Kent, England in 1915. As this was a place and time that had no affinity with Eastern mysticism, it is difficult to imagine where either his interest in or deep understanding of "spiritual" issues at such a young age came from. While still a young teenager, Watts won an essay competition offered by the British Buddhist Society, and before seeing out his teenage years, he was the editor of their scholarly journal. The clarity with which he discussed Buddhism, Zen and Taosim was evident even in his earliest teenage writings. These themes were elaborated many times across the dozens of books that he wrote before his death in 1973.

Until the late 1950s, Western culture had little interest in or appreciation of these Eastern spiritual philosophies, or "ways of liberation" as they are often called. The only vocation at the time which permitted people to explore spiritual issues was the clergy, and as a result Watts became an Anglican minister after migrating to America in the 1940s. During his time as a minister, he attempted to find common ground between the Judeo-Christian tradition and Eastern spiritual traditions. By the late 1950s, the strains of trying to generate this meld were too great. As society had begun to develop more openness to differing ways of viewing such issues, he left the clergy and became a "spiritual philosopher" for the remainder of his life. It was during this time that Watts was embraced by the socially disillusioned critics of that era, the beatniks, who in turn gave rise to the flower-children of the late 1960s. Practices such as meditation and yoga entered our culture as a result of this broad interest, and have retained a healthy following ever since.

When photos of the earth taken from space were first seen, it became evident to most that we live in a very beautiful and fragile eco-system, not an elaborate machine that can be tampered with and abused with impunity. In the 1980s, aspects of the cosmology from Eastern traditions found support from Western subatomic physics and books such as Fritjof Capra's *The Turning Point* became popular. The rise of environmentalism as a social movement and ecology as a field of study also supported a very different worldview to the traditional mechanistic paradigm of the West.

Embedded in the cultural and social changes that followed were a set of implications for personal philosophy and the experiencing of reality, as well as for psychology. Where notions of ecology extended into *social ecology*, a very different philosophy in regards to not just the nature of reality, but our place in this reality began to evolve. These notions have a long history not only in many of the spiritual traditions of the East, but also in the mystical elements of the religions with which we are more familiar in the West, such as Judaism and Christianity, as well as traditional paganism.

Over the last twenty years, an approach to psychology referred to as "Mindfulness" has emerged as an expression of these cultural developments. It borrows heavily from Buddhism in terms of meditation practice, and just as heavily from Western psychology in terms of an awareness of the role of thoughts in influencing our experience. John Kabat-Zinn, in *Full Catastrophe Living* describes a program that he and his colleagues at the

Stress Reduction Clinic of the University of Massachusetts Medical School developed over twenty years ago.[1] These Mindfulness programs have spread around the world and are usually available in such places as community mental health centers and services. They represent a continuation of the interest that people like Alan Watts inspired in Eastern mysticism decades earlier.

Mindfulness is the capacity to remain fully in the present moment without reacting to or judging it. We all have a natural tendency to label and evaluate our experience, and in so doing somewhat remove ourselves from the experience in preference to *thinking* about it. Fostering mindful awareness of the present moment, un-mediated by our mental processes, allows us to develop a greater acceptance of what is. With this acceptance comes a reduction of stress levels because a significant part of the stress is related more to our *views* of what is happening than to what is *actually* happening.

While it is important to approach such a program without too many expectations in regards to pain, chronic sufferers often report a decrease in their experience of pain as a result of participation. This makes sense, as regular meditation is known to settle down activity in the insular and anterior cingulate cortex, brain areas often associated with chronic pain.[2] Kabat-Zinn reports a study on the effects of the eight-week program on pain levels wherein 72% of chronic pain sufferers experienced a one-third reduction of their pain levels. Further, 61% of participants reported a halving of their pain levels as a result of participation in the program. Sometimes, participants report a total cessation of chronic pain, however the program conveners generally dissuade people from having this as an expectation in advance. Most of these improvements were found to hold over the ensuing years, however, only a minority of people were still actively practicing meditation four years later. Almost all past participants state that they still use an awareness of their breathing during the day, as fostered in meditation, as well as other informal mindfulness practices.

Over the course of eight weeks of instruction and practice in meditation and yoga, most people learn to relax to a deep level. The state of inner calm

---

[1] Kabat-Zinn (2009). *Full Catastrophe Living.*
[2] Davidson & Begley (2012) *The Emotional Life of Your Brain.*

which is often created is obviously conducive for a generally more relaxed frame of mind and approach to life. It naturally follows that if a person is becoming progressively more relaxed, their muscle tension is also decreasing over time and ultimately this will allow a greater flow of blood, and therefore oxygen, throughout the body. Such meditative and yoga practices entail exercising the parasympathetic nervous system—this is essentially the opposite of the Fight/Flight/Freeze response of the sympathetic nervous system. Many people call it the relaxation response. If chronic pain is resulting from the biological pathway of ischemia, then it stands to reason that people will find relief from this decrease of emotional and muscular tension through meditation. It is also possible that in learning to be more relaxed, people are also learning to be kinder to themselves, and less self-critical and demanding. This will aid in reducing pain, as less emotional and physical tension is being internally generated.

Regular meditation has been demonstrated to have positive effects on the brain structure and functioning in terms of boosting brain activity, coherency of brain wave patterns, and neural connections. Researchers have also found that meditation aids in the thickening of the brain structure associated with attention, sensory input and memory.[3] Bessel van der Kolk reports positive findings in brain analyses which researched the beneficial effects of meditation and yoga on trauma survivors. His findings suggest that the parts of the brain most central in overcoming the effects of trauma are stimulated through these practices. This may partially explain the popularity of meditation and yoga, and his finding that people suffering PTSD in the aftermath of the New York terrorist attack show a preference these approaches to emotional healing.

Meditation has also been found to decrease the emotional impact of pain.[4] The number of years over which a person has been meditating is important to this outcome, with reduced emotional impact of pain evident in those with the most years of meditation. People who don't meditate, and those who have been meditating for only a short time, both show greater brain activity in the anticipation of pain compared to long-term meditators.

---

[3] Grant (2009). *Change your Brain.*
[4] Brown & Jones (2010). "Meditation Experience Predicts Less Negative Appraisal of Pain". *Pain.*

The anticipation of pain is a significant problem for most people in chronic pain as they have learned to expect pain as a result of certain actions or bodily positions.

Pain anticipation itself is an emotionally stressful experience, and can often have as much impact on mood as does the actual pain. Zen meditation has also been found to reduce the perception of pain amongst people who are highly practiced in this method. Canadian research found that Zen meditators experienced an 18% reduction in pain intensity when compared to non-meditators. The slower rate of breathing amongst meditators whilst being subjected to painful stimuli was viewed as one of the possible pathways to reduced pain perception, as slower/deeper breathing has been associated with reduced perceptions of pain.[5]

As with other excellent approaches to psychotherapy, there is no reason to assume that chronic pain will *cease* for most people in the short term just by virtue of learning to meditate daily—Kabat-Zinn's reports confirm this. Personally, from some of the books I discovered in my father's library as a damaged 18 year old, I began to meditate. I have no doubt that it helped me emotionally and psychologically in a wide range of ways, and enabled me to overcome some aspects of my trauma. I suspect that the practice allowed me to loosen out the 'guitar string' of my central nervous system, and become a more relaxed person. However, after many years of meditating twice daily, I still remained in chronic groin pain until I learnt about its hidden psychology.

As detailed above, reduced emotional distress and perception of pain has only been observed in long-term meditators. That meditation is essentially healthy and worthwhile on a whole range of issues is beyond dispute.[6] However, if the goal is to reduce pain as soon as possible, meditation will often disappoint as the benefits are mostly seen from long-term practice. But, as it does offer a range of other benefits there are only good reasons to start a regular meditative practice. By beginning now, you will ultimately become a long-term meditator who can better manage pain and distress.

---

[5]   Grant & Rainville (2009). "Pain Sensitivity and Analgesic Effects of Mindful States in Zen Meditators." *Pain*.

[6]   see http://bit.ly/KenPopeMeditationResearch, which presents citations for over 100 research articles on meditation, all of which were recently published.

There are many resources available to teach you how to meditate, but a simple place to start is with sitting still and just noticing the rise and fall of your belly as you breathe deeply. See if you can do this for five minutes at a time to begin with, and slowly increase the length of time in which you focus on your breath. It may be helpful to visualize your breath coming in and out of your lungs, or to feel the sensation of the air entering and leaving your nostrils. Some people add to this with counting each out breath, or just repeating to themselves "one" every time they breathe out. Meditation need not be any more complicated than this simple practice.

The right understanding

Like other very useful practices, unless meditation is coupled with an understanding of what is responsible for producing the pain, it is less likely to lead to reductions in chronic pain in the short term. However, it is questionable as to whether people should settle for a reduction of pain when many can achieve an elimination, or at least a radical reduction of it.

"The right view," or "right understanding" is one of the Eight Noble Truths as described by the Buddha. This entails the right way of looking at life, nature and the world—an understanding of how reality works. The research cited throughout this book suggest a certain view of human functioning that is supported by evidence from various scientific quarters. The success of people using *The Hidden Psychology of Pain* supports the notion that the right understanding is required to overcome chronic pain.

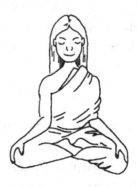

On a grand scale, wisdom and ultimately "liberation" can result from right understanding when combined with the other components of the Eightfold Path (such as right speech, right intention, right action, right livelihood, right concentration, right effort, and right mindfulness). On a more mundane, day-to-day level, right understanding can greatly aid in the reduction of your pain.

Without the right understanding of what produces chronic pain, it is likely that many people will experience a slight reduction of pain from daily meditation, as well as a generally calmer mind. However, it is unlikely that many people will actually *overcome* their pain. As such, I view the meditative practices of Mindfulness programs as being excellent adjuncts to *The Hidden Psychology of Pain,* and in combination with the right understanding, Mindfulness meditation can lead to wonderful outcomes. The irony is that these positive outcomes are more likely when you give up on a desire to achieve *any* particular outcome from meditation, and simply engage in the activity without an agenda of any kind.

Ultimately, the purpose of Mindfulness programs is to teach you to be more accepting of what *is*. The meditative practice can be taken and applied to all aspects of life, wherein ideally you can live and engage with the world in a more mindful or conscious manner. Each activity, from, participating in conversations to walking down to street, to washing the dishes, is an opportunity to live in a more conscious or aware manner if you simply focus on what it is that you are doing. Thus, the single point of attention as cultivated in meditation is applied to all of life's activities, so normal life provides the same opportunity for a calm centeredness as does formal meditation. Rather than living in our heads, in regards to what we think should be happening, or what we anticipate will happen, mindfulness fosters an awareness of what *is* happening. And what is happening is only ever happening in the present moment.

The Power of Now

Eckhart Tolle is a German spiritual philosopher who has reached millions of people around the world, helping many to find a way of creating inner peace. His first book, *The Power of Now* became an almost instant best seller and he continues to give his simple message to people from all walks of life. My view is that he is presenting the same message as Alan Watts did, however in a more straightforward manner for a more instant gratification age. Watts was a wordsmith who kept his audience spellbound with his wonderful use of language, but his message was couched in terms that were sometimes difficult to grasp. A reader of Alan Watts has to be patient with both him/ herself, as well as with Watts, in order to fully get an understanding of his messages.

Both Watts and Tolle present what Aldous Huxley referred to as "the perennial philosophy." This can be thought of as a "mystical" appreciation of reality via direct experience that is out of the ordinary, and unmediated by our common sense views of the world. Huxley suggests that the direct experience of the interconnectedness of all aspects of reality has always occurred for humans, but has historically been understood in terms of religious and/or spiritual experiences: a state of grace, being in the presence of God, cosmic consciousness, "oceanic" awareness, Christ-consciousness, peak experiences, Buddha nature etc.[7]

Each of the world's great religions have had mystics on their fringes who attempted to cultivate a direct experience of reality, in which the sense that one is an isolated pocket of consciousness in a disconnected world is seen to be no more than a social fabrication—a common illusion. Rather than spending their lives talking about religion and worshiping, their path has been to assist themselves and others to directly experience the universe as a totally interconnected web, with the individual being just one intersection in time and space on that web. They have developed many practices to assist in this awareness, which usually involve contemplation, meditation, and sometimes chanting, music and dance. The Eastern spiritual traditions are easily understandable in these terms, however people are often unaware that the religious traditions of the West also contain spiritual mystics, some of whom were persecuted as heretics. Some Christians and theologians also make sense of Jesus as a radical Jewish mystic, who also incurred the wrath of the religious establishment for challenging the orthodoxies of the time.[8]

---

[7] Huxley (1945) *The Perennial Philosophy*. Harper & Collins. New York
[8] Thiering (1992). *Jesus the Man*.

In his popular books, Eckhart Tolle presents the perennial philosophy for a new age and a new audience. In doing so, he wisely draws on many examples from the religious and spiritual traditions of the West, as well as those of the East. He is able to present various new interpretations of the important messages in the New Testament stories, interpreting Jesus as a profoundly wise person. In doing so, he manages to succeed at what Alan Watts set out to do when he became an Anglican minister—to find the common ground between the traditions of both the East and the West.

I have distilled what I view as the most important messages of both Watts and Tolle from a psychological perspective, and have seen these notions have a profound effect on people's lives.

Irene, a woman I saw several years ago, began our counseling process by telling me that she had tried all that psychology had to offer, and it had been found severely wanting. She did not think there was anything that I could do to assist her, as her depression was resilient to all treatment approaches tried in the past. Having just read *The Power of Now,* I decided to run the ideas by her, as it was clear that none of my usual psychological approaches were likely to work.

As Irene was a member of an evangelical Christian church, I was cautious in not wanting to present this approach to her from a spiritual perspective—she already had one, and was not on the market for another. Consequently, I felt the need to describe it to her in purely psychological terms. Despite her opening statements about the futility of counseling, she was quite receptive to what I had to say. When I saw her again two weeks later, Irene was a transformed person. She was no longer stressed and anxious, no longer downcast in mood or self-isolating in her behavior.

Beyond the immediate positive impact Tolle's ideas had on me, I now had experience of its power to bring about substantial change in others. As such, I have been confident in presenting this approach to clients ever since. What follows is a psychologist's interpretation of this different way of viewing psychological and spiritual reality.

It appears that our mind requires an ongoing degree of drama to keep it busy and entertained. Where new information and stimuli is not available from the environment, our mind/brain will generate it internally. The more emotional "juice," whether it be distressing or not, the better. Is this a natural function of the mind/brain? It appears that our brains have an almost insatiable need for seeking out new stimuli and gathering new information, especially in regards to future events.[9] Information gathering creates a response in the neurons responsible for feelings of pleasurable anticipation, and so is reinforced by the pleasure that follows. This insatiable need for more information appears to be a fundamental characteristic of the human mind/brain. Our mind/brain can also be thought of a danger sensing organ. Our cave man ancestor who was too optimistic to bother with the rustling in the bushes probably didn't live long enough to pass on his genes. We are the descendants of those who were negative and fearful enough to take the rustling in the bushes seriously. We are exquisitely sensitive to danger, and the mind/brain's tendency to look out for negative possibilities is part of our neurological "tool box".

Having a brain structure that allows us to form abstract concepts, to develop language and to anticipate the future is, however, a double-edged sword. It allows us a high level of consciousness and creativity such that, unlike many other animals, we are somewhat freed from mindlessly following instinctive behavioral patterns given by our genes. This flexibility in our behavior increases the species' chances of survival, as it gives us a high level of adaptability with which to respond to challenges. It creates the sense of choice in life, or free will that we appreciate. This is easily contrasted with other species that do not appear to exercise much choice in a vast range of important behaviors.

Humans seem to be the most conscious of all beings on the planet, and as far as the evidence suggests so far, in the universe. Alan Watts stated that as the universe is long-necked and spotted in the form of giraffes, it is *conscious* in the form of humans. We are *how* the universe "does" consciousness. But having a high level of consciousness due to our ability to abstract from what *is* also entails a high level of *self*-consciousness. For many of us, this reaches such an extent that our self-consciousness becomes a form of intense pain, rather than a source of pleasure in being alive.

While dogs do not have a high level of consciousness or awareness, they do "being a dog" very well. Once into maturity, when food or sex is available, they will chase either; and when it is not, they will sleep. You will never see a dog stressing about the prospect of not getting fed tomorrow night. When

---

[9]   Carter (2009). *Mapping the Mind.*

the food is presented they will devour it with great gusto, and not give a thought to either last night's or tomorrow's meal. With our greater brain power, while eating today's meal, we can be well aware of last night's dinner (and be either pleased or disappointed) as well as tomorrow's meal (and be fearful or excited). We can actually enjoy what we are eating now but ruin the experience by stressing about whether the next meal will be as good as this one.

This is a simple example of such a common human experience that it is justifiably called "the human predicament." Our mind/brain allows us to do all sorts of phenomenal tricks and possess many skills; however, it can also be the source of many of our greatest miseries.

We have the capacity to conceptualize things that are not currently present and real, e.g. a friend who is not in front of us, or something as ethereal as the economy. With this capacity for abstract and conceptual thought, our mind/brain is able to take us away from the real world and into the conceptual world of thought. In fact, this is what it is doing with us most of the time. How much of your time do you spend thinking about either what has already passed or what may come to pass? If you are a relatively normal human you will spend most of your life engaging in thoughts about the past and the future. Tolle makes sense of this reality in reference to "the ego" as a function of our mind.

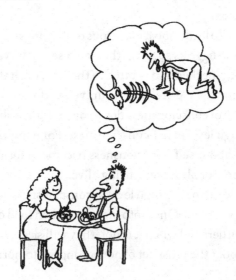

Yes, but what will tomorrow bring?

346

Our ego, or our sense of who we are, is what the mind creates. It is based on the story that we have developed about ourselves, and reflects many of the experiences that we have had. Ask a person who they are and they will usually tell you where they have come from and what they have done. It is experiences that generally give us this sense of who we are, and this is reflected in the story that each of us has about ourselves. This story is the collection of our experiences, and when all added together, can be thought of as our ego. Obviously, the past is very important in this story, but so is our anticipation of the future.

It seems that our mind will want to do almost anything other than be in the present moment. One of the reasons for this is that when you stop to really look at what is going on right now, there is rarely a problem. Most present moments are actually quite acceptable and drama-free. Obviously, this is not always the case as dramas do occur in relationships at home as well as at work; accidents do happen in real time, and sometimes we will be sick or in pain. But for the most part, most of our present moments are relatively alright.

Our mind/brain is an organ designed and evolved to aid our survival.[10] This requires a constant scanning of what could be wrong, so that we can take appropriate action. This priority, and it's obvious evolutionary value, is what keeps us looking for what is wrong, even if we have to search the past or the future for it. This makes the present moment (when there is usually not much going wrong) somewhat boring. Because our ego requires emotional juice, it has a tendency to jump away from the present moment and either go back into the past or project into the future.

Either way, whether it be focused on the past or the future, our ego tends to attach more importance to our *story* than to our actual *experience*. In dredging up a negative past event, our ego is able to generate feelings of resentment and bitterness, guilt and self-recrimination as well as anger. Our story will reveal that either we did something bad or something bad was done to us. Often, our mind will expand the story of what happened to us in the past and use this to make predictions about what will happen in the future. "As my boss has always spoken to me with a lack of respect, my guess is that he will do so again today." On the basis of such a story

---

[10] Carter (2010) *Mapping the Mind.*

about the future, our mind/brain is able to generate feelings of anxiety, fear, nervousness, trepidation, etc.

Stop and listen to the internal chatter that fills your head most waking hours. If you are a relatively normal human, you will find that your mind is in an almost constant state of small dramas, self-generated by re-hashing your story of the past, and/or projecting your story into the future. Associated difficult feelings will accompany these stories and you will spend much of your time feeling a combination of regret/bitterness/anger on the one hand, and fear/anxiety/tension on the other. It is not unusual to alternate between these distressed feelings in a veritable whirlpool of distressed emotion. Again, as this appears to result from the apparently unique human ability to abstract from what is actually happening, our remarkable brain structure is responsible for both our greatest achievements as a species as well as our self-generated misery. This is the human condition.

Distressed emotion, whether it be past-based anger and its variants, or future-based anxiety and its variants, can be viewed as analogous to other forms of pain. The capacity to feel physical pain is a blessing in disguise. How long would we last if we were unable to feel acute physical pain when our body tissue is being damaged? The average infant only learns to avoid hot, sharp or hard things as a result of running fowl of them.

It appears that even babies' brains are equipped to respond to some basic stimuli like large objects, perception of depth and the sound of deep bass notes. But we generally learn to develop new behaviors and change other behaviors as a result of, amongst other experiences, the long process of getting hurt. In so doing, we learn how to look after our safety and how to avoid pain. In addition, without an ability to experience physical pain it is possible that we could be injured and fail to take appropriate action to look after the injury.

Clearly, having the ability to feel pain is adaptive—it helps us to live. Of course, this natural ability to feel pain only really becomes a serious problem when the "system" isn't working properly, i.e. as with chronic pain, when we feel pain all the time, and long after the required healing has occurred.

We can think of emotional pain as being similar in many ways to physical pain. In both cases, pain acts as a warning system—something like a smoke detector. Physical pain is telling us that there is something very important to our well-being that we need immediately attend to. We don't need to think about it, but are wired in such a way that we will take action on feeling the pain as a reflex response. Likewise, emotional pain is alerting us to something that we need to take action on.

When you recognize that you are feeling distressed, try to "tune in" to the emotions more. Upset feelings begin as bodily sensations such as tightness in your chest or throat or butterflies in the stomach. Spend some time listening to what your body is telling you. What is the nature of the distressed emotion? You may simply start by noticing that you feel somewhat vexed but are not certain what this relates to. Remain still and spend time investigating it further, focusing on your physical sensations as clues. The distress will tend to be in relation to either something that has happened or something which you anticipate will happen.

Distressed emotions are likely to be a variation of one of the following basic feeling states: fear/anxiety, anger, sadness, boredom, shame, disgust. There are many more, of course, but they are generally elaborations of these basic ones. Rather than attempting to put the upset aside, allow yourself to go further into it in order to ascertain what it is about. It is highly unlikely that you will feel distressed for no reason. The times when upset feelings may occur for no apparent reason might even relate to the ingestion of recreational or prescription drugs that are producing an adverse side effect, or a bacteria or virus that your system is battling, even if you are unaware of this battle going on, or another undetected health problem such as thyroid disorders.

If, for no apparent reason, the distressed emotion remains over an unusual period of time (and you will really need to be totally honest with yourself about what "no apparent reason" means—e.g. it could be about the job or relationship problem that you are too frightened to admit to, much less address), then you should request a thorough medical check-up with your GP. Hopefully, after having excluded these types of health issues you will be able to develop a sense of what your upset is truly about.

The next step is to view this emotional pain in the same way as I have suggested you view acute physical pain: as a warning system. It is there to tell us to pay attention to something as a matter of urgency. When you begin to step on a four-inch nail, the purpose of the initial pain is pretty obvious. If you pay attention to the message, you will take your foot off the nail and thereby avoid causing serious injury to your foot. When it comes to emotional pain, the purpose is usually less clear. However, an evolutionary perspective would suggest that if the ability to feel emotional pain did not serve any purpose that had adaptive value, it would have been weeded out eons ago. It makes sense to view your emotional upset as yet another biological smoke detector. It is alerting us to something that we really need to pay attention to, or we will suffer even more. But what could emotional pain be alerting us to?

Emotional pain is drawing our attention to the fact that our mind/ brain is in the process of constructing a new problematic story, or adding yet another chapter to an already developed story. To the extent that we continue to go with the story, our emotional pain will also continue, and will most likely increase.

Any story that our mind creates about a past negative event will bring us to feel one or more of the following: anger, resentment, bitterness (about what was done to us); or regret, guilt, shame (about what we did). Stories about positive past events are not problematic and won't lead to distressed emotions, but rather will generate feelings of pride, pleasure, appreciation, etc. As these are not distressing, there is no need to view them as warnings.

The distressed feelings are alerting us to the fact that *our mind is taking us away from what is real* and towards what is not real. Memories about past events are no more reflections of what *is* currently happening than are footprints left on the beach. Any event that happened in the past is no longer happening now. You are not *now* a small child being berated by a schoolteacher or parent. You are not *now* experiencing the humiliation of the boss ridiculing you last Friday. Perhaps these events did happen, but are not happening now. Likewise, the idea that you may get fired when you turn up to work on Monday is not something that is happening now (unless it is that particular Monday).

Any story about the future, like any story about the past is merely a *thought-form*. It has a reality, but this reality is no more than in the form of minute brain cells firing in certain patterns to produce particular thoughts. See if you can conjure up the image of a pink elephant. Now make it a ferocious angry looking pink elephant. Do you feel frightened by it? Probably not, as you can easily recognize it as being merely a thought-form. Again, its reality is limited to tiny brain cells firing in a certain pattern to produce the image. Every thought you have about the past and every thought you have

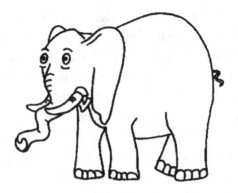

Imagine your own scary pink elephant

about the future has as much literal reality as the pink elephant. They only exist in your head as a form of thought. Others *may* agree with your version of history (or not), but this simply means that the story (thought-form) they have in their head coincides with the story you have in your head (or not). While this type of consensus is important for normal social discourse, it only has relative as opposed to absolute importance or validity. It is relatively important that your memory of an event coincides with others; however, in terms of what matters ultimately in life, it is less important whether you all agree that you met last Tuesday rather than last Wednesday.

Our stories of the past are *relatively* important but they can easily become incredible burdens that weigh us down so much that we may perish underneath them. Have you met people who are so attached to and burdened by their story of the past that they are simply unable to find pleasure in the present moment? Most people suffering varying degrees of PSTD would seem to fit this description; however, there is an important difference. Undigested memories of traumatic events are more "bodily memories" than they are stories. Due to the psychological digestive capacity being overwhelmed by the traumatic event, these experiences get dysfunctionally stored away in the body rather than becoming a story in the mind. Traumatized people are very easily brought to an extreme physical response when triggered by current cues to their distressing experience. This is not a product of the mind or ego creating a story, but a product of their bodies re-experiencing the trauma, generated by undigested distress in their mind/brain. As such, PTSD can be better thought of as an experience of the body rather than a story of the ego.

Processes like EMDR, cognitive imaginal techniques and EFT can help the experience to cease being a lived experience in the body, and in the process to then become a story. Once it is a story (literally, meaning a memory for the first time, rather than a lived experience in the body) the person then has a choice of what they will do with it. Be crushed by the story, or become free of it? This discussion is relevant to either of these options. If you are being crushed under the weight of trauma, get some competent help with it, preferably via an EMDR practitioner who has done the required training. Once becoming clear of the serious effects of PTSD, you will then be in a better position to make use of what Tolle, Watts and Mindfulness have to offer.

In regards to predictions of a problematic future that our mind makes, only one outcome is possible if we take the prediction seriously. We will be anxious. When our mind creates a story that involves misfortunes about what we think will or may happen, our mind has posed a problem that has no solution. If my car tyre is punctured when I leave work this afternoon, the solution to that problem will lie in the combination of the resources and the restrictions of the situation itself and what I can bring to the situation. If I bring with me a knowledge and physical ability to change a tyre then this is highly relevant to the ultimate solution of the problem. If the situation itself brings with it the resource of having an inflated spare tyre in my car and a jack, then these are resources needed for a solution. What if it has been raining heavily and the jack simply sinks into the mud on the side of the road rather than lifts my car? This is a limitation inherent in the situation. My knowledge, that a flat piece of wood under the jack will prevent it from sinking, may combine with the luck of finding a suitable piece of wood on the ground nearby.

As stated, the solution to the problem lies in a combination of who I am in the situation and the resources/limitations of the situation itself. When my mind is generating a story of how bad it will be if I have a flat tyre this afternoon, it is posing a problem that literally can't be solved. Why not? Because who I am in the situation (a necessary component of the solution) is not yet there in the situation. I am here, in this present moment situation imagining how bad it will be if that does happen. As such, the problem can't be solved, as I am not there to solve it (not to mention the fact that the situation itself is not even here yet). When we have unsolvable problems, and if we take them seriously, various forms of anxiety are the result. The problem is of course that we are trying to cross bridges before we get to them.

I have presented a reasonably trivial problem as an example but the same principle holds true regardless of the nature of the problem. More real world examples may be such situations as 'What will happen if I my spouse leaves me and takes the kids?' Our mind may oblige in answering the question with, 'You will lose the relationship with your kids, be financially crippled and wind up a bitter, depressed and lonely person.' When in the grips of the anguish associated with this glum story, it is very easy to forget that any projection into the future is simply a prediction, or a hypothesis.

Physicists are very familiar with the nature of predictions. They may not be willing to state, 'If you drop a pen, it will hit the ground.' Like most other scientists, physicists are more likely to give you a level of *probability* of the pen hitting the ground. Between the letting go of the pen and it hitting the ground, any number of other factors *could* intervene to stop what seems inevitable. The engine of a jet flying overhead could fall off and crash through the roof, meaning that the floor no longer exists for the pen to hit. Theoretically, an asteroid could hit the planet in that second with the same result. An explosion could occur on the floor below such that the floor rises up to hit the pen. While none of these things are *likely*, any of them *could* happen. As such, scientists describe outcomes in terms of probabilities with levels of confidence in their predictions. A physicist may say that she is 99% certain that the pen will hit the floor if you let go of it; however, even just the fact that the experiment is dependent upon a human deciding to let go of the pen introduces a level of unpredictability—you may decide at the last moment to not let go of the pen. Who's to know?

The point is that anything which we believe will happen is at best a prediction. There may be a very high probability of that prediction being correct. However, this does not detract from the reality that it is merely a prediction, a guess as to what might happen which may or may not come to pass. Any hypothesis about what *may* happen is clearly not about something that *is* happening. It is future-oriented, and as mentioned, the future is not entirely predictable because of all the potential factors. Regardless of whether your guess turns out to be right or not (e.g. whether you spouse does leave you and takes the kids, or not), the guess is nothing more than just another thought-form. Like the pink elephant, it has no more reality than a bunch of microscopic neurons firing in a certain pattern. If the thought-form is about the future, it is always about something that may or may not happen.

As with the prospect of having a flat tyre, what you do about that problem will only result from a combination of who you are in the situation and the resources/limitations of the situation itself. The "answer" cannot be found in any thought-form, as the problem itself is still just a possibility, and not an actual reality (unless it is happening in the present moment). You can't solve a problem unless you are in it, and any problem that *may* happen is not a problem that *is* happening. Anxiety will arise within you as you are attempting to grapple with an *unsolvable* problem. We can only solve problems that are real, not ones that aren't actually happening.

Your feelings of anxiety, nervousness, fear or tension are your psychological alarm system that all is not right. The difficult emotion is alerting us to the need to look at what is happening right now, or the problematic story that our mind is creating. As with the physical pain that will follow if you lean on a barbeque hot plate, this emotional pain is telling you to do something differently. That is the purpose of either type of pain.

The "something different" that you need to do is to look at the story which your mind is creating. The actual specifics of the story aren't terribly important. What is important is the mere fact that your mind is creating a story which is problematic. It is generating a guess as to what bad thing will happen. It is taking you away from what is real and towards what is clearly not real. As already stated, the problematic story, being a future thought-form, is a prediction and not a statement about what is currently happening. As such, it has no more reality than the pink elephant you can imagine.

When you realize this, and you recognize that your anxiety is coming from the story that your mind is creating about the future, you have brought your awareness/consciousness to the situation. When you become aware of this reality, you have become more conscious, and subsequently less unconscious. As long as we are lost in our stories of both the past and the future, we are living in an unconscious state, lacking awareness of the only reality there ever is, i.e. the present moment.

Soon, tomorrow will just be another "now." Likewise, when you think of the past, you are only thinking about it now, as you are never actually in the past. All we ever have is a series of "now moments" that keep on unfolding. Both the past and the future are no more than thought-forms that can only exist in the present moment.

This awareness, that your mind is generating a story, creates a gap between "you" and what your mind is doing. This gap is your consciousness. When you become aware of this, it is like a fish that becomes aware for the first time that it is swimming in water. Until this moment, we tend to be so engrossed in our story that our sense of who we are is usually located *within* the story: 'I am the person who is going to be left by my spouse and ruined.' If you are not the story (this is all that has happened to me and all that I guess will happen), then who are *you*? You are the *consciousness* that becomes aware that this is just a story.

As Alan Watts suggested, humans are the universe "doing" consciousness. Tolle suggests that the universe is a process that is moving towards greater consciousness. It is the same consciousness that becomes aware that you are hot or cold, or hungry, or tired. Our essential nature is consciousness, and not the stories that our mind tricks us into believing we are. Like the universe itself, our life journey seems to be one of moving towards greater awareness or consciousness, from the small amount of it we have when born to a hopefully larger amount we may have when we die. This progress can be seen in various stages of life, where children have more awareness than babies, teenagers have more awareness than children, and ideally adults will have more awareness than teenagers.

Becoming aware that you are not your story allows you to come back to what is real: the present moment. As stated earlier, most present moments don't contain the happenings which we tend to fear. For most of us, most of the time, the statement 'I am not currently being left by my spouse' is accurate. When you pull back to what actually is, rather than get lost in what was or what might be, you will be pleasantly surprised by how un-problematic most present moments are (not all present moments though, as bad things do sometimes happen in real time). Most of the things we fear are not happening right now, and may never actually happen. Or if they do happen, it is usually in a way quite different to how we expected. It is common for people to spend days or weeks fearing an upcoming event only to find that when it is actually happening, it is unfolding in a different way to how they imagined.

When you realize that your mind, via the *story*, has taken you away from the only reality that there is (i.e. the *now*), then you have a choice. You can choose to take the story seriously and remain anxious—or not. You are reminded by this "burst" of consciousness that your mind has just taken you away from what is real to what is not real. At this point, it is possible to take two or three deep breaths to anchor yourself in your body. Your body is able to act as an anchor in the present moment as it only ever exists now, and not in some future time. A deep breath allows you to become more aware of the present moment via your body, and less in the story which your mind was creating.

Many people report that at this point they are able to let the anxiety fall away. It has served its purpose as a warning as to what is going on. Seeing that you are not the story allows you to come back to the present moment, which is usually less problematic than our imaginations predict. We are always actually in the present moment, whether walking down the street, talking with a friend, or arguing with someone. These are all opportunities to be aware of the present moment. Meditation can help with this, as it is a ritualized focus on the present moment. However, the point of mindfulness is that we can be as aware of the moment with just one breath as much as we can with twenty minutes of focused breathing. There is only ever one breath and one moment. (You can see a brief point form "cheat-sheet" on this process in Appendix 9)

The suggestion here is that you would benefit from listening less to what your mind or ego or story has to say, and simply focus on what is actually happening in the present moment. Alan Watts was fond of suggesting "lose your mind as many times as possible each day in order to retain your sanity!"

Psychological & clock-time

Some people may object that this is simply impractical. If we don't plan for the future, bad things will happen. On many issues this is certainly the case. If I fail to get my car certified as road-worthy by a mechanic before the date when my registration is due, I will fail to get it registered. It is worth putting in the forethought and effort involved now to prevent this predicted event from happening. This scenario reveals the difference between "clock-time" and "psychological-time."

Our society is largely governed by the somewhat arbitrary movement of the clock. Most of us eat and start work at particular times, whether it suits our body's natural rhythms or not. If we choose to live in this culture, rather than a non-industrialized culture, then we choose to live with this adherence to the clock. We need to remember that this notion of time is itself just a thought-form. Our measures of time, minutes and hours are just social conventions with no inherent value, other than to allow society to function more smoothly.

Where non-industrialized people will see the passage of time in nature's cycles to allow them to plan for the future, industrialized society is unique in its slavery to the more arbitrary movements of the clock. In our society, things often have to be done by a certain time or by a certain date. This requires that if we want to avoid negative consequences, we must comply. I don't want to be fined for driving an un-registered car. This is a practical issue and is relevant to clock-time. Even non-Western hunter-gatherer people will know that if they fail to take X action now (e.g. when the waters are warmer), Z will not happen, and their lives may depend upon Z's result. While it is possible to get highly distressed about clock-time, it is not the main problem which beguiles humans.

Psychological-time is more the bane of our existence. It is the extra layer of distress that we may add to not getting our car registered on time: 'I will be fined and lose my license because I won't be able to afford the fine. Then without a license, I'll lose my job, and with no income, I won't be able to pay the mortgage, so my partner will leave me and take the kids, and I'll become a hopeless wreck.'

In this example, we can see how a sensible clock-time requirement has been added to by psychological-time, making the scenario even more distressing. The additional distress is unlikely to help you do what you need to do in order to get your car registered on time. At its extreme, this type of storytelling can immobilize a person to the point where they can't do what they need to, and bad results are more likely to follow.

You may actually need to take action now in order to prevent a bad situation from happening. If you can reduce the sense of psychological-time, and instead just deal with the clock-time, you will be in a better state to do what needs to be done. In regards to relationships, warnings of impending doom are often there for months or years before one partner leaves. It is not unusual for one partner to tell the other in many ways that they need to change this or that attitude or behavior, as they will not put up with it forever.

It would be foolish to ignore these warnings by telling yourself that you don't have to deal with what isn't yet happening, that s/he may never leave you, it is only a story, so you can just continue as usual.

You do need to tune in to what your partner (or any other reliable aspect of the world) is telling you now. You may need to make some changes now, and do something different now. Will it prevent a predictable separation? No one can really tell whether the separation will ever happen, or if it can be prevented. But you can deal with what is happening right now by making the necessary changes to be more adaptive to the current situation. Eliminating the psychological-time will help with this, as it will decrease anxiety and fear. This may allow you to be more adaptive and put your best foot forward rather than have your actions forced and constricted by fear.

What relevance does all this have for chronic pain? If you are laboring under a tendency to use a lot of psychological-time, you will be internally generating a great deal more stress than is necessary. This can accumulate to such a point that you feel overwhelmed by life in general. You may feel hopeless and helpless, which may feed into an already negative self-concept and low mood. This will increase your muscular tension, which may exacerbate an already present blood and oxygen deprivation in muscles and nerves. As such, chronic pain may be further perpetuated, and something of a vicious cycle easily created.

The concept of a "pain pattern" was discussed in earlier chapters. It is very common for chronic pain sufferers to not just be experiencing physical pain, but also experience a pattern of heightened levels of anxiety and fear of a grim future; helplessness/hopelessness about their inability to make a difference, leading to depression; anger at their misfortune of having an injury and at the fact that no treatment has thus far helped; grief over what they have lost in terms of jobs, relationships, and self-concept as healthy and vital, as well as enjoyed activities. The opportunities for emotional distress with chronic pain are almost endless and it seems that they can all feed back into the problem, making the pain worse and worse with each increase in emotional distress.

In all these variations of emotional distress, you will see stories operating: 'I was set for promotion before I got injured, and now I may never work again'; 'We had the best relationship, and now it will never recover'; 'I have been ripped off and abused by my employer and the insurance company'; 'I will probably need looking after for the rest of my life'; 'I may wind up crippled from this'; 'I will have no quality of life—things will just get worse.'

Many of these statements may reflect misinformation which people have been given by well-meaning but badly informed health professionals. Most people who are in chronic pain are *not* on the verge of being crippled for life. As *The Back Book* and decades of research make clear, most chronic pain does not indicate substantial damage to the spine.

These horror stories may also reflect people's actual experience. Maybe you really were set for a promotion and then you lost your job because of the pain. However, each of these statements are also stories about what is either no longer real, or what may never be real. They are also thought-forms, like the pink elephant. Learning about The Hidden Psychology of Pain can help you to challenge the problematic stories of future physical collapse and ensuing disaster, and you can take this a step further by practicing the suggestions in this chapter.

Icon of suffering

An additional message that Tolle provides to his readers is a way of dealing with intense suffering. For nearly two thousand years, our culture used the story of Jesus as its main way of making sense of a confusing and often painful world. Most of the "great stories" from the world's various cultures include messages about how to cope with suffering. In the East, Buddha developed an entire philosophy around acceptance and non-attachment as method of alleviating suffering. In the West, the story of the crucifixion of Jesus was for countless generations our culture's way of making sense of suffering. Regardless of its historical accuracy or religious associations, it is well worth exploring for its inherent wisdom.

With the exception of the last couple of generations, if it were possible to ask Westerners over the last two thousand years "What is *the* icon of suffering?" you would have been told "Jesus on the cross." This stark picture represented inescapable pain and suffering, and in many ways we can all relate to it. The standard theology states that Jesus was both divine and of the flesh, very able to experience real physical and emotional pain. In that sense, we can relate to him as we can sympathize with his intense suffering—we are all suffering on the cross.

Before and during the process of being crucified, Jesus was tormented and tortured in just about every way imaginable. He was betrayed by his own followers, held up for execution by his own people, and then physically flayed, beaten and humiliated. His body experienced the most intense agony, as did his heart and spirit. Finally, nailed on the cross, his escape was impossible. He was physically trapped and doomed to die a horrible and painful death.

Most of us have been broken by life in some way, shape or form. For some of us, it will be the tragic deaths of loved ones, for others it will be trauma from wars or natural disasters or accidents; and for others it will be extreme emotional torment or physical pain. Sometimes, when I meet clients whose stories are so extremely painful, I am reminded of Jesus suffering an awful death, hanging on the cross with no ability to change his circumstances. People will often have an understandable resistance to what is happening to them—a resounding *"NO!"* to their experience.

One book of the Bible, Mathew (27:46) depicts Jesus on the cross as a man in sheer agony, beseeching God with words that represent a massive *"NO!* This shouldn't be happening to me."* Jesus states, "My God, my God. Why have you forsaken me?" This can be read to mean "Why are you allowing this terrible agony to happen to me?" In this statement is an understandable rejection of all the pain and torment he is experiencing. As his rejection of agony continues, so does the agony intensify. This is a man in utter torment, being physically and emotionally destroyed by what is being inflicted upon him. As stated, most people who have been alive long enough can relate to this to some extent. In our own way, we have all given a resounding *"NO!"* to unwanted emotional and physical pain.

It is not my role or right, nor that of anyone else, to tell these people that they need to drop their resistance to suffering. However, the crucifixion story offers a way of coping with inescapable pain. John (19:30) states that Jesus' last words, before he peacefully slipped into death was "It is finished," and Luke (23:46) quotes Jesus as saying "Father, into Your hands I commit my spirit." These words demonstrate an acceptance of that moment, and with that acceptance comes peace rather than more torment. *"It is finished"* reflects a very different emotion than *"Why have you forsaken me?"* It reflects a resignation to what patently *is*—an understanding of the futility of struggling against an obvious reality. Jesus was nailed to a cross of wood and hung up to die. There was nothing he could do about this. He was left to suffer the pain of ordinary men and women.

Having been trapped in a car wreck for several hours while suffering intense pain and knowing that I was bleeding badly, possibly to death, gave me some small appreciation of his predicament. Many other people could relate to the anguish of Jesus via their own story of intense emotional or physical suffering. Some people are trapped in painful situations or realities of what has happened to them or their loved ones. While trapped in the car wreck, there were periods when I would struggle against what was happening to me, thrash about trying to free myself, and call out to God to get me out of this mess and to save me. I would like to say that I found the wisdom of acceptance that Jesus did, but the fact is I didn't. My experience did not go as far as dying with the peace that Jesus found through acceptance, as I did have the good fortune of not dying whilst trapped.

The crucifixion is an ancient cultural story of how to deal with intense suffering. How does this relate to you and your suffering? Whenever we internally resist what is, and our basic stance is *"NO!"* to the reality of pain of any type, just like Jesus on the cross, we intensify our agony. When we wriggle and writhe to get the "me" out of the experience, as though it could be done by an act of resistance or will, we add more power to the pain. We have a sense of what *should* be happening rather than what is happening, and our preference is definitely with the should-story rather than with the reality. This should-story is yet another fabrication of the mind, and again has no more reality than the pink elephant. It is an alternate reality, and to the extent that it differs from what *is*, will only produce more suffering.

The way out of suffering is not by clinging on to a belief in the should-story, but through accepting what is. Acceptance of various forms of suffering, including pain, is a much more effective coping strategy than trying to control the situation through a *"NO!"* stance. Acceptance can help reduce anxiety, fear and depression, and ironically enough, it can also decrease the pain. Again, much of our suffering will also come from stories about how horrible it is going to be as a result of _____, which our mind will generate in abundance.

How many times have you had the experience of a bad night's sleep, lying in bed worrying about how awful you are going to feel the next day only to find later that while you didn't like being tired, you actually coped with the reality of the day? When you take the psychological add-on out of the equation (the mind-generated story of misery), you are likely to find that you are more able to cope with what is actually happening. We seem to have an ability to absorb pain, but this ability is diminished when we forcefully resist reality.

It is from this recognition of the power of acceptance that Mindfulness programs can be very effective. The way through suffering is by entering it—noticing it, being with it, allowing it. That is, being open to whatever this moment brings. Kabat-Zinn suggests that people in pain ask themselves,

> "How bad is it right now, in this very moment?" If you practice this, you will probably find that most of the time, even when you are feeling terrible, when you go right into the sensation and ask, "IN THIS MOMENT, is it tolerable? Is it okay?" the chances are you will find that it is. The difficulty is that the next moment is coming, and the next, and you "*know*" they are all going to be filled with more pain.[11]

Remember that any "knowing" about the next moment is no more than a prediction, a thought-form. Past history allows us to make reasonable predictions about what will happen next. Based on your experience you *may* be able to accurately predict that the pain is going to get worse and harder to cope with. However, never forget that no matter how reasonable a prediction is, it is still just a prediction. A prediction is merely a thought-form, not a reality.

The truth is that you cannot actually know what the next moment will bring. You may have a brain aneurism and die before you hit the ground, in which case the pain in your back does not get worse. Or you may notice that without additional tension, through just accepting what is rather than emotionally resisting it, the pain actually begins to diminish and not worsen as you had expected. It is this guess ("the pain will get worse") that can generate so much anxiety in the present moment that the pain-inducing muscular tension may increase, and pain tolerance may decrease. With acceptance, a better way of coping can be found.

---

[11] Kabat-Zinn (2009 p.295). *Full Catastrophe Living.*

If you remain open to each moment with an accepting attitude, you will discover that new moments bring new experiences, as things rarely stay the same. There is a saying in Buddhism, "If you don't like what is happening, just wait. All things change."

Before reaching a point of acceptance you may need to go through denial and then anger as natural responses. Most things that we put energy into resisting are not huge calamities; they tend to be more mundane, small scale issues. Psychologist Richard Carlson referred to this in his best-selling book *Don't Sweat the Small Stuff, and It's All Small Stuff!* With large losses, allow yourself the space and time to go through the process of shock, denial and anger first before allowing acceptance to emerge. With small-scale issues, see if you can practice fostering an acceptance of reality. Ultimately, reality will win out anyway, so you may as well save your energy and time by trying to accept rather than reject it.

With enough conscious practice on small issues, you may be in a better position to accept the reality of seriously bad events that may occur in the future. Acceptance does not mean liking what is, or necessarily passively allowing it. You may choose to take action over realities that you can have some impact on. For example, I choose to have an inflated spare tyre and a jack in my car in case I do have a puncture. You will have more energy available to do the things you need to if you are not unnecessarily wasting it on insisting that reality not be what it patently is. Having an inner acceptance is more likely to allow you the clear perception and thinking required to take the appropriate action if or when the need arises.

What is *not* being suggested here is doing battle with your thoughts, or the story that your mind is creating. See if you can simply develop the practice of becoming aware of the upsetting emotion, noticing the story that is associated with the distress, and coming back to the present moment. None of this involves entering into a dispute or struggle with the story. Simply note that this is what your mind is doing again because it is what minds tend to do. Arguing with thoughts gives them an importance which they often don't deserve, and usually heightens their strength as well. With practice, you will be able to simply observe the thoughts or stories without attaching any importance to them. Just view them as being similar to clouds that may float past in the sky. There is no need to see your favorite childhood dog in a cloud shape, or the face of a hated primary school teacher. Just see the clouds without interpretation, and without attaching any particular importance or meaning to them. Observing your thoughts or stories can be much the same. There is no need to engage in debate, or pull them apart, or attach importance to them, or interpret them, as they are just thought-forms or stories. Recognize them for what they are, and then come back to the present moment with a deep breath.

Acceptance & Commitment Therapy

A more recent variation of cognitive behavioral therapy, Acceptance and Commitment Therapy (ACT) combines this mindful acceptance with traditional cognitive therapy approaches.[12] ACT was devised by Steven Hayes, Professor of Psychology at the University of Nevada, and represents part of what has been referred to as the "third wave" of behavior therapy. His popular book, *Get out of Your Mind and into Your Life* was a number one self-help book in America, and for a time even outsold *Harry Potter* on Amazon.com.

Hayes created something of a controversy within psychology, as his approach is often at odds with standard CBT, despite it also being a form of cognitive-behavioral therapy. Along with other related approaches of the third wave, ACT attempts to broaden psychological flexibility. In his presidential address to the Association for Behavioral and Cognitive Therapies Hayes stated, "The third wave reformulates and synthesizes previous generations of behavioral and cognitive therapy and carries them forward into questions, issues, and domains previously addressed primarily by other traditions, in hopes of improving both understanding and outcomes."

Unlike standard CBT, which instructs people to argue with and challenge their dysfunctional or irrational thoughts, ACT instructs people to just notice and accept their thoughts and feelings in the manner described above. This is particularly relevant for negative thoughts/feelings as well as physical states such as pain.

As Tolle suggests, "you" are really the consciousness that becomes aware of various aspects of experience. ACT also encourages people to identify with

---

[12] Hayes, Strosahl & Wilson (2003). *Acceptance and Commitment Therapy.*

the inner observer, referred to as the "self-in-context." This is a recognition that the sense of ourselves as being an isolated pocket of consciousness (our ego) is an illusion which takes us away from the fact that each individual is part of a much larger web of life. As we can only understand a fish's behavior in the context of the water in which it is swimming, we can only understand human experience in the context of our environments, or the larger web.

Within ACT, human problems are thought to arise from our tendency to over-identify with our thoughts (referred to as "fusion with thoughts"); judging and evaluating our experience rather than just accepting it; avoidance of experience when it does not comply with our thoughts of how reality should be; and reason-giving, or elaborate rationales for behavior. These common psychological tendencies take us in a direction of psychological rigidity and away from our core values, which are generally better guides for our actions and way of life.

The main principles of ACT are learning to accept thoughts, feelings, memories for what they are (thought-forms), and not what our ego would have us believe they are; developing an ability to simply accept these thought-forms, even when they are negative, troublesome or painful; remaining present to the current moment, rather than being lost in thoughts about either the past or the future; developing and accessing the "transcendent" sense of self as the observing consciousness which remains constant, regardless of various experiences which come and go; developing a sense of one's inner core values which are most relevant to a genuine sense of self; and a commitment to goals which are set according to one's values, and sticking to the process of achieving these.

Based on research evidence, ACT is considered an empirically validated treatment for depression. It has demonstrated preliminary research evidence of effectiveness for a variety of problems including chronic pain, addictions, smoking cessation, anxiety, psychosis, and workplace stress. Researchers have shown that the attitude of acceptance can explain improvements in functional outcomes for people suffering chronic pain.[13]

---

[13] Vowles et al (2007). "Acceptance and Values-Based Action in Chronic Pain: A Study of Treatment Effectiveness and Process." *Journal of Consulting and Clinical Psychology*.

Some pain management clinics offer ACT programs. Where the books and ideas of people such as Alan Watts and Eckhart Tolle address a broad range of human experience, ACT pain management programs are taking the components specifically applicable to chronic pain and training participants in their application to this problem. In addition to learning to accept rather than control, avoid or suppress negative feelings and pain, participants are encouraged to identify and pursue core values regardless of the pain. A range of experiential exercises, metaphors and demonstrations are used to assist people to develop this ability.

This is a great advance in the cognitive-behavioral treatment of chronic pain. However, as with other excellent therapies, to be maximally effective, I would suggest it needs to be approached with *The Hidden Psychology of Pain* in mind. Many therapies which are excellent in their own right can become more effective in treating chronic pain when they are combined with the ideas presented in this book. As stated at the beginning of this chapter, learning to adjust to chronic pain as untreatable and permanent is often an unnecessary response as many people can actually eliminate the pain.

In concluding this book, I would ask you to always keep in mind that the problem with chronic pain is *not* that it is untreatable or even mysterious. Clearly, chronic pain is highly treatable from a depth-psychology perspective for a great many people. The problem is that the wrong paradigms have been applied to it for too many decades, i.e. a purely bio-mechanical approach in medicine, and a purely mechanistic and shallow approach within psychology. To the extent that these approaches actively deny or ignore the role which psychology in general, and unconscious factors in particular, play in the production and maintenance of chronic pain, the problem is likely to remain in epidemic proportions in our society.

In order to address this epidemic of chronic pain, a paradigm shift is needed within all of the treating professions. In order to successfully overcome your chronic pain, your own paradigm shift is also needed. My hope is that this book can be a useful step in that process.

APPENDICES

APPENDIX 1

Pain Questionnaires (I)

i) **Pain Catastrophizing Scale.**

RATING	0	1	2	3	4
MEANING	Not at all	To a slight degree	To a moderate degree	To a great degree	All the time

NUMBER	*When I'm in pain . . . .*	RATING
1	. . . I worry all the time about whether the pain will end	
2	. . . I feel I can't go on	
3	. . . It's terrible and I think it's never going to get any better	
4	. . . It's awful and I feel that it overwhelms me	
5	. . . I feel I can't stand it anymore	
6	. . . I become afraid that the pain will get worse	
7	. . . I keep thinking of other painful events	
8	. . . I anxiously want the pain to go away.	
9	. . . I can't seem to keep it out of my mind.	

NUMBER	When I'm in pain	RATING
10	. . . I keep thinking about how much it hurts.	
11	. . . I keep thinking about how badly I want the pain to stop.	
12	. . . There's nothing I can do to reduce the intensity of the pain.	
13	. . . I wonder whether something serious may happen.	
	TOTAL SCORE	

ii) Pain Vigilance and Awareness Questionnaire.

RATING	0	1	2	3	4	5
MEANING	Never					Always

NUMBER	STATEMENT	RATING
1	I am very sensitive to pain	
2	I am aware of sudden or temporary changes in pain	
3	I am quick to notice changes in pain intensity	
4	I am quick to notice effects of medication on pain	
5	I am quick to notice changes in location or extent of pain	
6	I focus on sensations of pain	
7	I notice pain even if I am busy with another activity	
8	I find it easy to ignore pain (reverse your score for this item before adding it in the box)	
9	I know immediately when pain starts or increases	

NUMBER	STATEMENT	RATING
10	When I do something that increase pain, the first thing I do is check to see how much pain was increased	
11	I know immediately when pain decreases	
12	I seem to be more conscious of pain than others	
13	I pay close attention to pain	
14	I keep track of my pain level	
15	I become preoccupied with pain	
16	I do not dwell on pain (reverse your score for this item before adding it in the box)	
	TOTAL SCORE	

APPENDIX 2

A neurological understanding

While a neurological approach to the understanding of chronic pain is not the main focus of this book, some basic background in brain biology is inescapable as neurology tells us a great deal about the true nature of chronic pain. Although this book focuses primarily on the psychology that is relevant to chronic pain, it is obvious that all we experience is mediated through the brain and the rest of the central nervous system. This is as true of pain as it is for any other experience. Simply put, without a brain and spinal cord (together referred to as the central nervous system), we have no experience at all—painful or otherwise. As such, some basics of neurology are essential to making sense of what happens in our bodies and brains when we experience pain. At various places throughout this book are references to different parts of the brain and the role they play in our experience of pain, as well as the role which they may play in the resolution of pain. This discussion will help you make sense of these references.

Biological scientists, David Butler and Lorimer Moseley present a very sound explanation of the physiology and neurology of chronic pain. They go into the physical 'nuts and bolts' details to a minute degree, but also acknowledge the essential role which psychological factors like emotions and pain beliefs play in the maintenance of chronic pain. *The Hidden Psychology of Pain* does not attempt to replicate their physiological level of analysis—this can best be gained by reading their book.[1] Both their, and the more psychological approaches, are echoing the same message, albeit from different directions and disciplines—both physiology and psychology are fundamentally important in the production and maintenance of chronic pain, as humans are clearly both physiological and psychological beings.

---

[1] Butler & Moseley (2003) *Explain Pain.*

There is no inherent contradiction between these two approaches—they are merely two sides of the one coin—a reflection of the mind/body split espoused by Decartes hundreds of years ago. It is possible, with the greater awareness of mind/body holism, for these approaches to converge. *Explain Pain* and *The Hidden Psychology of Pain* represent physiologist's and psychologist's respective attempts to overcome the artificial distinctions between mind and body. Each discipline will approach it in a manner which may be different, but these differences can ultimately be complementary and inform each other.

For simplicity, you can think of the brain as being around the size of a coconut, shaped like a walnut, and loosely resembling a cauliflower with its undulating surface and stem (although in the brain, the stem sits further towards the back than in a cauliflower). The consistency of the brain is similar to cottage cheese or firm jelly. It can be conceptually divided in a range of ways: the brainstem; the cerebellum near the brainstem (often referred to as the "little-brain"); the cerebrum (the part we see when thinking of the brain) which sits on top of the brainstem and cerebellum; the two hemispheres of the neo-cortex (the outer part that is visible in an un-dissected brain); the various lobes of the cerebrum (temporal, parietal, occipital, and frontal lobes); and the corpus callosum, a thick bundle of around eighty million nerve "tentacles" which join two hemispheres of the cerebral cortex and allow them to be in constant communication.

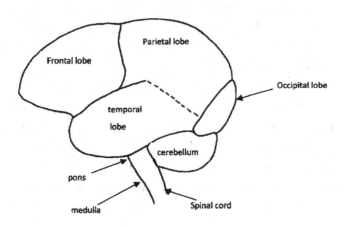

Major divisions of the brain

If the brain is sliced down the middle (severing the corpus callosum) and the two halves come apart, you will see, as well as some chambers, a range of brain modules which look like lumps and tubes, some of which can resemble nuts, grapes, even insects and seahorses. These components are grayish and contain many brain cells which connect with other brain cells via a complicated criss-crossing of strands or tentacles (axons) coming from them. Each brain module is replicated in each hemisphere of the brain (apart from the pineal gland, which sits at the center of the brain base), so although we talk about them as singular, they are actually one of a pair. As with all parts of the brain, each of these brain components have specific functions and communicate with other functional areas and components to enable both simple and complex actions. Some brain modules have a wide range of functions and are involved in many aspects of our experience.

On the outer surface of the brain, imagine wrapping a formal dinner serviette into a range of folds, bumps and valleys. This serviette represents the cortex. The number of layers of cells in the cortex differs, with the neo-cortex having six layers. Neo-cortex is Latin for the "new-brain", as it is the most recent development in the evolution of the human brain. Areas of the cortex which have less than six layers of cells are the archicortex and the paleocortex, both of which take in parts of the emotional limbic system. The cortex ranges in thickness from around 2mm to around 5-6mm, and if spread out would have around 500 square inches of surface area. This outer "bark" of the brain contains around 10-20 billion or more nerve cells, held together by 80-100 billion glial cells that support the brain cells (which are referred to as neurons).[2] It uses around 1 ½ pints of blood every minute, and burns around 400 calories each day.[3]

The cortex is the grey matter which we see in photos of an intact brain. It is made up of layers of brain cells, while the deeper white matter of the brain (within the outer grey bark) is made up of the nerve tentacles (axons) which come from these cells. The axons are covered in a white myelin sheath, giving them a different color to the cell bodies. These nerve tentacles (dendrites which receive nerve impulses, and axons which send the nerve impulses to other neurons) interconnect the brain cells with other neurons

---

[2]   Carter (2010). *Mapping the Mind.*
[3]   Hannaford (2005) *Smart Moves: why learning is not all in your head.*

in various parts of the brain, and also with other parts of the body. Via axons and dendrites, each neuron connects with around 7000 to 10,000 other neurons. Millions of these connections are made and unmade every second.[4] Some neurons are long and thin, some are star-shaped and reach out in all directions, and others look more like deer antlers.

The neurons communicate with each other through the passage of electrical currents from the axon hillock at the base of the nerve body and along these tentacles, forming pathways as patterns of interconnection between the neurons involved. The firing of single neurons is not enough to generate even a twitch. It is only when neurons manage to excite their neighbors, and this flow-on effect continues to other neighboring neurons, that a pattern of activity arises sufficient to create thoughts, perceptions, feelings and actions. Millions of brain cells are involved to produce even the most simple of thoughts.

The axons and dendrites of each neuron don't actually touch, as there is a microscopic space between each of these connections, referred to as a synaptic gap. As the electrical charge is unable to cross this gap, the release of brain chemicals (neurotransmitters) from the end of the axon is stimulated by the electrical charge which has been sent from the axon hillock near the base of the cell body.

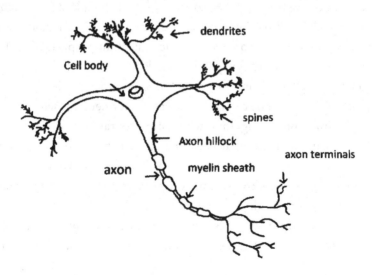

---

[4]   Butler & Moseley (2003) *Explain Pain.*

Currently, hundreds of neurotransmitters have been identified, and more are expected to be found yet.[5] Some have an excitatory function, leading to more activity in other neurons, and others have inhibitory functions which dampen down the level of neural activity. The most important neurotransmitters are thought to be serotonin (with an effect on mood, sleep, pain, appetite and blood pressure); acetylcholine (controlling activity in brain areas connected with attention, learning and memory); noreadrenaline/norepinehrine (inducing physical and mental arousal, as well as heightening mood); glutamate (used for forming links between neurons involved in learning and long term memory); enkephalins and endorphins (endogenous opioids that reduce emotional stress, decrease pain, and depress physical functions like breathing); oxytocin (the "love hormone," which creates a sense of oneness with others).

Such neurotransmitters are secreted by around thirty different types of cells. The chemicals cross the synaptic gap to be absorbed in specific receptor sites on the dendrites of the neighboring neurons—think of the receptor sites as being like locks which are opened by specific keys (neurotransmitters). The absorption of these chemicals can trigger an electrical current, which travels up the length of the dendrite where, if enough electrical charge has been received, the cell's axon hillock will fire and send the electrical impulse along to the next neurons via the axons, and so on. A single axon, which has multiple branches taking the impulse away from its cell body and towards other brain cells, can electro-chemically activate multiple parts of the brain and generate thousands of synaptic terminals.

Each brain cell has around seven to ten thousand possible connections with other brain cells. The total amount of such connections within a brain are simply mind/brain boggling, with estimates ranging as high as over a *million billion* connections. It is estimated that this amount of possible connections is *greater than the number of atoms in the known universe.*[6] Such numbers give the brain the ability to process one thousand new bits of information every second.

It is the neo-cortex which is the most plastic or adaptable part of the brain, and where most of the higher thinking functions come from—those

---

5   Carter (2010) *Mapping The Mind.*
6   Hannaford (2005). *Smart Moves: Why Learning is Not All in Your Head.*

functions which separate humans from lower forms of animal life, e.g. our ability to philosophies, to engage in complicated problem solving, as well as the development of self-awareness which evolves from language. It is the neo-cortex which is thought of as being the "human brain," whereas the deeper structures are older in an evolutionary sense, being shared by other forms of life.

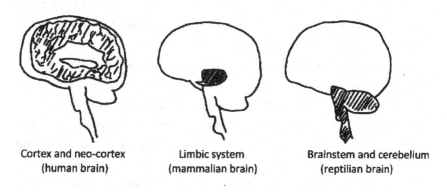

Cortex and neo-cortex	Limbic system	Brainstem and cerebellum
(human brain)	(mammalian brain)	(reptilian brain)

The three evolutionary stages and areas of the human brain

Deeper within the brain are modules which constitute parts of the limbic system, where emotions are generated. This emotional system within the brain is thought to have first emerged in mammals, so is often referred to as the "mammalian brain." Along with even deeper brain areas, the limbic system has a profound effect on our experiences as it is extremely connected to the cortex and feeds a great deal of information upwards to it. As with the multi-tasking nature of many brain areas, although the limbic system is central to our emotional experience of life, it has a range of other related functions, such as information processing and the laying down of long-term memories.

The most ancient part of the brain is the brainstem. As it is thought to have evolved more than 500 million years ago, and is shared by primitive forms of life, it is often referred to as the "reptilian brain." The brainstem is made up from the nerves that run up from the body via the spinal column, and therefore carry information from the body into the brain. The cerebellum, at the base of the back of the brain, is also viewed as being part of the reptilian brain, and is involved in motor coordination and some mental functions.

Parts of the limbic system, the entire brainstem and the cerebellum are sub-cortical, meaning that they are found in brain areas below or deeper within the brain than the neo-cortex. As such, they are thought of as being *un*conscious, as no conscious thought is involved in their actions.

The most conscious part of the brain, in fact the place where we become conscious of thoughts, bodily sensations and emotions, is the frontal cortex, behind the forehead. The pre-frontal cortex is the only part of the brain which is free from sensory information processing duties, and springs to life whenever we have thoughts.

As chronic pain is a very emotional experience for sufferers, it is important to have an awareness of our mind/brain's construction of feelings. The limbic system is where our mind/brain gathers information from bodily cues, combines it with information about the specific situation, as well as with learnt information from the past, and constructs a particular feeling about the circumstance itself—joy, sadness, anger, guilt, exhilaration, etc. The limbic areas of the brain give our experiences their emotional quality, and it is the frontal cortex where we become aware of these feelings.

The limbic system is comprised of a collection of brain structures located in the temporal region of the midbrain and parts of the brainstem region. It also has nerve projections into other parts of the neo-cortex. In places, elements of the limbic system form the inner border of the cortex itself, while other parts are deeper than the cortex, and are thus sub-cortical. This "mega-system" consists of a range of structures including the amydala, the hypothalamus and the hippocampus amongst others. It integrates many of the brain's subsystems so as to give us an emotional flavor to our experiences. It is also involved in learning and long-term memory, as these are important to emotions as well. Some neuroscientists suggest that via its projections into the pre-frontal cortex, the limbic system is implicated in the "executive" functions of the brain as well, such as impulse control and appreciating consequences of actions, etc.[7] Conversely, it appears that the pre-frontal cortex is also highly involved in emotions, so the neat distinction between the emotional parts of the brain and the thinking parts of the brain may just be more a convention than a reality.[8]

---

[7] Norden (2007). *Understanding the Brain.*
[8] Davidson & Belgey (2012) *The Emotional Life of Your Brain.*

Being our emotional center, the limbic system is highly involved in the often cited "fight/flight/freeze response" associated with survival-instinct emotions such as fear, anxiety or anger. The brainstem works in conjunction with the limbic system, as well as the thinking cortex, to assess the safety or danger of a situation. (This is discussed in more detail in Chapter 14). However, our sense of pleasure and joy is also derived from the limbic system. As memory is important in emotions, the limbic system is also central to both learning and long term memories—we need to call on our memories to decide if we like or dislike a TV series. Learnt messages from experience, memories and emotions all combine to give us movement towards certain actions, so the limbic system is also important in motivation—will I read a book or watch TV?

The perception and transmission of pain is controlled by structures of both our peripheral and central nervous systems. When body tissue is injured, a series of chemical reactions known as inflammatory responses are triggered, and nerve receptors (nociceptors—located in most body tissues) in the skin are stimulated. The pain may begin with skin tissue damage, but the processes underpinning the experience of pain are more in the central nervous system, and ultimately in the brain. These particular nerve fibers come in two types: A-delta fibers (stimulation of these fibers are related to the sensation of sharp, acute, localized pain), and C-fibers (stimulation of these fibers are related to dull, ache-type pain). Some of these nerve fibers respond to mechanical forces, like a bang or a pinch. Others sense changes in temperature; and others respond to chemical changes, either from outside the body (e.g stinging nettles) or inside the body (e.g. oxygen deprivation of muscles, or lactic acid).

The pain signals are transmitted by the nociceptors to the sensory neuron dendrites of *interneurons*. The dendrites and cell bodies of these sensory neuron cells sit outside of the spinal cord, and are referred to as 'second order neurons', or as 'messenger nerves' as their only job is to pass on the message of alarm. Here, the pain signals are transferred and carried upward along the spinal cord to specific sites in the brain, the first place being the thalamus. The brains of people show a general set of actions in the construction of pain, however there are individual differences in the exact brain actions, and also on different occasions within the one person.

The thalamus and midbrain receive the nerve messages where they are then transferred to the insular cortex and the anterior cingulate cortex (the ACC), the frontal lobes of the neo-cortex, and the limbic system where an emotional sense is made of the pain. We can however perceive pain without an involvement of these higher cortical brain areas. Just pain messages reaching the thalamus (lower in the brain than the cortex) is enough for us to experience pain—we don't need to think about it to know that we hurt. However, if we are to make sense of the pain in terms of where we feel it (e.g. in the foot), the quality of the pain (sharp), and the meaning of the pain (I have stood on a nail), the higher cortical areas need to become involved. Areas such as the ACC, the insular, the frontal lobes and the limbic system are all involved in allowing us to realize what has happened and to take appropriate action.

Despite the above description, we don't actually have pain receptors, pain nerves, pain pathways or pain centres in the brain.[9] Rather, pain is "constructed" by the brain in response to a wide range of nerve messages which reach it. The spinal cord, in receiving nerve messages, is told "increased temperature in my area". The nerve messages don't say "pain" to the brain, only "danger". The brain then needs to construct an impression of the nerve messages it receives in order to arrive at a certain sense or meaning of them. Not only messages from tissue damage is taken into account. The general context of the situation, the meaning ascribed to it, and the ramification of the experience are all taken into consideration by many areas of the brain working in concert to arrive at a particular experience or conclusion.

The danger messages relayed by nerve fibres usually do not result in the experience of pain, as these are going on most of the time, however most experience of pain usually begins with these messages. Thoughts are also very able to activate danger signals in your brain, without danger signals being relayed from any part of the body. Some sufferers of chronic pain can aggravate their pain simply by thinking about doing an offending action, or by watching another person lift a weight. It is even reported that simply imagining an offending movement can cause inflammatory swelling for some sufferers.[10]

---

[9]   Butler & Moseley (2003) *Explain Pain.*
[10]   Ibid.

Where pain is chronic rather than acute, it is much more likely to involve the brain areas higher than the thalamus, where our brain decides that pain is the fitting perception to have. The combined stimulation of these brain sites allows us to determine the texture and intensity of the pain, evaluating its emotional impact, linking it to memories and giving it meaning. The meaning is important, as being hit by a bullet in a battle (perhaps allowing you to go home and therefore survive the war) is going to get a different emotional response to being hit by a bullet on a hunting trip. This difference in meaning will have an impact on our experience of the ensuing pain. These brain processes also give us a motivational factor in regards to pain, which usually entails doing something about it. The necessary information is also sent to our somatosensory cortices, enabling us to remove our hand away from a flame, or avoid another bullet without having to think and plan the action.

The insular cortex, after receiving the nerve messages from the thalamus and midbrain, judges the sensation in regards to its seriousness—an impression is formed as to the degree of pain experienced. This is the part of the brain that becomes active when we simply imagine a particular type of pain. It is also active in response to a range of other non-pain related experiences, such as the passive listening to music. The insular is concerned with monitoring the body's boundaries and information from the internal organs. It plays an important role in not only the experience of pain, but also in the experience of several emotions including sadness, fear, anger, disgust and even happiness. As these feelings begin as physiological states in the body, the insular is centrally involved in receiving the internal bodily experiences such as muscle tension, heart rate and breathing from subcortical areas; combining them with the emotional flavor of the limbic system; and then informing the higher cortical areas of the prevailing 'state of mind', where we become conscious of the feeling.

The next brain region of central importance to the experience of pain is the ACC, a part of the middle pre-frontal cortex. It is located in the area between the emotional limbic system and the thinking neo-cortex. In addition to registering emotional pain from social experiences, the ACC registers pain from physical injuries. The ACC can be thought of something like a collar around the corpus callosum, which is the bundle of nerve fibers that connect the left and right hemispheres of the brain. In evolutionary terms, the ACC is older than the neo-cortex, and is joined to the limbic structures beneath by thick neural connections. It receives information from the many neural pathways that run up from these unconscious deeper-brain areas, as well as down from the cortical areas that process thoughts. As such, it has a large role to play in the melding of emotional reactions with thoughts and judgments. The ACC has an involvement in a range of functions from heart rate regulation to emotions, as well as rational decision making functions. It also provides a feedback loop that alerts us to errors so we can take corrective action. Finally, the ACC generates self-willed action and plays a central role in creating the sense of "I." As such, it is essential to the feeling of aliveness.

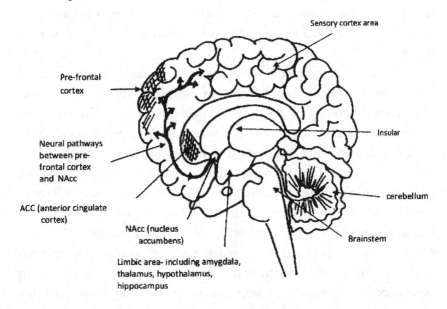

Pain relevant areas of the brain

Like the insular and the thalamus, the ACC is consistently activated with pain experiences, and chronic pain causes a high level of activation in both the insular and the ACC. As these brain areas are involved in thinking and emotions, the neurological evidence suggests that thoughts and emotions have a large role to play in making one hypersensitive to the pain.

As noted biologist Robert Sapolsky states in his best selling book, *Why Zebras Don't get Ulcers*, the brain is not a simple pain-ometer, giving us certain levels of "ouchness" in response to certain stimuli. Rather, our brain is a sense making organ which arrives at a certain conclusion regarding what we should be experiencing in relation to the nerve impulses, the social context of the situation (a battle or hunting), and the subsequent meaning of the experience. From these combined factors our brain decides if we experience pain, the quality of the pain, and how much of it we feel.[11]

Rather than just being an acute pain that doesn't end, chronic pain entails pain signals that are *repeatedly* generated. The related neural pathways can undergo physio-chemical changes, making them hypersensitive to the pain signals and more intense as this remodeling continues. With time, and repeated stimulation of the brain in this way, the pain signals can eventually become embedded in the central nervous system. In a sense, the nervous system has *learnt* to be in pain, like a memory constantly reminding the person of a pain from an injury that occurred long ago.

Recent research reported in *Nature Neuroscience* has revealed where this brain-wide learning of chronic pain derives from.[12] When the neurological activities of people with the same physical injuries and levels of pain were compared in a longitudinal brain imaging study, it was found that 85% of people who ended up experiencing chronic pain had a distinctive pattern which was not shared by those whose pain only became short-term. In particular, a heightened level of communication between two brain areas, the frontal cortex and a structure referred to as the nucleus accumbens (NAcc), were observed in those whose pain became chronic. The NAcc, located near the head of the ACC, is thought to play an important role in reward, pleasure, laughter, addiction, aggression, and fear. It also 'teaches' the rest of the brain how to evaluate and react to the outside world. When the experience is a painful one, the NAcc teaches the brain to develop chronic pain. The NAcc is able to do this as it sends out nerve projections to various brain structures, including the pre-frontal cortex. It also receives input from the pre-frontal cortex, as well as from the limbic system. The more these parts of the brain communicate with each other, the more pain sufferers are likely to develop chronic pain. As such, the emotional sense which the limbic

---

[11] Sapolsky (2004). *Why Zebras Don't Get Ulcers.*

[12] Baliki et al (2012)"Corticostriatal functional connectivity predicts transition to chronic back pain". *Nature Neuroscience.*

system adds to the pain experience becomes highly influential on the rest of the brain via the NAcc.

Recent neurological research conducted at the McGill University Health Center has demonstrated that the protein enzyme PKMzeta is central to building and maintaining pain-memory by *strengthening* the connections between the neurons involved in the pain experience. The neuronal process described above keeps reverberating when the connections between the specific neurons involved are reinforced by PKMzeta.[13] When the pain for a sufferer has become chronic, persistent changes in the sympathetic and parasympathetic nervous systems, as well as the hormonal, immune and movement systems are observed. The combined effect of persistent changes in these systems lead to the constant activation of brain areas associated with pain.[14]

Whenever you experience pain, either acute or chronic, the brain processes described above are happening. This must still be the case when you are experiencing pain which may have an unconscious psychological factor behind it, as the pain is still a physical and emotional experience. To suggest that Max's pain (from Chapter 1) was related to the emotional dilemmas relating to his childhood sexual abuse is in no way to suggest that his nociceptors, interneurons, thalamus, insular, NAcc and ACC were not involved.

Physical pain related to psychological factors still have biological pathways which generate the experience of pain via the above nerve and brain processes. Inflammatory responses can be created in body tissue just by the power of thoughts. Nerve receptors are very able to be stimulated in response to chemical changes brought about by oxygen deprivation in muscles and nerves. These messages are then sent up to the brain where a sense is made of them, and pain is constructed from the information received. The discussion of the neurology of pain is just as relevant to Max as it would be if he were hit across the back with a heavy lump of wood. The nature of what has happened to the afflicted body area is different, however the role of the nerves in conducting pain messages to the brain, and the

---

[13] Laferriere et al (2011). "PKMzeta Is Essential for Spinal Plasticity Underlying the Maintenance of Persistent Pain." *Molecular Pain.*

[14] Butler & Moseley (2003) *Explain Pain.*

brain then making sense of these messages is the same. Obviously, the sense which Max made of his pain, and the overall social context which included his feelings towards his brother, played a large role in his brain's construction of the chronic pain he felt.

Research with hypnosis and pain reveals that the brain's emotional/interpretative response to a painful stimulus can be dissociated from the amount of pain signals which are travelling up the spine to the brain. Brain imaging studies show that the pain perceiving areas of the brain can still be active when the painful stimuli is being applied, but under hypnosis the person can report that they experience no pain at all. This is because nerve pathways going down from the neo-cortex to the spinal cord can actually block the transmission of pain information and prevent it from entering the brain for interpretation. This neural pathway can allow chemicals such as endorphins to "flood" the area, making the neurons less excited, and therefore less likely to send the nerve message onwards. This probably explains such phenomenon as the placebo-effect, surgery without anesthetic while under hypnosis, and the experience of soldiers not noticing serious injuries during battles.

Clearly, the emotional and social sense made of the pain has an overriding function when compared to the nerve stimulation associated with the pain. Our brain processing of pain is a lot more complex than being a simple pain-ometer. This observed reality creates the possibility of cognitive and emotional factors being implicated in both the experience of pain and in pain reduction. *The Hidden Psychology of Pain* is an approach to using this observed reality to alter the cognitive and emotional factors relating to pain, and thereby alter the chronic pain experience itself. While it is a psychological approach (rather than a neurological one), there is still a neurological reality to what is happening when people use this approach in overcoming chronic pain: we are never physical or psychological, but are always both.

APPENDIX 3

Anatomy of the spine

While this book is deliberately not about spinal anatomy, some basic introduction is useful in that this can dispel some harmful myths that still permeate the discussion on back-pain. The points made about back pain can generalise across to other types of chronic pain.

The spine is a flexible column made up of vertebrae (small bones) with a bundle of nerves that take messages to and from the brain—this is referred to as the spinal cord. The vertebrae in the lower parts of the spine (coccyx and sacral) are fused, but not in the other areas of the spine. The vertebrae are joined and held together by muscles and ligaments, which are elastic body tissue. Each vertebra has bony parts jutting out to which muscles are attached.

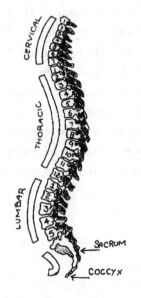

The purpose of the spine is to support the body; to help the body and limbs to move; and to protect the spinal cord. There are five main sections of the spine, each having different functions with different weight-bearing and movement burdens. From the bottom of the 'tail bone' upwards, they are the:-

- coccyx
- sacrum or sacral spine (hip area)
- lumbar spine (lower back)
- thoracic spine (upper back)
- cervical spine (neck).

Vertebrae are surrounded by ligaments and muscles. In between the vertebrae are small shock

Structure of the spine

384

absorbing 'cushions' called discs which contain a jelly-like substance surrounded by a membrane. Danger nerve signals can be activated in discs as their outer layer does have a nerve supply. However, the nerve supply to discs are not as rich as the nerve supply to the surrounding muscles and ligaments. As such, injured discs may be slow to result in hurt, with inflammation and pain often experienced 8-12 hours after the injury.

Although not fragile structures, discs can be damaged by trauma or by general 'wear and tear' from normal body use over a lifetime.

They can rupture, so that the membrane containing the jelly-like substance breaks; they can become squeezed, such that they protrude out between the vertebrae—a bit like a balloon containing water when it is

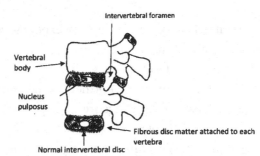

The disc is made up of fibrous tissue attached to the vertebra above and below

squeezed through your fingers. This is referred to as a herniated disc, often mislabelled a 'slipped disc'. Although a popular term this is an anatomical impossibility as the disc membrane is attached to each vertebra. It is not a 'thing' which can slip anywhere, as it is a tough fibrous container which is attached to the bone above and the bone below. Bulter & Moseley (2003) state that the bulges, herniations, even the squeezing onto a nerve, or the release of chemicals may irritate nerves, but do not necessarily alarm the nervous system. Therefore, there is no necessity that such disc damage must result in either acute or chronic pain. Discs are able to slowly heal from damage to a certain extent, but they will always carry the signs of injury.

The lower back carries most of the weight burden and it is also the area in which people are most likely to have pain. The next most likely area of the spine to have pain is the neck, which obviously has little weight burden in comparison. The reason why little attention will be paid to the anatomy in this book is that, despite the conventional wisdom, it seems to be largely unrelated to chronic pain, as opposed to acute pain. This seemingly odd statement is the topic developed throughout this book.

APPENDIX 4

Standard medical treatments for chronic back pain

As a sufferer of pain, you may have experienced many of the interventions listed here and might therefore already be familiar with some of their advantages and disadvantages.

Drug treatments are one of the conventional medical therapies for chronic pain. Such painkilling drugs are 'non-specific', meaning that they generally dull the reception of pain signals in the central nervous system, but do not target specific pains. The commonly used drugs include:—paracetamol and other analgesics; codeine and other opiate pain killers which are derived from narcotics; and non-steroidal anti-inflammatory drugs (NSAIDs). Some people report that all of these drugs can give relief for acute and chronic lower back pain, but a high proportion of people (perhaps as high as fifty percent) can experience adverse side effects such as constipation, drowsiness and addiction. Any medication that induces sleepiness, such as the narcotic based ones, can be counterproductive as excessive sleep and rest is the opposite of what a person in pain needs in order to get better.

NSAIDs aim at decreasing both pain and inflammation, and are the most commonly prescribed painkillers. The Cochrane review (scientifically rigorous summaries and analyses of the results of clinical trials of health care interventions published by the Cochrane Library in the UK) has found evidence that NSAIDs do provide some short term pain relief, as much as analgesics like paracetamol or aspirin do. However, most pain sufferers are looking for long term relief. In addition, various NSAIDs can produce adverse side effects such as gastrointestinal problems including ulcers and internal bleeding, renal toxicity and adverse effects on hypertension control.[1]

---

[1]   Barnsley (2010) "The significance of chronic back pain". *Medicine Today.*

Some drugs, such as benzodiazepines like Valium, can be prescribed as muscle relaxants for the relief of acute back pain, however there is little evidence for benefit with chronic back pain. As with narcotic based medications, these drugs can be counterproductive because they also can produce drowsiness as well as a range of other symptoms. In addition, as the central nervous system will desensitise to such drugs, their effects wear off over time and the person needs to keep increasing the dosage level in order to get the same relaxant effect. This is a recipe for addiction as well as subsequent problems in withdrawal.

Pain relieving injections are often given in medical attempts to alleviate chronic pain. These injections can be administered in the facet joints on each side of the vertebrae, using either corticosteroid or anaesthetic drugs; epidural injections of a local anaesthetic drug into the space next to the spinal cord; and caudal injections into the membrane over the spinal cord near the base of the spine. Like most other medical interventions, there is no evidence that corticosteroid injections into painful lumbar zygapophyseal joints are of any benefit when compared to local anaesthetics alone.[2] And there is no reason why anaesthetics would be considered an option for *lasting* pain relief, as the effects clearly wear off with time. In fact, there is mixed evidence as to whether any type of fluid injected into the spine is effective, even in the short term. Adverse side effects such as pain at the injection site, infection, nerve damage and haemorrhage can result from such injections. No evidence exists that spinal injections can provide permanent relief of pain in the lower back.[3]

Anti-depressants for pain?

Some antidepressants have been prescribed as a potential reliever of back pain, however the evidence in their favour is poor as there no demonstrated increase in people's ability to function. In America, at least 50% of antidepressants are prescribed for people who are not depressed, and chronic pain is one of the main non-depression reasons for these prescriptions.

---

[2] Barnsley (2010) "The significance of chronic back pain". *Medicine Today.*
[3] Ibid.

Controlled studies have not consistently reported antidepressant efficacy in alleviating chronic pain in general.[4] A team of Cochrane Researchers set out to assess the state of evidence for antidepressants in the treatment of chronic pain. They compared the results of 10 studies which compared the levels of effectiveness of antidepressants with placebos. The lead author of the study, Dr Donna Urquhart of Monash University reported, "We found no clear evidence to support the clinician's prescription of antidepressants in reducing pain and depression for patients with chronic low back pain".[5]

In addition, a large amount of people (estimates vary between 30%-60%) are likely to suffer adverse side effects from the newer generation of antidepressants, the Selective Serotonin Re-uptake Inhibitors (SSRIs), as well as the Selective Serotonin Noradrenaline Re-uptake Inhibitors (SSNRIs). These adverse side effects can ironically enough include worsening depression, anxiety, panic, agitation, and even *bone and joint pain*. Tricyclic antidepressants (TCAs) have been used at doses lower than typical for treating depression, however these can often cause drowsiness and subsequent inactivity as well. Like SSRIs, TCAs also have the potential to cause adverse effects and drug interactions.[6]

Surgery may be considered to remove disc material from a 'slipped disc' that is causing sciatica or other nerves symptoms (referred to as a discectomy), however it is rarely considered a viable option for most people suffering uncomplicated back pain. This is due to the lack of clarity of physical causes actually needing intervention (beyond what is often seen in the pain free population), as well as to poor outcomes. A laminectomy can be performed to correct the bony spurs of arthritis, removing protruding bits of bone and the nerve 'decompressed'. A surgical fusion may be performed when there is a forward slippage of a vertebra, referred to as spondylolisthesis. Most medical authorities argue against the use of surgery for the vast majority of people in chronic pain—this would not be the case if surgery was a highly successful intervention.

---

[4] http://www.sciencedaily.com/releases/2008/01/080122203148.htm
[5] Urquart (2008) "No clear evidence that antidepressants assist in the management of chronic low back pain". *Science Daily*.
[6] Ibid.

APPENDIX 5

The value of physical therapies?

Most people in chronic pain will have either tried a wide range of physical therapies only to eventually give up in despair, or will eventually arrive at that point. Physical therapies are provided by a range of health practitioners including general practitioners, chiropractors, osteopaths, orthopedists, neurologists, neurosurgeons, rheumatologists, and a range of other body therapists who provide hands-on treatments such as massage. This disparate group are unified in the basic belief that the spine and its surrounding musculature can be easily injured due to their deficiencies, and is therefore in need of corrective physical intervention.

People may very well feel better in the short term as a result of any number of physical therapies: however, there is simply no proof that in the long run such approaches result in a sustained reduction or elimination of chronic pain. To feel better in the short term may be a welcome improvement, however my experience of people in chronic pain is that they want a long-term solution to what is by definition a long-term problem—not something that will just make them feel better for a few days at a time. Despite this, physical therapies are our culture's main way of dealing with chronic pain.

I am not suggesting in any way that people who offer physical therapies in the absence of supportive evidence are doing so in an unethical manner. One could not call the chronic pain epidemic a scientific fraud, nor can one reasonably think of the physical therapists who service this epidemic as engaging in some kind of conspiracy.

The creation of the chronic pain epidemic is a process of social construction in which both the lay population and the service providers each play their own role. It is simply not a process that has been informed or governed by science. Rather, it has been informed by patients' emotional needs and treatment providers' needs to provide a service, and to act with some certainty despite not knowing the real causes.

Most physical therapists and GPs are sincerely motivated in their desire to reduce suffering, and many no doubt do believe that they are succeeding. Ultimately, their sincere desire to help can absorb the information which science is revealing. When it does so, more help will be available to those suffering. However, it may require that physical therapists change their role with chronic pain sufferers to being one of an educator and provider of reassurance rather than a manipulator of the anatomy.

Research does support the contention that physical therapies can be effective in helping with *acute* pain resulting from a recent injury. When it comes to pain that has been experienced for more than three months, there is simply no evidence that any form of physical treatment actually works. People may feel temporarily better as a result of the physical therapy bringing blood and oxygen back into the pained area; and they may also feel emotionally better as a result of having some kind and gentle attention. In addition, most physical therapist counsel their patients to some degree, even if they are largely unaware of it or wouldn't refer to their advice and reassurance as counseling. Kind psychological and physical treatment is particularly important when sufferers experience little kindness or even touch in their normal lives.

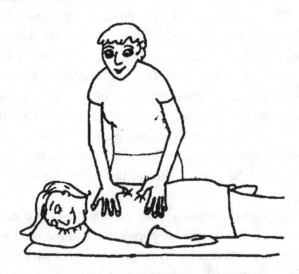

Physical therapy meets a psychological need

Touch provides a range of benefits to our emotional, physiological and neurological states.[1] On an emotional level, touch is important as it can express reassurance. It can lead to secretions of neurotransmitters such as dopamine, oxytocin as well as endorphins. Stress hormone levels can be reduced, the immune system bolstered and depression lessened with kind touch. It is obviously extremely important, especially if people are getting little touch as part of their daily experience. These factors can all lead to short-term improvements in how sufferers feel both emotionally as well as physically. But if this is the only treatment they receive, it is likely that a year down the road, their pain will remain essentially unchanged despite minor fluctuations provided by short term effects of the physical therapy.

My groin pain certainly felt better after lying on the blocks provided by the chiropractor. I managed to replicate this treatment at home with the blocks which I made for myself. However, the pain never went away with physical interventions. The only way to eliminate the pain was to get to the hidden psychology behind it.

When claims of effectiveness of physical therapies are studied across large samples of sufferers, the evidence of improvement in pain simply disappears. Edzard Ernst, a Professor of Complimentary Medicine at the Peninsular Medical School in the UK, states in a recent edition of *New Scientist* that there is some evidence that chiropractic adjustments are *about as effective* as other standard treatments.[2] The problem is that standard treatments, such as physiotherapy, are for the most part ineffective in treating chronic pain. Ernst's research team analyzed the data from the more credible studies on chiropractic and concluded that "spinal manipulation is not associated with clinically relevant specific therapeutic effects."[3]

In regards to the value of physiotherapy interventions, Professor of Physiotherapy Paul Hodges revealed the following state of evidence.[4] Both high and low velocity manipulations of the spine, the types which either physiotherapists or chiropractors do, have been shown to have some positive impact with *acute* pain but no positive impact on chronic back pain.

---

[1]   Arden (2010) *Rewire Your Brain: Think Your Way to a Better Life.*

[2]   Ernst (2009) Opinion Essay—*New Scientist*

[3]   Ibid.

[4]   Hodges (2004) "Exercise and Bone Strength/physiotherapy". ABC Radio National Health Report.

There is no evidence that massage has a strong effect on chronic pain. The only available evidence on massage suggests that it can have a small and transient effect, especially with acute pain from a recent injury. As stated earlier, even small and transient effects can be very welcome to sufferers, so many people will value massage. However, there is no evidence that it will help people to largely reduce or eliminate chronic pain. Traction has not been found to produce positive outcomes with chronic back pain. There has been no systematic evaluation of the value of magnets in the management of pain, and as such no credible evidence exists. TENS machines, which stimulate skin, nerves and muscles with mild electrical currents, have been demonstrated as ineffective in treating chronic back pain.

As can be seen, all of the approaches which constitute "standard treatments" (see also the discussion of medical drugs and surgical interventions in Appendix 4) have been found *ineffective* when it comes to chronic pain. Any of the above mentioned interventions may be helpful with the short term pain related to an acute injury—and *none* of them have been demonstrated through research to effectively help with chronic pain.

The lack of evidence for physical treatments of chronic pain has largely escaped the attention of the "rehabilitation bureaucracy" which is mostly made up of physiotherapists. As such, physical therapies will still be regularly prescribed as a matter of course, and often funded by insurance companies and governments, despite their lack of proven effectiveness. People will continue to seek out these interventions in desperation due to unrelenting pain, and because these interventions continue to be marketed as effective treatments when they are not.

This review of the evidence is not to say that people who report benefits from physical treatments are either delusional or lying. But, when large numbers of people are studied statistically, there are so few who claim a lasting benefit that the positive results are more a matter of random luck or a placebo effect than attributable to the treatment itself. If there were more people in a sample of one hundred who reported positive outcomes to a particular therapy, then this would be reflected in a statistically significant finding that such treatment produces positive results above the rate of chance. But the results of studies performed simply don't confirm this possibility. A positive outcome would also have to be compared against a placebo treatment with no known value, as the positive result may have come about purely as a result of expecting the treatment to work. A treatment effect may also be operating, whereby the person experiences the benefit of receiving kind attention with the physical intervention itself actually being irrelevant to the outcomes.

If you are clearly getting better, it could be possible to continue with physical therapy at the same time as incorporating *The Hidden Psychology of Pain*. But be aware that small improvements could be resulting from a placebo effect (in which case the improvement won't last), or just by virtue of appreciating being treated with kind touch (in which case the improvements also won't last, simply because it is not addressing the root cause of the problem). If you are appreciating the kind touch, and as such are unwilling to let go of the physical therapy, perhaps work at changing how you perceive the therapy. It may not actually be doing anything to assist in eliminating the pain beyond the effects of kindness, however just focus on the nice experience of kind touch without seeing it as a treatment for a serious physical disorder that requires physical treatment. It may also be worth working out how to get more kind touch in your life without having to pay a therapist for it, as this is a normal human need from which we will suffer in its absence.

If you retain an awareness of *The Hidden Psychology of Pain*, it is possible for you to continue receiving benefit from treatment provided by a physical therapist. The proviso would be that you approach this treatment with the expectation that at best, it will bring blood and oxygen back into the pained area. It may therefore provide some alleviation and help you to feel better emotionally. If you approach physical therapy with the idea that you have a serious physical condition requiring hands-on treatment, then paradoxically you are more likely to remain in pain. This is simply because such a belief, being strengthened by the physical therapy itself, is the exact purpose of the pain—to monopolize your attention, to have you focus on the physicality of your experience, to have you worry and ruminate over the pain, and to expect and hope that physical treatment will work. This is why your mind/brain has created the pain: to distract your attention away from the deeper psychological causes. As long as you retain your focus on the physicality of the pain (aided with physical therapy), then the mind/brain's strategy is working perfectly. You will remain in physical pain and be distracted from the psychological pain indefinitely.

Research shows that people in chronic pain want to receive hands-on treatment as it feels good to be carefully handled when in pain. Ironically, physical therapy meets a psychological need rather than a physical need. The situation is similar to patients demanding antibiotic treatment for the common cold. The antibiotic is likely to make the person feel emotionally better, because they figure they have got the treatment they need, but it is not likely to do anything physical to help with the cold.

In Australia and the UK, physical therapists are able to provide chronic pain sufferers with essential information, reassurance and support, rather than with just physical manipulation. As Medicare, insurance companies or the NHS, and not the patients themselves are often paying for most of the services, physical therapist have more opportunity to "defy" the patient's demand for hands-on treatment, and provide what has actually been demonstrated to work—just information.

In third party funded health services, the purely physical treatment approach to chronic pain is more likely to be balanced with psychological approaches such as information, support and reassurance. People who want to entertain the psychological possibility, while also entertaining the standard physicalist view, generally fail to get better. In my own practice, I have seen many people who show this pattern. Part of them wants to accept what I am telling them, as it logically holds together and seems to relate to their experience. However, another part of them wants to believe that the next physical therapy will be the one to provide a cure. Invariably, they remain in pain. The only time physical therapy is supported by the scientific evidence is in regards to *acute pain* from a recent injury. With such injuries, the evidence would suggest that you either rest the sore area for a short time or pursue short term physical therapy (be advised by your physician).

Physicians and physical therapists can best assist their patients by restricting their hands-on services to only those who are in acute pain, and to provide accurate information and reassurance only to their patients who are in chronic pain. Such services meet a genuine need in the community. At any one time, many people are suffering from acute pain and do need physical therapy assistance. As such, physical therapists are extremely valuable and can always play a very important role in the treatment industry.

As an analogy, counseling is essentially useless as a "medical" intervention for people suffering from brain tumors, particularly if the goal is to cure the tumor. People may feel better about talking with a psychologist about their condition, may appreciate the psychologist's kindness, and it may help them to cope with an unpleasant reality. But no amount of counseling is likely to "solve the problem" of the brain tumor in any medical sense—it is simply the wrong intervention.

As we live in a culture that constantly reminds us of the supposed fragility of the spine (e.g. chiropractic warnings to not sit on a wallet in your back pocket), there are persistent invitations to focus on the physicality of pain and ignore the underlying emotions. Standard physical therapy is likely to just add to this overall focus on the physical and further distract us from looking at emotions. Discussing the mind/body condition of RSI, Dr Lucire writes,

> Physical treatments cannot represent rational activity in the alleviation of the condition, as physical remedies are irrelevant to the resolution of the conflict or need which is at the base of the symptom. At the same time, such disease-focused remedies reinforce false beliefs about the body. One might further argue that their administration discourages attention to the real cause of the problem, the need or conflict combining with the belief and opportunity that the doctor provides.[5]

This section would not be complete without mentioning my experience with a physical therapy called Structural Integration, or "Rolfing". Years before I came across the role which hidden psychology plays in chronic pain, I had developed a "frozen shoulder syndrome", where any movement of my right arm became painful and constricted for several months. A friend, who had trained as a Rolfer, treated my shoulder with this approach, and the pain resolved over the next few days. John Sarno reports that he used to refer his chronic pain patients to Rolfing practitioners who worked at his clinic, and often saw very positive results from this approach. He only ceased with advocating this treatment as he saw that, as with most other physical therapies, patients who received the treatment were reinforced in their physical focus on the pain, and thereby failed to completely recover.

---

5   Lucire (2003). *Constructing RSI: Belief and Desire.*

As stated earlier, if you are able to develop and maintain an awareness of chronic pain's hidden psychology, it is theoretically possible for you to benefit from a therapy like Rolfing, and not simply reinforce the "smoke screen" which chronic pain is. The extent to which you succeed in striking the right therapeutic balance (between a psychological focus and a physical focus) is in your hands.

APPENDIX 6

The evolution of psychology

A brief history of psychology shows that as an academic discipline, it developed towards the end of the 19th century in the new experimental laboratories of Wilhelm Wundt in Germany and William James in America. At around the same time, Sigmund Freud was busy developing his career in Vienna, applying therapeutic approaches to the treatment of psychological problems. If he was practicing today, he would be referred to as a neurologist, but his school of psychology came to be known as psychoanalysis. It is best seen within its socio-historical context and can be viewed as an expression of the European intellectual mindset of the time. *Crime and Punishment*, written by Dostoevsky in 1866, reveals that the notion of a subconscious or unconscious mind predated Freud's writings by decades. Such ideas were in fact part of the European culture for a long time before Freud turned it into a focus of scientific inquiry. Many renowned European philosophers throughout history, going as far back as the ancient Greeks, and no doubt the pagan cultures of prehistory, saw the significance of the unconscious. This awareness is also seen in non-European cultures around the world and throughout history as a general facet of their cosmology, rather than just being confined to their versions of medicine or psychology. By the late 19th century, the broad notion of psychology having a role to play in illness, including both emotions and the unconscious, was reasonably well established. The medical precursors to Freud go back considerably further, as evidenced by Benjamin Collins Brodie's theories of "hysteria" to explain bone and joint disease in the 1830s, and Robert Brudnell Carter's 1853 suggestion that hysterical conditions arise from the patients inability to cope with emotions.[1]

---

[1] Lucire (2003). *Constructing RSI: Belief and Desire.*

Nineteenth century neurologists Charcot and Janet also wrote extensively on such issues in relation to hysteria, and provided Freud with much of the groundwork and inspiration for his career. Freud did however take these and a range of other psychological notions and melded them into a new theory of psychological functioning as well a new method of therapy. Where psychology in universities was essentially a new research enterprise in the late 19th century, the application of psychology to human problems was, for the most part the application of psychoanalysis. As psychoanalytic approaches to psychology were using notions of the subconscious or unconscious mind as a corner stone of their model, the term "depth-psychology" was introduced to reflect a deeper delving than mere surface level thoughts and feelings. The assumption is that, as with icebergs, the part of the mind that we are consciously aware of (like the visible tip of the iceberg) is only a minor part of the overall mind or psyche. The greater part of the mind is viewed as being below the level of conscious awareness (as the majority of the iceberg is below water level).

The power of psychoanalysis in applied psychology held sway for many decades and spawned generations of "neo-psychoanalytic" theories and practices. But depth-psychology never had psychology all its own way.

During the 1920s, American psychologist John Watson took Russian physiologist, Pavlov's experiments with classically conditioned dogs a step further by applying the principles to human behavior. In so doing, he began another school of thought within psychology which came to be termed "behaviorism," as it focused purely on behavior.

While behaviorism became a very powerful force within academic and experimental psychology, especially in America, psychoanalysis for the most part remained the "king" of applied psychology (as opposed to academic psychology). It was primarily what psychologists and psychologically oriented psychiatrists did to help people in distress. Behaviorism represents psychology's most extreme application of the mechanistic mindset to its subject matter, humans. It adopted the model of science suggested by Newtonian physics, and as such, defined out of bounds for a scientific psychology anything that could not be objectively observed and therefore measured. Consequently, the new focus was exclusively behavior. As the mind could not be seen or measured, it was no longer the subject matter of academic psychology within the behaviorist paradigm. The same held true for other non-observables such as emotions, motives, psychological drives, thoughts and beliefs. Where some behavioral psychologists still acknowledged the presence of such phenomenon (just not within their "scientific" psychology), others dismissed the very existence of any such psychological factors altogether. Psychology reached the ridiculous point where it had ceased to even acknowledge its own subject matter: the psyche.

It is interesting that despite this extreme stance of behaviorism, there were some American psychologists working with people in distress during the 1930s who recognized that it was preposterous to pretend that humans didn't have minds, thoughts and beliefs. Psychologists such as Gordon Allport and George Kelly were early representatives of what would later be called cognitive psychology. As far back as the Great Depression, they insisted that any psychological research or interventions with people must also take into account the mental maps or 'schemas' that people use to make sense of their experience.

The behaviorists were not to be outdone, however, and in the 1940s were reinvigorated by the work of experimental psychologists B.F. Skinner. He boosted the mechanistic view, suggesting that all human behavior could be understood in terms of the patterns of reinforcement in stimulus-response relationships. The term "radical behaviorism" came into being to describe Skinner's approach. Again, psychology demonstrated its tendency towards taking an idea that can explain certain aspects of human experience and expanding it to cover *all* aspects. For example, Skinner reasonably suggests that we may continue putting money into a vending machine, as this behavior is rewarded by a can a fizzy drink which we find pleasurable. The coin-giving behavior has been reinforced by the pleasurable reward of the drink, and is therefore more likely to happen again. This may be a reasonable proposition when we are talking about putting coins into a vending machine, but the further we go away from simple behaviors and towards the more complex behaviors which distinguish humans from other forms of life, the more inadequate this explanation becomes.

Again, while this type of radical behaviorism was dominating academic and research psychology, especially into the 1950s and 60s, psychoanalysis and its newer variations were still the predominant form of psychological treatment. The need to incorporate an awareness of the cognitive (thinking) aspects of human experience into psychology was gaining momentum in academic psychology as a result of the excessive claims of behaviorism.

Seeing the inadequacy of a psychology focused purely on behavior, academic psychology began to incorporate the cognitive aspect to behavioral theory, resulting in contemporary cognitive-behavioral psychology. Along with Kelly and Allport, Canadian psychologist Albert Bandura was one of the academic and research leaders who insisted on the need to incorporate the internal cognitive processes involved in the learning of new behaviors. He developed what became called "social behaviorism" to explain the social learning processes of complex behaviors. This was an advance over the simplistic notions of strict behaviorism, in that it presented a more realistic picture of how we learn complex behaviors from watching those around us. Aaron Beck and Albert Ellis also developed an emphasis on people's thinking styles in their approaches to helping those in psychological distress. These two people had a profound effect on applied psychology, as this is the type of psychological therapy which most psychologists are today practicing.

Until the advent of Rational Emotive Therapy (Ellis) and Cognitive Behavior Therapy (Beck), the behavioral components of therapy were viewed as being separate from the thinking components. It was then recognized that even strictly behavioral therapists were in fact engaging people on a thinking level, and even strictly cognitive therapists were assisting people to behave differently. With time, this artificial distinction between cognitive and behavioral interventions has all but disappeared, now resulting in a broad cognitive-behavioral paradigm.

The behavioral element of CBT is an emphasis on developing a set of daily activities which have the potential to create pleasure as well as a sense of mastery and achievement. This can give people a much needed emotional boost. As stated earlier, the cognitive element of CBT is the notion that distress is not caused by actual events on our lives, but by our interpretations of these events. As such, CBT combines the need to develop different behaviors with the need to critically review, and where necessary, challenge the types of thoughts we have about situations and events. The ideal is that the client and the therapist work collaboratively, as something like co-researchers, treating the client's thoughts as hypotheses that can be tested and challenged in a scientific manner in relation to actual evidence. For example, the idea "I am a loser" can be tested for its accuracy, and hopefully changed in light of the evidence. If the person has ever succeeded in an aspect of life or developed positive skills, then this evidence would argue against the negative belief.

The final school of thought in psychology to have a major impact is humanistic psychology, which also arose in response to the excesses of behaviorism. It introduced a focus on the uniqueness of humans as goal-seeking, conscious beings who are moving towards a sense of wholeness, not just organisms responding to environmental stimuli or instinctual impulses. Humanistic psychology, under the leadership of psychologists like Carl Rogers and Abraham Maslow, created a different understanding of human experience and an approach to counseling that emphasized the necessary conditions for therapeutic change. As cognitive-behavioral psychology and humanistic psychology rose to prominence in the 1960s and 70s, a new raft of therapeutic approaches were popularized, and psychoanalysis began its decline into relative obscurity.

Psychoanalysis was rightly criticized for a range of shortcomings, including its lack of scientific rigor as well its apparent bias against women (does anyone seriously still want to argue that "penis envy" is a real phenomenon?) It has been viewed as a reflection of turn of the century middle class Viennese values, and therefore of questionable value in this very different era. In addition, it often took years of therapy before any progress could be seen, and as such, fostered a dependency on the therapist. But the more that it became relegated as yesterday's therapy, the more the baby was thrown out with the bathwater. Many pearls of wisdom that were based on decades of observation were discarded in favor of both the more "scientific" cognitive-behavioral, and the "here and now" humanistic paradigms. Depth psychology became something that people studying fine arts, cultural studies and even politics were more likely to examine than were psychology students.

Australian cartoonist and social commentator, Michael Leunig, in *The Lot in Words*, provides a good example of depth-psychology awareness in the arts. Another example of psychoanalytic ideas in the arts is *Writing in Restaurants*. In his book, American playwright David Mamet makes sense of theatre and the craft of acting from a psychoanalytic frame of reference. Robert Rowland Smith, in *Breakfast with Socrates* shows how contemporary philosophy has more of an interest in psychoanalysis than does psychology.

Discussions about psychoanalysis have become an unusual experience for most students of modern psychology, to such an extent that you now have a better chance of a well-informed psychoanalytic discussion with someone in the arts or philosophy, and even the theatre, than with someone in psychology.

There are a range of reasons for psychology having turned its back on psychoanalysis. Most of these relate to the social, cultural and political context in which Freud operated. Also, with psychology's desire to become more scientific over the 20th century, there was too much subjectivity in psychoanalysis to be tolerated. But perhaps the greatest "crime" committed by Freud was the about-face he took on the issue of the sexual abuse of children. In the early stages of his career, Freud took the reports of sexual abuse of his female patients at face value, giving them the credence they deserved. Were he to have continued with this acceptance of such reports, Western culture could have inched closer to a proper dealing with the issue. In a later stage of his career, Freud reformulated his theory of allegations of sexual abuse, coming to view them as mere fantasy, and even "wish-fulfilment" of his patients. That is, he denied the actual reality of the sexual abuse, and instead chose to present such allegations as figments of his patient's imaginations. In so doing, Freud not only missed a rare opportunity to put the sexual exploitation of children on the early 20th century social agenda, but he also set this possibility back for nearly a century. It was not until the 1980s that the sexual abuse of children became a topic of social discussion. Until then, our culture had suffered from a mass denial and repression of awareness relating to this abuse of children. One has to question how much Freud's lead on the issue, denying the reality, contributed to the forced silence which ruined so many people's lives.[2]

---

[2] As a practicing psychologist, I am horrified by the amount of clients I have (males as well, but usually females) who report to having been sexually violated as children and young people. It may be a skewed perception from working closely with a non-representative sample of people, but my impression is that the sexual abuse of children has been prevalent in our society. Rather than recognize this and deal with it, our culture chose for most of the 20th century to deny the reality and to force the whole issue underground. This was only challenged by the brave souls who raised the topic in the public arena in the 1980's and onwards. My only hope is that with this raised awareness, leading to programs such as protective behaviors being taught in schools, the prevalence

Referring to psychosomatic studies looking at irritable bowel syndrome (IBS), Robert Sapolsky demonstrates a contemporary view of Freud's approach: "These studies tended to focus on a lot of psychoanalytic gibberish (there, now I'll get myself in trouble with that crowd)—some hoo-ha about the person being stuck in the anal stage of development, a regression to the period of toilet training where going to the bathroom gained great acclaim and, suddenly, diarrhoea was a symbolic reach for parental approval. Or the approval of the doctor as a parental surrogate. Or something or other . . ."[3]

As stated, many of Freud's notions can be seen as highly dated and of limited use, however even Sapolsky, who has written a brilliant book about the stress-disease connection, throws the depth-psychology baby out with the Freudian bathwater, as does much of our culture. No doubt, such health conditions as IBS have a range of highly complex biological factors. However, the current understanding of its cause could be greatly aided by re-introducing some depth-psychology notions, whilst not needing to revert back to Freud's complete model of the psyche. In a later section, Sapolsky does acknowledge that after nearly a hundred years, few other intellectuals are considered important enough to still merit regular criticism, as is Freud.

CBT is the undoubted current 'emperor' of psychology, and follows from the importance given to conscious thoughts. We typically use styles of thinking which can prove less than helpful, e.g. black or white thinking wherein situations are viewed as all bad or al good, rather than as shades of gray, or emotional reasoning where because I feel that someone hates me, it means they *do* hate me. These are standard examples of what are referred to as thinking errors. The job of CBT is to correct these thinking styles, with the assumption that a person's mood will lift if they are thinking in a more rational style which is supported by evidence.

As stated, it is hard to deny an element of truth in this formulation: however, it is another thing again to suggest that these are the root source of all our psychological problems. CBT is often criticized as focusing too much on the role of surface-level conscious thoughts to the exclusion of

---

of molestation is slowly reducing. Personally, I would be happy to become unemployable as a psychologist if one day we lived in a society that cherished children and genuinely protected them from all forms of abuse and neglect.

[3] Sapolsky (2004) Why Zebras Don't Get Ulcers. (p.83)

unconscious thoughts, feelings, memories and urges—as such, it can be viewed as shallow and superficial, resulting in only temporary therapeutic changes. It has also been criticized as simplistic, mechanistic, reductionist, and not as well supported by outcome evidence as its enthusiasts claims. Despite its apparent shortcomings, CBT has been the psychology flavor of the month for several decades now. Its adherents can at times take on a religious type zeal, often claiming that it is the only useful approach to take with any and all human problems. This enthusiasm is often maintained in the face of conflicting evidence, which suggests that the emperor is in fact less well clad than what he would like to believe. [4] [5] This zeal for CBT, particularly when it is to the exclusion of other useful approaches, demonstrates that psychology is just as able to operate in a 'folk' manner as is medicine, rather than in an evidence informed scientific manner.

[4] King (1999) "Depression: Do We Really Know What We Are Doing?" *Psychotherapy in Australia.*

[5] Cuijpers et al (2010) "Efficacy of cognitive–behavioural therapy and other psychological treatments for adult depression: meta-analytic study of publication bias". *The British Journal of Psychiatry.*

APPENDIX 7

Sample of research demonstrating structural pathology in pain-free populations

The following begins with studies that used more primitive assessment technologies, and moves towards more contemporary studies that use the most advance means of detecting structural pathology. A plethora of research supports the basic contention that most structural abnormalities, which are viewed as being responsible for chronic pain, also exist in high proportions within the pain free population.

- Studying the role of cervical nerve root deformities with apparent nerve compression and subsequent pain, Fox, Lin, Pinto and Kricheff (1975) examined myelograms of 231 people (where a dye is injected via a small needle inserted through the skin into a part of the spinal column, showing up the spinal cord and nerve roots). From these assessments, they concluded that 76 of these people had nerve root deformities, and the remainders did not. The results show no correlation between this structural pathology and the experience of pain. In fact, they concluded "We agree with McRae who stated that *any patient over 30 years of age*, no matter what symptoms or signs he presents, is apt to have posterior cervical disk protrusion demonstrated, if he happens to have a myelogram" (Fox et al 1975, p. 361. italics added).

- In a similar vein, Magora & Schwartz (1980) report extensive research conducted with a sample of 1244 people, 800 of who experienced lower back pain, and 444 of who experienced no pain at all. All subjects in the study were examined for structural abnormalities of the spine using neurological and orthopaedic state examinations and X-rays. These researchers found no evidence of a relationship between lower back pain and the incidence of conditions that have been assumed to cause such pain such as spondylolysis, degenerative osteoarthritis, transitional vertebra, or spina bifida occulta. That is, the structural abnormalities of the in-pain group did not differ in any way to the structural abnormalities of the no-pain group. Each were just as likely or unlikely to have the same structural abnormalities, suggesting that the abnormalities are irrelevant to chronic pain.

- In a study using CAT scans as the diagnostic tool for structural abnormalities in the spines of people with no history of back trouble, Wiesel, Feffer, Citrin and Patronas (1984) found that in the over 40 age group, there was an average of 50% abnormal findings with diagnoses of stenosis, herniated disc, and facet degeneration occurring most frequently. When the under-forty age group were included in the statistics, the prevalence of structural abnormality in the lumbar spine averaged out to 35.4%. These abnormalities were found in people with no back pain.

- Boden, Davis, Patrona & Weisel (1990) studied the MRIs of 67 individuals who had never had low-back pain, sciatica, or neruological claudication. They found that amongst subjects who were less than 60 years of age, 20% had a herniated nucleus pulposus, whereas in the over 60 year group 36% had a herniated nucleus pulposus and 21% had spinal stenosis. Abnormalities were found in 57% of this age group, despite these people not being in pain. All but one of the 80 year old subjects had disc degeneration or bulging on at least one lumbar level, while this was found in 35% of all subjects aged between 20 and 39. Clearly, the risk of harmless structural pathology of the spine is age related. No wonder it is referred to as 'grey hair of the spine'.

- Jensen et al (1994) took MRI scans of the lumbar spines of 98 people who were asymptomatic of pain. Only 36% of the subjects in the study were found to have normal discs at all levels, ie. no structural pathologies. The remaining 64% of people with no back pain were found to have intervertebral disc abnormalities (ie. bulge, protrusion) and nonintervertebral disc pathologies, while 38% of them had these structural abnormalities at more than one level of their spine. In addition, they found that the prevalence of disc abnormalities differed little with physical activity score. These researchers concluded that "the discovery by MRI of bulges or protrusions in people with low back pain may frequently be coincidental".

- Stadnik and colleagues (1998) also used MRIs to examine structural abnormalities in a study of 36 people without low-back pain or sciatica. They found that 81% of these people had bulging discs or focal disc protrusions, but no pain.

- In a more recent predictive study in which people with identifiable abnormality of their discs or spinal canal were followed up 7 years later, Borenstein and colleagues (2001) conducted MRI scans on their subjects. They found no evidence that the existence of structural pathology was predictive of who later experienced lower back pain. That is, people were just as likely or unlikely to wind up in back pain whether they had structural pathology of their spine 7 years earlier or not. In addition, people who had the longest lasting low-back pain did not have the greatest degree of structural abnormality of their spine in the original scans. Again, the presumed relationship between chronic pain and structural abnormalities was just not found.

Deyo (2002) points out that 'the disease management paradigm', in which specific therapies are devised to address specific anatomic or physiological abnormalities, has worked well in general medicine. However, when it is applied to issues of chronic pain or ill health, obvious failings are apparent.

The medical treatment of chronic pain has moved away from empirically treating symptoms based on scientifically generated information, such as that presented above, to simply 'modifying pathophysiologic conditions' in relation to presumed physical causes. As these findings reflect, Deyo (2002 p.1444) concludes that, "Anatomic abnormalities can be readily identified by imaging studies, but most of these abnormalities are common even in healthy people". Echoing experts such as Professor Sarno, he goes on to state that,

> ". . . as we learn more about the evolution of chronic pain syndromes, evidence suggests that mood disorders, perceptual styles, and cognitive, social and even financial factors may help determine who develops back pain and who becomes disabled by it."

APPENDIX 8

EFT on a Page

(adapted from www.emouniverse.com)

<u>THE BASIC RECIPE</u>

The Setup . . . Repeat 3 times this affirmation:

*"Even though I have this.,
I deeply and completely accept myself"*.

while continuously rubbing the Sore Spot or tapping the Karate Chop point.

The Sequence . . . Tap about 7 times on each of the following energy points while repeating the Reminder Phrase (the part of the Setup Phrase that you filled the blank with) at each point.

(eye brow) (under eye) (chin) (under arm) (thumb) (mid finger) (karate chop)
EB, SE, UE, UN, Ch, CB, UA, BN, Th, IF, MF, BF, KC
(side of eye) (under nose) (collar bone) (below nose) (index finger) (baby finger)

The Gamut Procedure . . . Continuously tap on the Gamut point while performing each of these 9 actions:

(1) Eyes closed (2) Eyes open (3) Eyes hard down right (4) Eyes hard down left (5) Roll eyes in a circle (6) Roll eyes in other direction (7) Hum 2 seconds of a song (8) Count to 5 (9) Hum 2 seconds of a song

The Sequence (again) . . . Tap about 7 times on each of the following energy points while repeating the Reminder Phrase at each point.

EB, SE, UE, UN, Ch, CB, UA, BN, Th, IF, MF, BF, KC

Note: In subsequent rounds The Setup affirmation and the Reminder Phrase are adjusted to reflect the fact that you are addressing the _remaining_ problem.

APPENDIX 9

Process for staying in the present moment

- Be aware of feelings of anxiety, worry, fear, etc
- Recognize that these feelings are our body's alarm system—they are telling us something very important that we need to tune into.
- These feelings come from the thoughts that our minds are engaging in—they must always be about things that *haven't yet happened* (and may never happen).
- The feelings are alerting us to the need to look at our thoughts—that's what they are there for.
- What problematic story about the future is your mind creating?
- Recognize that this story is no more real than a pink elephant—it is just a bunch of thoughts, ideas. It has no more reality than a series of brain cells 'firing' in a certain pattern. That is the extent of its reality.
- When you realize this, and recognize that your anxiety is coming from this story about the future which your mind is creating, you have brought your awareness/consciousness to the situation.
- This awareness creates a 'gap' between you and what your mind is doing. This gap is your consciousness.
- As soon as this gap is created, you can see that your mind has taken you away from what is real (Now) to what is not real and may never happen (i.e. the future). We can never know what will happen as it is all just guesses, predictions.
- Take 2-3 deep breaths to anchor yourself back into your body. Your body is only ever aware of Now, and come back the only reality—Now. You may need to do something about what is happening Now.

APPENDIX 10

Testimonials from the Hidden Psychology of Pain clients

<u>Helen's story</u>

On moving from the city and looking to the green countryside to sooth my ailments (chronic pain and mental anguish), I thankfully made an appointment with the psychologist, Dr James Alexander—really, just someone to talk to. I received two blessings.

The first was being introduced to *The Hidden Psychology of Pain*, which ultimately enabled me to fix my back problems. I had been told by one of Sydney's top experts that the best I could do was to learn to live with the ongoing pain. At the time, I had been learning and teaching meditation and Tai chi for years, however the pain had remained present and persistent. Within days of having a true understanding of what was happening in the muscular tissue in my back, the pain was gone. The problem was emotional in nature and my mind had decided to shield me from my emotional problems by creating pain in my back. Knowing the fact of blood and oxygen deprivation allowed me to tell my mind to send oxygen to these areas of my back, and the pain stopped completely.

The second blessing was EMDR therapy, which has directly fixed the enormous emotional anguish and pain I was living with daily (PTSD). I did not realise that the emotional flash backs, recurring distressing memories, increased anger, inability to control mood swings or concentration problems, and the constant avoidance of thoughts and feelings were not normal. I thought it was just something I had to learn to control. My father had the same issues, so was I just like him? We both had a problem with anger and substance abuse, and we would both jokingly say that we were self-medicating. This turned out to be true.

In May 2010 I quit smoking tobacco and marijuana, and I also quit coffee and alcohol. To say this was difficult would be an understatement. After three months, I was an emotional mess, but instead of going back to my old well-established addictions, I chose to go back to the psychologist and began EMDR therapy once a week for about 6-8 weeks. Slowly, my world changed and it became much easier to deal with my life, my memories and my emotions. I am not so directed by intense emotions including uncontrollable rage, and morbid grief. I feel as if now I stand in the light at the end of the tunnel. I give thanks daily for both of these blessings—not having physical or emotional pain. This has given me room to live my life.

Note: 'Helen' had received chiropractic and physiotherapy treatment in her thoracic area, however this aggravated the pain. An osteopath told her that the pain was likely to be 'of internal origin'. Chinese medicine and acupuncture made no difference. An X-ray revealed mild thoracic scoliosis with some disc narrowing and spondylitic change at T8/9. The doctor, who assessed her at a prestigious pain clinic, a Consultant in Pain Management, wrote in a report to her GP that,

> "I think it is feasible that the pain arises from the T8/9 intervertebral disc. Unfortunately, if this is the case, there is no direct interventions that are likely to be helpful and symptomatic treatment is the only option available".

This specialist advised Helen to simply get used to being in pain, and to seek treatments that may alleviate it such as a TENS machine. Helen had grown up with a range of upsetting and traumatic experiences which she carried within her. Several years before I met her, her son had died and she had remained grief stricken as well as in extreme physical pain for years. As she reveals, Helen responded well to both *The Hidden Psychology of Pain* and to EMDR.

Richard's story

Initially I attended Dr James Alexander's rooms to address my depression. During the course of my visits the subject of pain arose. I was, at the time, experiencing severe pain across the top of my back which I'd assumed was as a result of a shoulder "reconstruction". The result of this pain was that I was unable to sleep through the night, waking up with severe pain which no amount of twisting, turning or other adjustment of posture would remedy. I would eventually sleep due to being exhausted only to awaken an hour or so later with the pain – this process was repeated for a number of years.

James introduced me to 'The Hidden Psychology of Pain', explaining that pain like mine was likely to be coming from emotional issues that had not been resolved. He also asked me if I would be interested in trying some therapy which involved tapping on certain points of my body – this was supposed to assist in the treatment of the pain. My initial, though perhaps not voiced, opinion was that this would be unlikely to make any difference. I was wrong.

After a number of sessions I found that using this technique, along with some relaxation CDs he provided, I was able to enjoy a full night's, pain free sleep. I have enjoyed this luxury now for around 18 months or so. There is no sign that the pain will return, it is now a distant (and might I add vague) memory. In my experience, not only has the pain "disappeared", but the memory of it has almost been lost.

I have recommended the Hidden Psychology of Pain to other pain sufferers, but have had no feedback to date. Perhaps this is due to the scepticism with which people treat such "oddball" treatments, and their reticence to participate. There is nothing "oddball" about this approach – it works, is simple and should, I believe, be promoted heavily. Freedom from pain without the use of drugs is what we all want, and it should be more prominent.

James also introduced me to EMDR therapy. This was used to address the emotional issues that were behind my chronic pain. I found this therapy extremely helpful in my overall recovery. The results were beyond anything I could have hoped for. My emotional issues are well under control, and this result can be laid squarely at the feet of EMDR.

I can thoroughly recommend this approach. I have benefited from it and now enjoy sleep without pain, and a more relaxed life.

Thank you James for your being innovative in your treatment, patient in your dealings with me and my troubles, and proving to me that I can regulate my feelings.

Rebecca's story

This is the experience of Rebecca, a 20 year old university student who was highly disabled by months of extreme pain in her knees and back. It followed years of similar physical problems, and many attempts at physical therapy. At the beginning of the psychological process, her pain was deeply entrenched, and the prospect of it remaining untreatable was a terrible possibility for her.

I was diagnosed with Os-good Schlatters by a physiotherapist when I was about 11. It is a minor growth problem whereby the muscles growing around the bone, and the bones (femur/tibia) are growing at different rates and therefore the patella is not moving correctly in the knee joint thus causing pain and inflammation. My treatment for this was to work on strengthening the quadriceps (particularly the OM) and some stretches. I also wasn't allowed to use stairs or engage in any high impact activities like running.

By early high school, this problem seemed to have spontaneously resolved. I was doing a lot of athletics then. At 14 I began having problems again, and without seeing a physio, chose to stop all high-impact activity. I had some problems during late adolescence, but never anything major. I simply noticed that sometimes walking around hills, and especially down our steep concrete driveway would hurt.

Then at the beginning of 2011, I started getting some back pain for the first time. This coincided with a high stress period where my mum was beginning a new relationship, and I was under a lot of pressure with my voluntary work. The back pain went away, probably because I chose to drop a subject at uni, and thus reduce the pressure on myself.

In mid 2011, I was doing a lot of voluntary work at a food co-operative. I spent a whole weekend working to cater an event, which involved lifting and moving heavy things around the co-op. I lifted a particularly large bag of grain and noticed it hurt my back. I didn't have any major troubles until a few weeks later when I started experiencing severe back pain. I saw a chiropractor who explained to me that there are both physical and emotional factors which can affect the health of the spine. However, she treated almost exclusively the physical factors, working to realign my spine. A couple of times she used muscle testing to determine whether there were other factors in play, including dietary and emotional factors. However neither of these

415

were explored deeply. While I definitely had improvements with my back while seeing her, those improvements were not lasting. I had recurrences of the pain which meant I had to see her weekly, or fortnightly at best. I ceased treatment when I went home over summer.

I also saw several physiotherapists about my knees. They prescribed for me a range of stretches (hamstring, calf) and exercises (gluteal lifts, OM clenches, quadriceps clenches). I did these for approximately 4 months, but without any success. Roughly the same exercises were prescribed by two other physiotherapists, with the addition of core strengthening exercises. Still, the inflammation in my knees particularly became worse, with an increase in swelling and redness so that I was icing my knees 2-4 times per day.

My back was not as bad as my knees during the two months that I was home over summer. But it still hurt with bending and lifting, and sometimes with extended sitting. Towards the end, I saw a physiotherapist who prescribed almost constant lying down. I noticed my back pain got worse after this—I think because I became more concerned about my back.

The pain in both my knees and my back was usually worse the more distressed I was about it. For instance, if I wasn't able to engage in a normal everyday activity which I usually would. At my grandparents, I was almost exclusively confined to my bedroom as it was the only place I could lie on a good flat mattress.

Sometimes I was surprised when I did things that I thought would hurt and didn't. For instance I got fed up with waiting for appointments and referrals over the Christmas period and decided to go to the emergency department at the hospital to try to get a referral. There, I did more walking than I'd done in a week, just around the hospital, but with comparatively little pain. This supports the thesis that there was nothing physically wrong with my knees, otherwise the pain would have behaved more consistently.

I started getting results with my knees and my back within one week of beginning to read the information you provided, and doing the online exercises. Particularly, I saw an almost immediate reduction in the pain and swelling in my knees. Now I still get some pain, particularly when beginning new activities. For example I did a yoga class and got back pain. However, I ignore this, continue with the activity, do some journaling and, generally the next time I do the activity, I get little or no pain. I think this supports the idea of conditioning.

I honestly don't know how to thank you enough for putting me on to these ideas. After seven months of pain, and two months of disability, in only four weeks I am back to normal. I'm riding my bike again, studying full time at uni, essentially doing everything I used to do, and also more.

As terrible as the pain was, getting over it psychologically has also given me the opportunity to address a number of other areas in my life which I was neglecting. Through the EMDR therapy, I have been able to look at a number of childhood events which I hadn't properly dealt with, and essentially reprogram my brain into adult mode. All of this has given me a dizzying sense of control over my own life—which I now realize I had been lacking.

So, thank you, thank you, thank you. All of this has really given me a new start at my life.

APPENDIX 11

Pain Questionnaire (II)

i) **Pain Catastrophizing Scale.**

RATING	0	1	2	3	4
MEANING	Not at all	To a slight degree	To a moderate degree	To a great degree	All the time

NUMBER	*When I'm in pain . . . .*	RATING
1	. . . I worry all the time about whether the pain will end	
2	. . . I feel I can't go on	
3	. . . It's terrible and I think it's never going to get any better	
4	. . . It's awful and I feel that it overwhelms me	
5	. . . I feel I can't stand it anymore	
6	. . . I become afraid that the pain will get worse	
7	. . . I keep thinking of other painful events	
8	. . . I anxiously want the pain to go away.	
9	. . . I can't seem to keep it out of my mind.	
10	. . . I keep thinking about how much it hurts.	

NUMBER	When I'm in pain	RATING
11	. . . I keep thinking about how badly I want the pain to stop.	
12	. . . There's nothing I can do to reduce the intensity of the pain.	
13	. . . I wonder whether something serious may happen.	
	TOTAL SCORE	

ii) Pain Vigilance and Awareness Questionnaire.

RATING	0	1	2	3	4	5
MEANING	Never					Always

NUMBER	STATEMENT	RATING
1	I am very sensitive to pain	
2	I am aware of sudden or temporary changes in pain	
3	I am quick to notice changes in pain intensity	
4	I am quick to notice effects of medication on pain	
5	I am quick to notice changes in location or extent of pain	
6	I focus on sensations of pain	
7	I notice pain even if I am busy with another activity	
8	I find it easy to ignore pain (reverse your score for this item before adding it in the box)	
9	I know immediately when pain starts or increases	

NUMBER	STATEMENT	RATING
10	When I do something that increase pain, the first thing I do is check to see how much pain was increased	
11	I know immediately when pain decreases	
12	I seem to be more conscious of pain than others	
13	I pay close attention to pain	
14	I keep track of my pain level	
15	I become preoccupied with pain	
16	I do not dwell on pain (reverse your score for this item before adding it in the box)	
	TOTAL SCORE	

APPENDIX 12

Placebo treatment?

Are the propositions put forward in this book, and the cases of seemingly miraculous healing presented, just a placebo effect? This is obviously a legitimate question to ask. Placebo effects are an under-appreciated but usually present factor in most health interventions. In fact, they are so prevalent that one would have to question the value of referring to them as 'effects' which operate separately from the therapeutic effects of the actual intervention. Placebo effects reflect a person's strong desire to overcome a particular problem, and often will be the catalyst to assist their whole organism to aid in the healing required. With a belief in the therapy, a range of psychological and biological factors can be initiated to assist the body's natural ability to heal. Wishful thinking certainly plays a role—why wouldn't it? Most people in chronic pain who I have ever met have wished to not be suffering. They bring this strong desire to every intervention tried.

Are placebo effects really a problem? When it comes to physical pain, I suspect that placebos can only be viewed as a problem when you take a view which sharply differentiates between the mind and body. This distinction can no longer be supported for the range of philosophical, scientific and therapeutic reasons detailed throughout this book. With most of the 'pain-industry' still operating within this distinction between mind and body, placebo effects are a problem because improvements with each new physical intervention usually do not last. Many people will experience short term improvements with new therapeutic attempts, such as physiotherapy or chiropractic manipulation. But their experience is usually reflected in the research findings—over a period of time, these interventions are unlikely to result in lasting changes, and they again find themselves in pain. This will keep on happening until the real causes of the pain are addressed.

As suggested in this book, the real causes are more psychological than physiological.

In determining for yourself whether The Hidden Psychology of Pain program generates nothing more than a placebo effect, consider the following. This approach will not work for a person suffering from a severed spinal column. Allan House in the UK has demonstrated that a similar approach to that suggested in this book has worked with people who are suffering from 'hysterical paralysis', but not for people with paralysis derived from catastrophic physical trauma. The only conditions that a psychological approach are likely to have a large positive impact on are conditions which have a large *psychological* component. A severed spinal column has no psychological cause—the person is unable to move because the required nerve pathways have been physiologically destroyed. No amount of psychotherapy will restore a person's ability to move if they have suffered this sort of damage. But people who have suffered paralysis for primarily psychological reasons have been cured of this affliction.

The fact that many people have been cured of their pain using ideas such as those presented in this book demonstrates that the condition was, to begin with, primarily psychologically generated. Detractors may want to disparage this healing by calling it a placebo effect, but in so doing, they are tacitly acknowledging that the condition is primarily psychogenic—which is the major proposition of The Hidden Psychology of Pain. The alleviation of pain is its own proof, as only conditions which have a large psychological component are amenable to psychological treatment, or to what may be disparagingly called a 'placebo effect'.

Ultimately, the acid test of any approach is whether or not the pain returns. However, even if there has been a reprise from the pain using this psychological approach, and it proves to be temporary, this exception to the normal pain pattern also demonstrates the points being made. For even a temporary alleviation of pain, something other than a structural abnormality must be responsible, as structural abnormalities, once basic healing processes have happened, usually do not vary. Discs never 'un-bulge' themselves as a result of new ideas which the sufferer has incorporated. When even a short term relief from pain has been experienced due to psychological intervention, then this can only be possible if the pain is itself largely psychogenic. The information gleamed from such an exception to the pain pattern is important, as it informs the sufferer as to what is actually going on—and such information is an essential component of the cure.

I believe, and I would suggest that much of the evidence presented in this book confirms, that our culture has a rich tradition in understanding mind/body health issues. This is reflected in the works of people like Freud, and several generations of 'neo-psychoanalysts', such as Franz Alexander and others, who followed his pioneering efforts; as well as more contemporary clinicians such as John Sarno and Stanley Coen. Such people have explored and embraced psychology's rich heritage, rather than simply settling for the current flavour of the month. Chronic pain is not a mystery, but its resolution requires that we challenge the prevailing view of humans as sophisticated machines.

Having experienced my own healing of pain, and seen it occur in countless other people, I have no doubt about the reality of what is proposed in this book. Become aware of the psychological factors, see the role which they play in producing physical experiences such as chronic pain, and you are well on your way to becoming pain-free. Address the psychological distress, and you are even further in your quest to become pain-free. If people want to call such a recovery a placebo effect, then I can only think that they have totally misunderstood the propositions of this book.

BIBLIOGPRAPHY

Alexander, F (1987) *Psychosomatic Medicine: Its Principles and Applications.* 2nd. ed., New York; London: Norton.

Andrade J, & Feinstein D. (2003). "Preliminary report of the first large scale study of energy psychology." www.emofree.com/research/andradepaper.htm.

American Academy of Pain Management. http://www.painmed.org/patientcenter/facts_on_pain.aspx

Arden, J (2010) *Rewire Your Brain: Think Your Way to a Better Life.* John Wiley & Sons, New Jersey.

Baliki, M., Petre, B., Torbey, S., Herrmann, K., Huang, L., Schnitzer, T., Fields, H., Apkarian, A. "Corticostriatal functional connectivity predicts transition to chronic back pain". *Nature Neuroscience*, 2012; DOI: 10.1038/nn.3153

Bandler, R, & Grinder, J (1975) *Patterns of the Hypnotic Techniques of Milton H. Erikson.* Meta Publications, USA.

Barnsley, L (2010) "The significance of chronic back pain." *Medicine Today.* Aug, Vol 11, No.8

Benor, D., Ledger, K., Toussaint, L., Hett, G & Zaccaro, D (2009) "Pilot study of Emotional Freedom Techniques, holistic hybrid derived Eye Movement Desensitisation and Reprocessing and Emotional Freedom Technique, and cognitive behaviour therapy for treatment of test anxiety in university students". *Explore: the Journal of Science and Healing.* 5, 338-340.

Bigos, S., Battie, M., Spengler, D., Fisher, L., Fordyce, W., Hansson, T., Nachemson, A., & Wortley, M.(1991) "A prospective study of work perceptions and psychophysical factors affecting the report of back injury". *Spine.* Vol 16, No. 2-6.

Borenstein, D., O'Mara, J., Boden, S., Lauerman, S., Jacobson, A., Platenberg, C., Schellinger, D., & Wiesel, S (2001) "The Value of Magnetic Resonance

Imaging of the Lumbar Spine to Predict Low-Back Pain in Asymptomatic Subjects." *The Journal of Bone and Joint Surgery.* Sep; 83-A(9): 1306-11.

Boden, S., Davis, D., Patronas, N., Weisel, S. (1990) "Abnormal magnetic-resonance scans of the lumbar spine in asymptomatic subjects. A prospective investigation." *Journal of Bone and Joint Surgery.* Mar; 72(3):403-8.

Breggin, P., & Cohen, D (2000) *Your Drug May Be Your Problem.* Da Capo Press, Philadelphia, PA.

Breggin, P. (2001) *The Antidepressant Fact Book.* Da Capo Press, MA.

Broom, B (2007) Meaningful Disease: how personal experience and meaning cause and maintain physical illness. Karna Books Ltd. London

Bridge, D. & Paller, K (2012) Neural Correlates of Reactivation and Retrieval-Induced Distortion. *Journal of Neuroscience,* 2012; 32 (35)

British Medical Journal (2006) "Acupressure Relieves Low Back Pain". Feb 17th.

Brown, C. & Jones, A. (2010) "Meditation experience predicts less negative appraisal of pain: Electrophysiological evidence for the involvement of anticipatory neural responses." *Pain,* DOI: 10.1016/j.pain.2010.04.017.

Brown, S (2009) *Play: How it Shapes the Brain, Opens the Imagination, and Invigorates the Soul.* Scribe Publications, Australia.

Buenaver, L., Quartana, E., Grace, E., Sarlani, E., Simango, M., Edwards, J., Haythornwaite, M., & Smith, M (2012). "Evidence for indirect effects of pain catastrophizing on clinical pain among myofascial temporomandibular disorder patients: The mediating role of sleep disturbance." *Pain,* DOI: 10.1016/j.pain.2012.01.023

Burton, A. (1995) "Psychosocial predictors of outcome in acute and subchronic low back trouble". *Spine.* 20 (6).

Butler, D., Moseley, L. (2003) *Explain Pain.* Noigroup Publications, Adelaide.

Carter, R (2010) *Mapping the Mind.* Orion House, London.

Cartwright, R., & Lamberg, L (2003) "Directing Your Dreams". *Psychology Today* (http://psychologytoday.com/print/20776)

Cherry, D (2009) "Managing chronic non-malignant pain". *Medicine Today.* 10(12):36-40

Cook, J (2010) Personal communication—email 7th September.

Cook, J (2002) "The Tendinitis Myth." ABC Radio National Health Report. 29th Apr. (http://www.abc.net.au/rn/talks/8.30/helthrpt/stories/s543389.htm)

Cuijpers, P., Smit, M., Bohlmeijer, E., Hollon S., and Andersson, G (2010) "Efficacy of cognitive–behavioural therapy and other psychological treatments for adult depression: meta-analytic study of publication bias." *The British Journal of Psychiatry*. 196, 173-178.

Dahl, J., Wilson, K., & Nilsson, A (2004) "Acceptance and Commitment Therapy and the Treatment of Persons at Risk for Long-Term Disability Resulting From Stress and Pain Symptoms: A Preliminary Randomized Trial." *Behaviour Therapy*, 35, p885–801.

Davidson, R., & Begley, S (2012) *The Emotional Life of Your Brain*. Hudson Street Press, New York.

Deyo, R (2002) "Diagnostic Evaluation of LBP: reaching a specific diagnosis is often impossible." *Archives of Internal Medicine*. Vol 162, No. 13, July 8; 1444-1447.

Deyo, R., & Weinstein, J (2001) "Low Back Pain". *New England Journal of Medicine*. Vol.344, No.5—Feb; 361-370.

Doidge, N (2007) *The Brain That Changes Itself*. Scribe Publications, Melbourne.

Donn, J., Mendoza, M., & Pritchard, J (2008) "AP probe finds drugs in drinking water." Associated Press National Investigative Team, March 10, 2008

Duncan, B (2010): www.heartandsoulofchange.com

Ecker, B. & Hulley, L (1996) *Depth Oriented Brief Therapy. How to be brief when you are trained to be deep- and vice versa*. Jossey-Bass Publishers, San Francisco.

Ecker, B., Hulley, L., & Ticic, R (2012) Unlocking The Emotional Brain. Routledge. New York.

Engel, G (1977) "The need of a New Medical Model: A Challenge for Biomedicine". *Science*. Vol.196, No.4286, 129-137.

Ernst, E (2009) *New Scientist*—Opinion Essay. 30th May, pp.22-23.

Ernst, E., Myeong Soo Lee, Tae-Young Choi (2011) "Acupuncture: Does it alleviate pain and are there serious risks? A review of reviews." *Pain*. 152 (4).

Eysenck, H (1985) "Personality, cancer and cardiovascular disease: a causal analysis." *Personality and Individual Differences*. Vol 6, No.5, p.535-556.

Eysenck, H (1991) "Science, Racism, and Sexism". *Journal of Social, Political & Economic Studies*. Vol 16, Summer, p.217-250.

Feinstein, D. (2008). "Energy Psychology: A Review of the Preliminary Evidence." *Psychotherapy: Theory, Research, Practice, Training*. 45(2), 199-213.

Feinstein, D (2010) "Rapid Treatment of PTSD: Why Psychological Exposure with Acupoint Tapping May be Effective." *Psychotherapy Theory, Research, Practice*. Vol. 47, No. 3, 385-402

Forgash, C., & Copely, M (2008) *Healing the Heart of Trauma and Dissociation with EMDR and Ego State Therapy*. Springer Publishing, NY.

Fox, A., Lin, J., Pinto, R., Kricheff, I (1975) "Myelographic Cervical Nerve Root Deformities". *Radiology.* 116: 355-361, August.

Freud, S (1961) *Beyond the Pleasure Principle.* WW Norton & Company.

Grant, J., & Rainville, P (2009). "Pain Sensitivity and Analgesic Effects of Mindful States in Zen Meditators: A Cross-Sectional Study". *Psychosomatic Medicine.* 71: 106-114

Grant, M (2009) *Change Your Brain, Change Your Pain.* Wyong, Australia.

Hannaford, C (2005) *Smart Moves: Why Learning is Not All in Your Head.* Great River Books, Utah.

Harris, R., Zubieta, J., Scott, D., Napadow, V., Gracely, R & Clauw. D (2009) "Traditional Chinese acupuncture and placebo (sham) acupuncture are differentiated by their effects on u-opioid receptors (MORs)". *Journal of NeuroImage;* 47 (3): 1077-1085

Hay, L (1988) *Heal Your Body: the mental causes for physical illnesses and the metaphysical way to overcome them.* Hay House Inc, California.

Hayes, S., Strosahl, K., & Wilson, K (2003) *Acceptance and Commitment Therapy: an experiential approach to behaviour change.* The Guilford Press, New York.

Healy, D (2004) *Let Them Eat Prozac: the unhealthy relationship between the pharmaceutical industry and depression.* New York University Press, New York.

Hodges, P (2004) "Exercise and bone strength/physiotherapy." ABC Radio National Health Report, 25th Oct. (http://www.abc.net.au/rn/healthreport/stories/2004/1225732.htm)

Hologram5 (2009) USA Today blog: http://www.usatoday.com/news/health/2009-08-03-antidepressants_N.htm

House, A (2005) "Blind through the mind—contemporary cases of hysteria". ABC Radio National. http://www.abc.net.au/radionational/programs/allinthemind/blind-through-the-mind—contemporary-cases-of/3442838

Huxley, A (1945) *The Perennial Philosophy.* Harper & Collins. New York.

Jensen, M., Brant-Zawadksi, M., Obuschowksi, N., Modic, M., Malkasian, D., & Ross, J (1994) "Magentic resonance imaging of the lumbar spine in people without back pain." *New England Medical Journal.* Vol 331, No. 2, July 14, 69-73.

Jernbro, C., Svensson, B., Tindberg, Y., & Janson, S (2012) "Multiple psychosomatic symptoms can indicate child physical abuse—results from a study of Swedish schoolchildren." *Acta Paediatrica.*101 (3): 324.

Kabat-Zinn, J (2009) *Full Catastrophe Living: using the wisdom of your body and mind to face stress, pain, and illness* (15th anniversary edition). Bantom Dell, New York.

King, R (1999) "Depression: do we know what we are doing? *"Psychotherapy in Australia.* Vol 5, No3. May.

Kirchheiner, J., Nickchen, K., Bauer, M, Wong, M-L, Licino, J, Roots, I., & Brockmoller, J. (2004) "Pharmacogenetics of antidepressants and antipsychotics: the contribution of allelic variations to the phenotype of drug response." *Molecular Psychiatry.* 9, 442-473.

Kirsch, I (2010) *The Emperor's New Drugs: Exploding the Antidepressant Myth.* Basic Books, New York. Kolling Institute of Medical Research. http://www.kolling. usyd.edu.au/research/pain-management-group/index.php

Kripke DF, Langer RD, Kline LE.(2010) "Hypnotics' association with mortality or cancer: a matched cohort study." *BMJ Open,* 2012;2:e000850 DOI: 10.1136/bmjopen-2012-000850

Kyung-Eun Choi, gizewski, E., Rampp, T., Dobos, G., Forsting, M., Musial, F.(2010) "Acupuncture changes brain's perception and processing of pain, researchers." Radiological Society of North America (November 30).

Laferriere, A., Pitcher, M., Haldane, A., Huang, Y., Cornea, V., Kumar, N., Sacktor, T., Cevero, F., & Coderre, T (2011) "PKMzeta is essential for spinal plasticity underlying the maintenance of persistent pain." *Molecular Pain.* 7 (1): 99.

Lane, J (2010). "Wolpe Not Woo Woo: A Biochemical Rationale for Using Acupressure Desensitization in Psychotherapy." http://www.energypsych. org/displaycommon.cfm?an=1&subarticlenbr=84

Lavelle, P (2005) "Back pain fact file". ABC Health Matters. (http://www.abc.net. au/cgi-bin/common/printfriendly.pl?/health/library/backpain_ff.htm)

Lehrer, J (2012) "The Forgetting Pill". *Wired.* March edition.

Linde, K., Allais, G., Brinkhaus, B., Manheimer, E., Vickers, A., White, A (2009) "Acupuncture for migraine prophylaxis". *Cochrane Database of Systematic Reviews.* Issue1.

Linton, S. J (2000) "A Review of Psychological Risk Factors in Back and Neck Pain". *Spine.* May 1;25(9):1148-56.

Lloyd, J (2011) "Antidepressant use skyrockets 400% in past 20 years". USA Today. 20th Oct.

Lockwood, D (1962) *I the Aboriginal.* Landsdown Publishing Pty Ltd, Sydney.

Lucire, Y (2003) *Constructing RSI: belief and desire.* UNSW Press, Sydney.

Lucire, Y (2011) http://www.lucire.com.au/

Lucire & Crotty (2011) "Antidepressant-induced akathisia-related homicides associated with diminishing mutations in metabolizing genes of the CYP450 family." *Pharmacogenomics and Personalized Medicine* 2011:4 65-81

Luo, Gangadharan, Kumar Bali, Xie, Agarwal, Kurejova, Tappe-Theodor, Tegeder, Feil, Lewin, Polgar, Todd, Schlossmann, Hofmann, Liu, Hu, Feil, Kuner, Kuner. "Presynaptically Localized Cyclic GMP-Dependent Protein Kinase 1 Is a Key Determinant of Spinal Synaptic Potentiation and Pain Hypersensitivity". *PLoS Biology,* 2012; 10 (3)

Magora, A., & Schwartz, A (1980) "Relation Between the Low Back Pain Syndrome and X-Ray Findings". *Scandinavian Journal of Rehabilitation Medicine.* 12:9-15.

Mamet, D (1986) *Writing in Restaurants.* Penguin Books, NY.

Maté, G (2003) *When the Body Says No: Understanding the stress-disease connection.* John Wiley & Sons, Inc. New Jersey.

McCory, E., De Brito, S., Sebastion, C., Mechelli, A., Bird, G., Kelly, P., & Viding, E (2011) "Heightened neural reactivity to threat in child victims of family violence". *Current Biology.*21 (23): R947-R948.

McCraken, L.M (1997) "Attention to Pain in Persons With Chronic Pain: A Behavioural Approach". *Behaviour Therapy.* 28: 271-284

Miller, S., Hubble, M., & Duncan, B (2008) "Supershrinks: what is the secret of their success?" *Psychotherapy in Australia,* Vol14, No.3. Aug.

Milne, G (2007) *Hypnosis and the Art of Self-therapy.* Geddes & Grosset, New Lanark, Scotland.

Moncrieff, J (2009) *The Myth of the Chemical Cure.* Palgrave Macmillan, UK.

Montgomery, R., & Evans, L (1985) *You and Stress: a guide to successful living.* Nelson Publishers, Melbourne.

Moss-Morris, R., Humphrey, K., Johnson, M., & Petrie, K (2007) "Patients' perceptions of their pain condition across a multidisciplinary Pain Management program: Do they change and does it matter?" *Clinical Journal of Pain.* Vol 23, No.7, September

Nachemson, A (1976) "The Lumbar Spine: and orthopaedic challenge." *Spine.* Vol 1, No.1—March; 59-71.

Norden, J (2007) *Understanding the Brain: course guidebook.* The Teaching Company, USA.

Pachana, N., O'Donovan, A., & Helmes, E. (2006) "Australian clinical psychology training program directors survey", *Australian Psychologist*, Nov 41(3): 168-178.

Petrie, K., & Weinman, J (2012) "Patients' Perceptions of Their Illness: The Dynamo of Volition in Health Care." *Current Directions in Psychological Science.*21(1). 60-65.

Phan, B (2012). "As Valentine's day approaches, cardiologist describes broken heart syndrome." *Science Daily.* http://www.sciencedaily.com/releases/2012/02/120207121928.htm

Porges (2011) *The Polyvagal Theory. Neurophysiological Foundations of emotions, attachment, communication, self regulation.* WW. Norton & Company, NY.

Proust, M (1921) "The Guermantes Way", Vol 5, Pt1, Ch2, In *Remembrance of Things Past.* Translated by R & C. Cortie (1988).

Ruden, R (2005). "Why Tapping Works: a sense of healing. The Neurobiological Basis of Peripheral Sensory Stimulation for Modulation of Emotional Response". (http://www.healingthemind.net/html/Why_tapping_works.html)

Russell, B (1961) *History of Western Philosophy* (2nd Edition). George Allan & Unwin Ltd, London, UK.

Sakai, C. S., Connolly, S. M., & Oas, P. (2010). "Treatment of PTSD in Rwandan genocide survivors using Thought Field Therapy". *International Journal of Emergency Mental Health, 12,* 41–50.

Sapolsky, R (2004) *Why Zebras Don't Get Ulcers.* St Martin's Griffin, NY.

Sarno, J (1991) *Healing Back Pain: the Mind-Body Connection.* Warner Books, New York.

Sarno, J (1998) *The Mindbody Prescription.* Warner Books, New York.

Sarno, J (ed) (2006) *The Divided Mind: The Epidemic of Mindbody Disorders.* ReganBooks,

Sarno, J., & Coen, S (1989) "Psychosomatic Avoidance of Conflict in Back Pain". *Journal of the American Academy of Psychoanalysis,*17(3), 359-376.

Schnurr, P., Friedman, M., Engel, C., Foa, E., Shea, T., Chow, B., Resik, P., Thurston, V., Orsillo, S., Haig, R., Turner, C., Bernardy, N (2007) "Cognitive Behavioural Therapy for Posttraumatic Stress Disorder in Women." *Journal of American Medical Association.* 297(8); 820-830.

Schofferman, J. (1992) "Childhood Psychological Trauma Correlates with Unsuccessful Lumbar Spine Surgery." *Spine.* Vol17, No. 6, June.pp138-144.

Scogin, F (2003) "The status of self-help administered treatments". *Journal of Clinical Psychology,* 59(3).

Selfridge, N & Peterson, F (2001) *Freedom from Fibromyalgia.* Three Rivers Press, N.Y

Seligman, M (1991) *Learned Optimism.* Random House, Australia.

Sezgin, N., & Ozcan, B (2009) "The effects of progressive muscle relaxation and Emotional Freedom Techniques on test anxiety in high school students: A randomised blind controlled study". *Energy Psychology: Theory, Research and Treatment.* 1, 23-29.

Shapiro, F (2012 a) *Getting Past Your Past: take control of your life with self-help techniques from EMDR therapy.* Rodale Inc, New York.

Shapiro, F (2012 b) "The Evidence on EMDR." The New York Times—'Health'. Thurs 22nd March. http://consults.blogs.nytimes.com/2012/03/02/the-evidence-on-e-m-d-r/

Shapiro, F., & Forrest, M.S (1997) *EMDR: the breakthrough "eye movement" therapy for overcoming anxiety, stress, and trauma.* Basic Books, New York.

Siddall, P.& Cousins, M. (1997) "Spinal Pain Mechanisms". *Spine.* 22(1)

Siegel, D (2011) *Mindsight: the new science of personal transformation.* Bantom Books, New York.

Smith, A (2007) http://www.smi-mindbodyresearch.org/index.htm). The Seligman Medical Institute.

Smith, R (2010) *Breakfast with Socrates: a day with the world's greatest minds.* Profile Books, UK.

Somerville, W (2004) "Cognitive Control Training for PTSD". Unpublished Manuscript, submitted as research for Doctor of Psychology Degree, School of Humanities & Social Sciences, Department of Psychology, Bond University.

Spengler, C., Eipert, F., Findsterbusch, J., Bingel, U., Rose, M., Buchel, C. (2012). "Attention Modulates Spinal Cord Responses to Pain". *Current Biology;* DOI: 10.1016/j.cub.2012.04.006

Stadnik, T., Lee, R., Coen, H., Neirynck, E., Buisseret, T, & Osteaux, M. (1998) "Annular tears and disk hermination: prevalence and constrast enhancement on MR images in the absence of low back pain or sciatica." *Radiology.* Vol 206, 49-55.

Stewart-Brown, S (2004) "Low Back Pain and Physiotherapy". ABC Radio National Life Matters 18th Oct. http://www.abc.net.au/rn/talks/8.30/helthrpt/stories/s1220113.htm

Stickgold, R (2002) "EMDR: A Putative Mechanism for Action". *Journal of Clinical Psychology,* Vol. 58(1), 61-75

Stickgold, R (2008) "Sleep-dependent memory processing and EMDR action." *Journal of EMDR Practice and Research,* Vol 2, No.4

Streltzer, J., Byron, M., Eliashof, M., Kline, A., Goebert, D. (2000) "Chronic Pain Disorder Following Physical Injury." *Psychosomatics.* 41:3, May-June.

Sullivan, MJL., Bishop, S., Pivak, J (1995) "The pain catastrophising scale: development and validation." *Psychological Assessment.* No.7, 524-532

Szabo, L (2009) "Number of Americans taking antidepressants doubles." USA Today http://www.usatoday.com/news/health/2009-08-03-antidepressants_N.htm

Takashima, A., Petersson, K., Rutters, F., Tendolkar, I., Jensen, O., Zwarts, J., McNaughton, B., and Fernandez, G (2006) "Declarative memory consolidation in humans: A prospective functional magnetic resonance imaging study". *Proceedings of the National Academy of Sciences.* Jan 17, Vol 103, No.3

Thiering, B (1992) *Jesus the Man. A new interpretation from the Dead Sea Scrolls.* A Bantam Book, Australia.

Ulett, G.A. (1992). "Beyond Yin and Yang; How Acupuncture Really Works." St. Louis: Warren S. Green and Co.

Urquhart, D. (2008) "No clear evidence that antidepressants assist in the management of chronic low back pain." *Science Daily* http://www.sciencedaily. com/releases/2008/01/080122203148.htm

van der Helm, E., Yao, J., Dutt, S., Rao, V., Saletin, J., & Walker, M (2011) "REM Sleep Depoentiates Amygdala Activity to Previous Emotional Experiences". *Current Biology,* Nov 23rd.

van der Kolk, B., Spinazzola, J., Blaustein, M., Hopper, J., Hopper, E., Korn, D & Simpson, W (2007) "A Randomized Clinical Trial of Eye Movement Desensitization and Reprocessing (EMDR), Fluoxetine, and Pill Placebo in the Treatment of Posttraumatic Stress Disorder: Treatment Effects and Long-Term Maintenance." *Journal of Clinical Psychiatry* 68:0.

Vincenzino, B (2010) "Corticosteroid injections for tendon injuries." Radio National Health Report. http://www.abc.net.au/rn/healthreport/stories/2010/308 4056.htm#transcript

Vowles, K., & McCracken, L. (2008). "Acceptance and values-based action in chronic pain: A study of treatment effectiveness and process". Journal of Consulting and Clinical Psychology, 76, 397-407.

Waddell, G., Aylward, M., & Sawney, P. (2002) "Back Pain, Incapacity for Work and Social Security Benefits: an international literature review and analysis." The Royal Society of Medicine Press Ltd, Oct.

Wiesel, S., Tsourmas, N., Feffer, H., Citrin, C & Patronas, N (1984) A study of computer-assisted tomography.I. "The incidence of positive CAT scans in an asymptomatic group of patients". *Spine.* Sep; 9(6): 549-51.

Young, J (1999) *Cognitive therapy for personality disorders: A schema-focused approach (revised edition).* Sarasota, Florida: Professional Resource Press.

INDEX

A

Acceptance 39, 152, 336, 361, 363-5, 427-8, 433
Acceptance and Commitment Therapy (ACT) 364
acid reflux 17
acupressure 236-7, 239-40, 243, 290, 426, 429
acupuncture xxvii, 236-43, 286-7, 293-4, 298, 413, 428-9, 433
acute pain xvii-xviii, xxvi, 47, 49, 58-60, 66, 68-9, 75, 83, 98, 110, 131, 141, 390-2, 394
adrenaline 97, 219, 284, 292
adverse effects 312, 386, 388
alcohol 41, 68, 102, 201, 213-15, 264-6, 276, 279-80, 313, 413
Alexander, F 425
allergies 1, 17, 124-5, 127
Ambien 279
ambivalent attachment 106, 114, 177
amygdala 99-100, 115, 202, 208-9, 217, 238, 284, 291-4, 433
anatomy iii, xxiii, xxvi, xxviii, 19-20, 27, 48, 51, 90, 92, 131, 384-5, 390
anger 15, 82, 93, 104-6, 111-12, 135-6, 152, 186-9, 192, 199-200, 216, 347-50, 363, 376-7, 412
anterior cingulate cortex 338, 378
antidepressants 196, 214, 266-7, 277-8, 311-13, 315, 321, 387-8, 428-9, 433

anxiety 44, 72, 82, 103-4, 116-17, 198-200, 218, 240-1, 244-5, 261, 283, 287-91, 293-8, 348-9, 354
arthritic i
asthma 1, 17, 105, 128
ATP 77-9
attachment style 113-15, 177-8
avoidant attachment 114, 177
axon 256, 373-4

B

Back Book 158-61, 164, 166, 359
Back pain xix-xx, xxii, 15, 26-8, 30-1, 47-50, 61, 67, 88-9, 158, 160, 162, 302, 426-7, 429-32
Beck, A 5, 308, 400
benzodiazepines 279, 387
bilateral stimulation 255, 324, 331-2
bio-psycho-social medicine 34-5
biological pathways xxvi, 14-15, 85, 95, 98, 111, 126, 144, 382
biology xix, xxiii, 54, 144, 201-2, 208, 217, 259, 310, 326, 370, 430, 432-3
blood xviii, 57, 63, 76-81, 83, 86-7, 92-3, 97, 153, 155, 163, 167, 209-10, 284, 288
boom-or-bust 167
brain 63-7, 114-19, 128-32, 208-13, 215-20, 222-8, 237-9, 242-7, 254-60, 264-7, 286-9, 291-7, 324-32, 344-8, 370-84

brainstem 100, 119, 209-10, 284-5, 292-3, 328-9, 371, 375-7
Breggin, P 426
Buddha 341, 343, 359
bursitis 16, 94

C

cancer xxiii, 18, 21, 58, 67, 86, 96, 177, 278, 280, 319, 427, 429
cannabis 215, 264-6, 276, 313
cardiac system 16
Carpal tunnel syndrome 17
Cartesian dualism 40
causality 48, 56
CBT 6, 38-9, 118, 162-3, 289, 297, 303, 305-8, 321-2, 364, 400, 403-4
Cherry, D 426
childhood iv, xxvi, 8, 10-12, 41-2, 67, 98, 100, 105, 112-13, 119, 122, 201-2, 245-6, 253
chiropractic xxiii, xxviii, 20, 31, 51, 60, 71, 391, 395, 413, 421
Christ 343
chronic fatigue xxii, 17, 36
chronic pain i-v, xv-4, 12-16, 25-33, 35-9, 41-53, 57-62, 66-8, 73-6, 107-9, 137-47, 157-66, 299-307, 365-6, 383-92
classical 21, 123, 125-8, 170, 277
clock-time 356-7
Cochrane review 386
cognitive-behavioral psychology 6, 38, 400-1
conditioning 28, 123, 125-8, 167, 170, 277, 417
conflict 15, 39, 42, 48, 59, 71, 88, 104, 116, 152, 192, 302, 326, 395, 431
consciousness 98, 100, 105, 116, 137, 175, 235, 295, 343, 345, 354-6, 364-5, 411
consolidation 99, 211, 433
cortisol 97
covert recollections 100, 202
crisis xvii, xxiii, 23

culture ii, xiii-xiv, xxi, xxvii, 22-5, 36, 53-4, 65-6, 134-6, 142-3, 198-200, 337, 357, 359, 402-3
CYP 312-13, 430

D

Decartes 371
dendrites 244, 256, 372-4, 377
depression i, iii, xxiv, xxvii, 12, 21, 39, 67, 195-9, 304, 310-13, 321, 387-8, 404, 427-9
depth psychology 303, 307, 401
dermatological xxii
desensitization 199, 289-91, 299, 317-19, 321, 323-5, 327, 329, 331, 333, 429, 433
diagnosis xvii, 28, 30, 51, 57, 61, 110, 132-3, 149, 204, 297, 427
disc 16, 26-8, 30, 41, 48-52, 60, 85, 88, 110, 155, 159, 385, 388, 406-7, 413
disorganized attachment 114
Doidge, N 427
dopamine 166, 288-9, 391
dream rescripting 225
dream seeding 225
dreams xxvii, 145, 208-9, 211-13, 215-16, 218, 221-9, 266-7, 279, 328, 426
drugs 10, 41, 67, 165, 195-6, 201, 215, 238, 266-8, 278-82, 308-9, 311-15, 322, 349, 386-7
dualism 21-3, 40

E

Eckhart Tolle 344
EFT xxvii-xxviii, 237, 240-3, 246-9, 251-3, 255, 257-61, 263, 270-2, 275, 277, 283, 287-91, 293-8, 331-2
ego iii, xxi, 346-7, 351, 356, 365, 427
elbow pain 17
Ellis, A 5, 400
EMDR iii-iv, xxi, xxvii, 205, 213-14, 220, 255, 293, 299, 317-25, 327-34, 352, 412-14, 417, 432-3

emotional trauma xvi, 3, 9, 149-50, 317
Emotions 25, 115
endorphins 166, 287-8, 374, 383, 391
energy psychology xxvii, 236-7, 240-2, 248, 260, 286-7, 289, 293, 297, 425, 427, 432
enzymes 311-14
epidemic xviii-xix, xxii-xxiii, xxvi, 3, 23, 25, 29, 55-7, 128, 137-9, 366, 389, 431
epinephrine 93, 97, 219, 284, 292
exceptions 66, 154-5, 157, 179-80, 250, 308, 314
exercise xiii, 26-7, 47, 97, 158-9, 166-70, 174, 189, 192, 196, 205, 210, 227, 268, 314-15
exposure therapy 199, 290-1
eye movement 199, 289, 299, 317-19, 321, 323, 325, 327, 329, 331, 333, 425, 432-3

F

fear 72, 99-100, 115, 119, 122-3, 141-2, 166-8, 180-1, 216-18, 291, 293-4, 327, 348-9, 354-5, 358
feelings 11-13, 38, 81-3, 102-6, 109-11, 113-19, 135-7, 151-2, 173-4, 192-3, 233, 245-6, 347-50, 364-6, 411-12
Fibromyalgia 17, 204, 221, 432
fight/flight/freeze 94, 251, 283, 288, 329, 339, 377
floatback 205
foot pain 94, 131
football xiv, 3, 11, 65, 107, 131, 138, 141
frequent urination 17
Freud, S 428
frontal cortex 108-9, 145-6, 209-11, 288, 291-2, 376, 379, 381

G

Galen 21
gastrointestinal xxii, 16-17, 386
genitourinary 16-17

GP 13, 50-2, 55-6, 60, 110, 123, 277, 314, 349, 413
Gut xviii, 126, 292

H

hand pain 17
heart disease 18, 58, 91, 96, 280
heart pain 92
heartburn 17
heat 77, 159-60, 173, 243
helplessness 11, 21, 82, 198, 216, 224, 286, 335, 358
Herniation 41, 51, 88, 385
herniations 88
hidden psychology i-v, xxii-xxiii, 10, 18-19, 31-2, 71, 87-8, 92, 143-4, 148-9, 161, 169-70, 315-17, 340-2, 412-14
hippocampus 99, 115, 209, 293, 376
Hippocrates 20-1
holistic i, 21, 289, 332, 425
hopelessness 21, 31-2, 286, 358
House, A 18, 428
hypnosis 6, 65, 79, 383, 430

I

IBS 403
immune system 16-17, 127, 274, 289, 391
Inflammation 57, 127, 155, 385-6, 415-16
injury xvi-xviii, 17, 43, 51, 56, 58-60, 62-3, 68-71, 108, 110, 130-2, 138, 155, 167, 348-9
insular 202, 239, 338, 378-80, 382
integrative medicine 219
irritable bowel 17, 36, 403
ischemia 76, 78-9, 81, 83-4, 86-9, 94, 120, 126, 167-8, 339

J

James, W xxi, 40, 303, 397
James, William 303, 397
Jesus 343-4, 359-61, 433

K

Knee pain 16

L

laryngitis 17, 133-4
Ligament xviii, 26-7, 47, 78, 85-7, 93, 243, 384-5
limbic system 99-100, 118-19, 210, 219, 246, 251, 284-8, 291-2, 294, 328-9, 372, 375-9, 381
low back pain 16, 28, 50, 61, 67, 142, 158, 160, 239, 388, 407, 426-7, 430, 432-3
Lucire, Y 429-30

M

MAO inhibitors 214
mechanistic 22-5, 40, 337, 366, 398-9, 404
medicine iii-iv, xvi, xix, xxi, xxiii, xxvi, 19-26, 28, 30, 32-6, 40-1, 47-8, 66-7, 149, 425-8
meditation 6, 41, 71, 97, 236, 268, 337-43, 356, 412, 426
memory 99, 115, 189, 197, 209-13, 219-20, 228-31, 233-5, 251, 320, 324-5, 328-30, 351-2, 374, 376-7
metabolizer 312
migraine 17, 239, 429
mind/body 15, 18, 40, 45, 126, 134, 144, 148-9, 175-7, 242, 319, 327, 371, 395, 423
mindfulness 40, 337-8, 342, 352, 356, 362
mirror box 64
Morris, D xxiii
multiple factors 67
muscle problems 83
muscles xviii, 15-16, 19, 26-7, 47, 58, 78-81, 83-90, 97, 128, 138, 153, 166-8, 284, 384-5
Musculoskeletal 57

myths iv, 19-20, 73, 75, 158, 162-3, 166, 384

N

neck pain 44, 79, 250, 429
nerve pain 85, 87-90, 92, 196
Nerves 87, 292
neurology xxviii, 19, 36, 125, 239, 242, 310, 325, 370, 382
neuron 373, 377
neuroplasticity 325
neurotransmitters 80, 262, 286, 288, 297, 373-4, 391
nightmares 200, 219-21, 226, 228, 260, 267, 279
NLP 189
noreadrenaline 217, 219, 292, 374
norepinephrine 94, 219, 288, 292, 298
Now i, 9, 13, 124, 133, 190-1, 194, 231, 233, 327, 342, 344, 350, 411, 416
nucleus accumbens 108, 145-6, 381

O

Osler, W 21
Osteoarthritis 16-17
overlay 15-16, 58-9, 68, 72, 75, 81, 127
overuse 57, 94, 132
oxygen 76-9, 81, 83-7, 90, 92-4, 97, 144, 153, 155, 163, 167, 210, 251, 284, 412

P

pacing 169-70
Pain questionnaires xxiv, xxviii, 367
paralysis 18-19, 74, 128, 422
personality 21, 42-4, 119, 136, 152, 182, 185, 427, 434
Petrie, K. 431
pharmacogenetics 278, 282, 311-12, 315, 429
physical therapy 19, 32, 142, 161, 172, 239-40, 390-1, 393-5, 415

physiotherapy ii, xxiii, xxviii, 20, 30-1, 51, 57, 93, 132, 157-8, 160-1, 391, 413, 421, 428
pinched nerve 16
placebo xxviii, 45, 162, 237-8, 259, 294, 297, 311, 321-2, 383, 392-3, 421-3, 428, 433
postural muscles 79, 81, 84
pre-frontal cortex 108-9, 145-6, 209, 288, 291-2, 376, 379, 381
Prozac 196, 214, 267, 321, 428
psychiatry 18, 32, 39, 196, 260, 308-11, 321, 404, 427, 429, 433
psychoanalysis 4, 15, 48, 88, 302-4, 308, 397-9, 401-2, 431
psychogenic 47, 62, 94, 102, 107, 131, 136, 143, 148, 153, 422
psychological overlay 15, 59, 68, 72, 75, 81, 127
psychology i-v, xx-xxiii, xxv-1, 3-10, 23-4, 34-41, 148-50, 159-63, 236-7, 239-42, 247-9, 301-10, 315-20, 323-5, 395-404
psychoneuroimmunology 94, 125
psychosocial xvi, xxv, 23, 34-5, 43, 45, 142, 426
psychosomatic 15, 32, 48, 62, 88, 147, 160, 165, 182, 202, 302, 403, 425, 428, 431
psychotherapy iii, xxvii, 42, 112, 153, 236-8, 247-8, 289-90, 293-4, 298-9, 303-9, 315-19, 323-4, 427, 429-30

R

Rage 186
rebirthing 6, 154
reductionist 21, 310, 404
relaxation 71, 97, 153, 260, 268, 275, 287, 289, 291, 339, 414, 432
REM sleep 208-15, 217-19, 278, 282, 433
repression 102, 145, 402
rescripting 225-6, 229-31, 235
responsibility iv, vi, 11, 73-4, 124, 182-5, 205, 264

rhinitis 1, 123, 126-7
Rolfing 395-6
rotator cuff 16, 94
RSI iii, xxi-xxiii, 24, 32, 49, 53, 55-8, 62, 94, 128, 132-3, 138, 395, 397, 429

S

Sapolsky, R 431
Sarno, J 431
schemas 116, 120, 144, 147, 178-9, 304, 399
sciatica 16-17, 388, 406-7, 432
scoliosis 16, 413
secondary gain 37, 62
secure attachment 114-15
self-analysis 174, 203
self-criticism 152, 185-6
serotonin 166, 196, 267, 288, 374, 388
sexual abuse 11, 41, 101, 106, 146, 246, 249-50, 252-3, 259, 382, 402
Shapiro, F 432
Sharpe, M xvi
shin splints 17
shoulder pain xxii, 16, 48, 50, 94, 105, 250
sinus 127
skin disorders 17
sleep iii, xxvii, 196, 208-15, 217-22, 224, 260-82, 288-9, 294, 334, 345, 361, 374, 414, 433
sleeping tablets 277-81
social workers 305, 316, 333
spina bifida occulta 16, 406
spinal stenosis 16, 406
Spine xvi-xvii, 41, 43-4, 112, 425-6, 429-32, 434
spondylolysis 16, 50, 406
spondylolysthesis 16
SSNRI 388
SSRI 196, 214, 267
Stilnox 279
stress xxvii, 21, 67-8, 93-4, 96-7, 137, 208, 217-20, 259-60, 283-5, 287-9, 310, 320-3, 338, 429-33

stress cardiomyopathy 93
structural pathology xxviii, 28, 48-50, 52, 55, 57, 61-2, 66, 68, 73, 84-5, 155-8, 164, 259, 405-7
Subconscious 98, 397-8
substances 67, 93, 186, 201, 214-15, 264-7, 276, 279, 311, 313, 315, 336
surgery 1, 41-2, 51, 65, 79, 84, 90, 92, 112, 129, 165, 383, 388, 426, 431

T

tall poppy syndrome 136
tendonitis 16-17, 57
tendons 47, 57-8, 78, 85-6, 90, 93-5, 132, 138, 243, 255-6
tension headache 17
thalamus 211, 238, 292, 377-80, 382
therapy iii-iv, 38-9, 112, 239-41, 289-91, 303-6, 317-18, 331, 333, 364, 390-6, 400-1, 412-15, 425-8, 430-2
thoughts 4-5, 7-8, 38, 81-3, 117-19, 235-6, 288, 319, 363-5, 373, 376, 380, 398-400, 403-4, 411-12
tingling 78-9, 89
TMJ 17
TMS 15-16, 58, 84, 86, 112, 146, 288, 300
Tolle, E 342-4, 346, 352, 355, 359, 364, 366
transitional vertebra 16, 406
Trauma iii, xxi, 41, 112, 195, 197, 199, 201, 203, 205, 207, 323, 327, 427, 431
Tricyclic antidepressants 214, 388
trigger points 85-7

U

unacceptable feelings 104, 173
Unconscious 96-7, 99, 101, 103-5, 107, 109, 111, 113, 115, 117, 119, 121, 123, 125, 127-9

V

van der Kolk 321-2, 339, 433
vertebrae xviii, 1-2, 8, 26, 49-51, 71, 89-90, 141, 149, 155, 384-5, 387
Vietnam veterans 199-200, 260, 320

W

Watts, A 336, 338, 343, 345, 355-6, 366
Weil, A 8
whiplash 16
withdrawal 260, 268, 280-2, 314-15, 387
wrist pain 94, 129
Wundt, W xxi, 397

Z

Zen 336, 340, 428
ZIP 197